T0220470

The World Health Organization

According to its Constitution, the mission of the World Health Organization (WHO) was nothing less than the "attainment by all peoples of the highest possible level of health" without distinction of race, religion, political belief, economic status, or social condition. But how consistently and how well has the WHO pursued this mission since 1946? This comprehensive and engaging new history explores these questions by looking at its origins and its institutional antecedents, while also considering its contemporary and future roles. It examines how the WHO was shaped by the particular environments of the postwar and Cold War periods (1948–1991), the relative influence of the United States and other approaches to health care, and its place alongside sometimes competing international bodies such as UNICEF, the World Bank, and the Gates Foundation. The authors reevaluate the relative success and failure of critical WHO campaigns, from early malaria and smallpox eradication programs to struggles with Ebola today.

MARCOS CUETO is a professor at the Casa de Oswaldo Cruz, a unit of Fiocruz, the main Brazilian biomedical institute, and is coeditor of the journal *História, Ciências Saúde – Manguinhos*. His book, coauthored with Steven Palmer, *Medicine and Public Health in Latin America: A History,* won the 2017 George Rosen award of the American Association for the History of Medicine.

THEODORE M. BROWN is a professor of history in the School of Arts and Sciences and of Public Health Sciences and Medical Humanities in the School of Medicine and Dentistry at the University of Rochester. He is an associate editor (history) of the *American Journal of Public Health.*

ELIZABETH FEE passed away on October 17, 2018. She was at that time the senior historian at the National Library of Medicine. She was a prolific scholar who authored, coauthored, and edited many books including the coauthored book with Theodore M. Brown, *Making Medical History: The Life and Times of Henry E. Sigerist.*

Global Health Histories

Series Editor:
Sanjoy Bhattacharya, University of York

Global Health Histories aims to publish outstanding and innovative scholarship on the history of public health, medicine and science worldwide. By studying the many ways in which the impact of ideas of health and well-being on society were measured and described in different global, international, regional, national and local contexts, books in the series reconceptualise the nature of empire, the nation state, extra-state actors and different forms of globalisation. The series showcases new approaches to writing about the connected histories of health and medicine, humanitarianism, and global economic and social development.

The World Health Organization

A History

Marcos Cueto
Casa de Oswaldo Cruz, Fiocruz

Theodore M. Brown
University of Rochester

Elizabeth Fee
National Library of Medicine

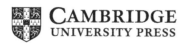

CAMBRIDGE
UNIVERSITY PRESS

CAMBRIDGE
UNIVERSITY PRESS

University Printing House, Cambridge CB2 8BS, United Kingdom

One Liberty Plaza, 20th Floor, New York, NY 10006, USA

477 Williamstown Road, Port Melbourne, VIC 3207, Australia

314-321, 3rd Floor, Plot 3, Splendor Forum, Jasola District Centre, New Delhi - 110025, India

79 Anson Road, #06-04/06, Singapore 079906

Cambridge University Press is part of the University of Cambridge.

It furthers the University's mission by disseminating knowledge in the pursuit of education, learning and research at the highest international levels of excellence.

www.cambridge.org
Information on this title: www.cambridge.org/9781108483575
DOI:10.1017/9781108692878

First published 2019

A catalogue record for this publication is available from the British Library

Library of Congress Cataloging in Publication data
Names: Cueto, Marcos, author. | Brown, Theodore M., 1942- author. |
   Fee, Elizabeth, author.
Title: The World Health Organization : a history / Marcos Cueto, Theodore M. Brown,
   Elizabeth Fee.
Other titles: Global health histories (Series)
Description: Cambridge, United Kingdom : Cambridge University Press, 2019. |
   Series: Global health histories | Includes bibliographical references.
Identifiers: LCCN 2018047191 | ISBN 9781108483575 (hardback) |
   ISBN 9781108728843 (pbk.)
Subjects: | MESH: World Health Organization. | Global Health
   https://id.nlm.nih.gov/mesh/D014943 | International Agencies–history
   https://id.nlm.nih.gov/mesh/D007390Q000266 | Health Policy–history
   https://id.nlm.nih.gov/mesh/D006291Q000266 | Health Services Administration–history
   https://id.nlm.nih.gov/mesh/D006298Q000266 | Disease Eradication–history
   https://id.nlm.nih.gov/mesh/D060740Q000266 | International Cooperation–history
   https://id.nlm.nih.gov/mesh/D007391Q000266 | History, 20th Century
   https://id.nlm.nih.gov/mesh/D049673 | History, 21st Century
Classification: LCC RA441 | NLM WA 1 MW6 | DDC 362.1–dc23
LC record available at https://lccn.loc.gov/2018047191

ISBN 978-1-108-48357-5 Hardback
ISBN 978-1-108-72884-3 Paperback

This book is dedicated to Corinne Sutter-Brown,
Ted Brown's beloved late wife who passed away
on September 6, 2017

Contents

Figures

Tables

Acknowledgments

We undertook this history of the World Health Organization more than ten years ago with initial support from the Rockefeller Foundation and the World Health Organization. It is important to emphasize, however, that this is not a commissioned or official history. After 2008, we had no financial links with the WHO or the Foundation, and we pursued this book project independently. At the WHO we received generous support from Ariel Pablos-Mendez, Thomas Prentice, Hooman Momen, Marie Villemin Partow, Reynald Erard, Tomas John Allen, Eugenio Villar, and Gaby Caro. Socrates Litisios, a former officer of the WHO and a colleague in historical study, also provided key advice at several stages of our work. Conversations with former officers and leaders in global health such as Halfdan T. Mahler, Ilona Kickbusch, Paulo Buss, Jo Asvall, and Michael Marmot clarified many events and ideas. Historians working on global health gave us inspiration, friendship, and useful critical comments. Among them were Jaime Benchimol, Sanjoy Bhattacharya, Anne-Emanuelle Birn, Iris Borowy, Gilberto Hochman, Paul R. Greenough, Randall Packard, Mariola Espinosa, Adam Warren, Patrick Zylberman and Gabriela Soto-Laveaga. The young and talented Brazilian historian, Gabriel Lopes, was extraordinarily helpful in expanding the references and developing the index. We would also like to thank the anonymous reviewers of the book manuscript who provided sound advice and very useful comments.

Several Cambridge University Press officers played a key role in the publication of this book: Michael Watson, Lucy Rhymer, Lisa Carter, Melissa Shivers, and Natasha Whelan. It is a great honor to be part of the Global Health Histories of the Press.

We are grateful to the archivists and librarians who made our work possible and to the institutions that provided images for this book. We also owe thanks to our home institutions: the National Library of Medicine for Elizabeth Fee, the University of Rochester for Theodore M. Brown, and the Casa de Oswaldo Cruz, Fiocruz for Marcos Cueto. Theodore Brown is also grateful to the research assistance provided by several University of Rochester students and colleagues, particularly Rodney Chau, Michael Healey, Susan Ladwig, and

Victoria Stepanova. In addition, Marcos Cueto would like to thank the Brazilian Conselho Nacional de Desenvolvimento Científico e Tecnológico (CNPq) and its Bolsa de Produtividade and express his gratitude for the generous invitations to be fellow at the Swiss Brocher Foundation in l'Hermance and the Robert F. Kennedy Visiting Professorship in the Department of History of Science at Harvard University. The final manuscript was completed at these institutions and discussed by the three of us in a number of meetings in Bethesda, Maryland where we benefited from the warm hospitality of Mary Garofalo.

This book is the result of the collective efforts of Marcos Cueto, Ted Brown, and Elizabeth Fee. Liz was an essential and central partner from start to finish of this project. Sadly, she passed away when the completed text had already entered the copyediting, layout, and production phases of publication.

Abbreviations

ABC	Abstinence, Be Faithful and Use Condoms (AIDS)
ACT UP	AIDS Coalition to Unleash Power
AIDS	Acquired Immunodeficiency Syndrome
AMRO	American Regional Office (World Health Organization)
ARV	Antiretroviral Drug
AFRO	African Regional Office
AZT	Retrovir
BCG	Bacille Calmette-Guérin (vaccine)
CCM	Country Coordinating Mechanism
CDC	Centers for Disease Control and Prevention
CIDA	Canadian International Development Agency
CIPLA	Chemical, Industrial, and Pharmaceutical Laboratories (India)
CVA	Children Vaccine Initiative
DALY	Disability Adjusted Life Year
DAH	Development Assistance for Health
DDT	Dichlorodiphenyltrichloroethane
DFID	Department for International Development
DOTS	Directly Observed Therapy
ELISA	Enzyme-linked Immunosorbent Assay (AIDS test)
EHA	Emergency and Humanitarian Action Division (World Health Organization)
EMRO	Eastern Mediterranean Regional Office (World Health Organization)
EPA	Environmental Protection Agency
EURO	European Regional Office (World Health Organization)
EPI	Expanded Program on Immunization
FAO	Food and Agriculture Organization
FF	Ford Foundation
FFF	Food supplementation, Female literacy, and Family planning
FCTC	Framework Convention on Tobacco Control
GAVI	Global Alliance for Vaccines and Immunization

GOBI	Growth monitoring of young children, Oral rehydration therapy, promotion of Breast feeding, and Immunization
GPA	Global Program on AIDS
HAART	Highly Active Antiretroviral Therapy
HEW	Department of Health, Education and Welfare
HP	Health Promotion
HRP	Special Program of Research in Human Reproduction
HSF	Department of Health System Financing
ICA	International Cooperation Agency
ILO	International Labor Organization
IHD	International Health Division (Rockefeller Foundation)
ITN	Insecticide-Treated mosquito Nets
IC	Interim Commission
IHR	International Health Regulations
IUD	Intrauterine Contraceptive Device
IPPF	International Planned Parenthood Federation
LGBT	Lesbian, Gay, Bisexual and Transgender
LRCS	League of Red Cross Societies
LNHO	League of Nations Health Organization
MEP	Malaria Eradication Program
MDG	Millennium Development Goals
MDR-TB	Multidrug-Resistant Tuberculosis
MMV	Medicines for Malaria Venture
NAM	National Academy of Medicine
NATO	North Atlantic Treaty Alliance
NGO	Nongovernmental Organization
NIH	National Institutes of Health
NCD	Noncommunicable Diseases
NTD	Neglected Tropical Diseases
OCP	Onchocerciasis Control Program
ODA	British Overseas Development Administration
OIHP	Office International d'Hygiène Publique
ORT	Oral Rehydration Techniques
OXFAM	Oxford Committee for Famine Relief
PAHO	Pan American Health Association
PASB	Pan American Sanitary Bureau
PEPFAR	President's Emergency Plan for AIDS Relief
PHC	Primary Health Care
PMI	President's Malaria Initiative
PPP	Public Private Partnerships
RBM	Roll Back Malaria
SARS	Severe Acute Respiratory Syndrome

SDG	*Sustainable Development Goals*
SEP	*Smallpox Eradication Program*
SPHC	*Selective Primary Health Care*
SARS	*Severe Acute Respiratory Syndrome*
STD	*Sexually Transmitted Disease*
SEARO	*South-East Asia, Regional Office (World Health Organization)*
TDR	*Special Program for Research and Training in Tropical Diseases*
TPC	*Technical Preparatory Committee*
TRIPS	*Trade-Related Aspects of International Property Rights*
UNAIDS	*Joint United Nations Program on HIV and AIDS*
UNICEF	*United Nations Children's Fund*
UNDP	*United Nations Development Program*
UNESCO	*United Nations Educational, Scientific, and Cultural Organization*
UNEP	*United Nations Environmental Program*
UNFPA	*United Nations Population Fund*
UNICEF	*United Nations International Children's Emergency Fund*
UNRRA	*United Nations Relief and Rehabilitation Administration*
USAID	*US Agency of International Development*
UHC	*Universal Health Coverage*
WHA	*World Health Assembly*
WHAM	*Women Health Action Mobilization*
WPRO	*Western Pacific Regional Office (World Health Organization)*
WTO	*World Trade Organization*
XDRTB	*Extensively Drug-Resistant Tuberculosis*

Introduction: The World Health Organization and the Dilemmas of the Cold War and the Post–Cold War Periods

This book is a narrative history of the world's principal multilateral health agency during its 70 years of existence (1948 to early 2018). According to its Constitution, the mission of the World Health Organization (WHO) was nothing less than the "attainment by all peoples of the highest possible level of health," without distinction of race, religion, political belief, economic status, or social condition. The book will offer a synthetic overview and assessment of how consistently and how well the WHO has pursued this mission and will identify the two perspectives that have marked its history and its changing place in global health.

During its first decades of existence, the United Nations' specialized health agency was the acknowledged international leader on matters of health and disease and was at the center of a global network of scientists, physicians, and health policy makers. The agency played a preeminent role in the political validation of international health as a field during the second half of the twentieth century and helped shape the notion of technical health assistance for developing countries. But toward the end of the 1980s, the agency was accused of inefficiency, lack of transparency, and irrelevance. The role of the agency as the coordinating authority for international health was seriously questioned, and it increasingly had to surrender to or compete with private and public organizations that staked claims in global health.

The WHO was officially created in 1948 after a protracted period of discussion and negotiation that began in 1945. Its creation marked a change in the history of international health because the WHO merged into a single organization four functions of previous international health organizations: centralized epidemiological surveillance, campaigns against epidemics, disease control, and the reform of health systems. The book will describe what the agency did in surveillance and epidemic intervention but will concentrate on the last two functions during the Cold War and post–Cold War periods. Among its disease-control programs were the unsuccessful attempt to eradicate malaria, launched in the mid-1950s, and the successful elimination of smallpox during the 1970s. An example of a major effort to reform health systems was Primary Health Care (PHC), promulgated at the Alma-Ata conference that took place in 1978.

One theme of this book is that the various programs initiated by the WHO embodied two very different perspectives that reflected the orientation of the organization itself. One was a socio-medical perspective and the other was a technocratic, biomedical perspective. These two perspectives have frequently been portrayed as opposites: horizontal and multi-sectoral vs. vertical and mono-focal. But as we will see, there were nuances in each one of them, and the two could overlap. The WHO Constitution's Preamble underscored the first perspective by presuming that diseases were caused and sustained socially and economically, with their control requiring a broad societal response. The second perspective presumed that epidemic diseases were basically biomedical events that needed technological interventions alone to tame them. Besides their narrow focus, technology-driven disease-control campaigns could also be faulted on the grounds that they sometimes carried with them remnants of the old "civilizing mission" mindset of the western colonial powers. This perspective was captured in a 1948 *Lancet* article that stated that the just-founded WHO had the "means of bringing the resources of science to vast populations now living in medical darkness."[1]

During the 1960s and 1970s, advanced industrialized countries began to lose their control over the World Health Assembly (WHA) as a by-product of decolonization and the growing number of newly independent, voting countries. The change in composition of the WHA had an impact on the presumptive mandate of the WHO, as the agency no longer automatically followed the wishes of the superpowers but now had to take into account the priorities and demands of developing nations unwilling to accept what was dictated from above. Two important instances of the influence of developing countries in the WHA were the inclusion of socio-medical dimensions in the smallpox eradication campaign and the introduction of a new program of Primary Health Care. The smallpox eradication program was not a purely vertical and authoritarian program but relied substantially on leaders and volunteers in local communities. Primary Health Care gained support because it promoted basic health system development and not merely vertical intervention. Supporters of PHC did not reject vertical programs per se but believed that they should be coordinated with health system components and not be budgeted by separate short-term funding.

Toward the end of the Cold War (around 1991 with the dissolution of the Soviet Union), the organization faced challenges from the wealthy nations that to a very large extent funded the agency. These nations increasingly

---

[1] "History at Geneva," *The Lancet* 255:2 (July 9, 1948), 17–19, p. 18.

questioned the legitimacy of the UN and its specialized agencies and supported neoliberal policies and health reforms. They also favored the biomedical perspective described previously and emphasized the role of the WHO in normative standard-setting and the provision of epidemiological information. The vicissitudes of the WHO during the 1990s, including poor central leadership, lack of coordination with regional offices, and a growing dependency on bilateral aid and private donors created the circumstances for organizational crisis and attempts at institutional reinvention.

In spite of losing resources and prestige and facing the challenge of reconciling the requirements of developing nations with demands for budgetary restraint by the industrialized countries, some WHO programs in its sixth decade made valuable contributions. Among the more notable were the promotion of essential drugs and access to antiretroviral treatment, successes with childhood immunizations, advances in the control of tobacco, and proposals made by a Commission on the Social Determinants of Health, formally reported in 2008. These latter proposals downplayed the role of technology, emphasized equity in access to health resources, promoted grassroots participation in health decision-making, and legitimated broader social demands aimed at improving the living conditions of the global poor. Yet at the same time, during its sixth decade, the WHO experienced a resurgence of technocratic ideas and practices and of neoliberal policies that promoted public-private partnerships, including alliances with the World Bank and with major private donors like the Bill and Melinda Gates Foundation. These partnerships (usually one or more private for-profit organizations and at least one public or not-for-profit organization) made contributions to the reduction of morbidity and mortality but normally relied on short-term and ultimately limited strategies. As a result of the coexistence of two different sets of practices, the WHO continued to witness conflicts about priorities and fragmentation in global health initiatives.

The primary sources on which this book relies are archives and libraries in Europe and the United States. We worked mainly in the Archives and Library of the World Health Organization in Geneva, Switzerland; the Wellcome Library in London; the League of Nations Archives in Geneva; the UN Archives in New York City; the Rockefeller Archive Center in Sleepy Hollow, New York; the Library of Congress in Washington, DC; the US National Library of Medicine in Bethesda, Maryland at the Arthur and Elizabeth Schlesinger Library on the History of Women in America at the Radcliffe Institute for Advanced Study at Harvard University; the Center for the History of Medicine of the Francis A. Countway Library of Medicine, also at Harvard; the Department of Rare Books and Special Collections of Princeton University Library; and the US National Archives in College Park, Maryland. We have also been able to examine materials at the WHO regional offices for Africa, the

Americas, the Eastern Mediterranean, and Europe. We regret that we have not been able to conduct research in the WHO regional offices for South-East Asia and the Western Pacific, but in the case of South-East Asia we were able to rely on a number of meticulously researched studies that partially filled this gap. For example, Amrith and Bhattacharya have provided exemplary studies, and the latter author has demonstrated how the smallpox policies of the 1970s designed in Geneva were embraced, contested, and sometimes sabotaged by local politicians, health officers, and physicians.[2] We have also relied on several excellent, primary–source based studies of specific people, projects, and programs.[3]

We have likewise drawn heavily on official and semi-official histories of the WHO, written usually by retired agency officers. These include four "ten-year" commissioned histories that cover the periods to 1957, from 1958 to 1967, 1968 to 1977, and 1978 to 1987. Although no author's name appears on any of these volumes, the first two were almost certainly written by Norman Howard-Jones and the latter two were definitely written by Socrates Litsios. Both Howard-Jones and Litsios were WHO officers, as were Neville Goodman and Yves Beigbeder who also contributed useful histories. Several of WHO's regional offices have also produced historical volumes, some published anonymously and others with an author's or editor's name. These studies sometimes fail to achieve consistent balance between facts and narrative overview and occasionally lapse into a celebratory tone, yet collectively they are rich sources of information and contain few factual errors. Litsios, in addition, has not only produced two memorializing ten-year volumes but has written a number of probing and critical studies on various aspects of the history of the agency.[4]

---

[2] See Sunil S. Amrith, *Decolonizing International Health, India and South Asia, 1930–1965* (Hampshire: Palgrave, 2006) and Sanjoy Bhattacharya, "The World Health Organization and Global Smallpox Eradication," *Journal of Epidemiology and Community Health* 62:10 (2008), 909–912.

[3] See Sung Lee, "WHO and the Developing World: The Contest for Ideology," in Andrew Cunningham & Bridie Andrews (eds.), *Western Medicine as Contested Knowledge* (Manchester: Manchester University Press, 1997), 24–45; Harry Yi-Jui Wu, "World Citizenship and the Emergence of the Social Psychiatry Project of the World Health Organization, 1948-c.1965," *History of Psychiatry* 26 (2015), 166–181; and Soraya de Chadarevian, "Human Population Studies and the World Health Organization," *Dynamis* 35 (2015), 359–388.

[4] World Health Organization, *The First Ten Years of the World Health Organization* (Geneva: World Health Organization, 1958); World Health Organization, *The Second Ten Years of the World Health Organization, 1958–1967* (Geneva: World Health Organization, 1968); World Health Organization, *The Third Ten Years of the World Health Organization, 1968–1977* (Geneva: World Health Organization 2008); and World Health Organization, *The Fourth Ten Years of the World Health Organization, 1978–1987* (Geneva: World Health Organization, 2011). For an anonymous regional history, see World Health Organization, Regional Office for the Western Pacific Region, *Fifty Years of the World Health Organization in the Western Pacific Region* (Manila: World Health Organization Regional Office for the Western Pacific,

Of the secondary literature in general, a comprehensive and insightful scholarly work is Randall M. Packard's *A History of Global Health: Interventions into the Lives of Other Peoples*.[5] Packard provides important insights into the workings of the WHO and its predecessor and competitor organizations and also synthesizes a wide range of scholarship on related topics. He utilizes, for example, work by Mark Harrison on nineteenth century health regulations which demonstrates how intertwined these regulations were with contemporary economic interests.[6] We also incorporate scholarship on international health agencies during the interwar period (1919–1939), relying on a pioneering collection of essays in a volume edited by Paul Weindling, and on the monograph on the League of Nations Health Organization (LNHO) by Iris Borowy.[7] Work on other international health agencies is also integrated, specifically Marcos Cueto's history of the Pan American Sanitary Bureau and Paillette's study of the *Office International d'Hygiène Publique*.[8] Packard relies as well on the scholarship of Amy L. S. Staples, whose book on crucial post–World War II multilateral institutions (the World Bank, the Food and Agriculture Organization, and the World Health Organization) studies the construction of the ideas and policies of economic development, modernization, and technical assistance for developing nations.[9] John Farley's biography of Brock Chisholm, the first director-general of the WHO, provides insights into the friction between Chisholm and the makers of US foreign policy. We

1988). For authored or edited regional histories, see Leo Kaprio, Regional Director Emeritus, *Forty Years of WHO in Europe* (Copenhagen: World Health Organization Regional Office for Europe, 1991) and Alexander Manuila (ed.), *EMRO: Partner in Health in the Eastern Mediterranean,1949–1989* (Alexandria: World Health Organization Regional Office for the Eastern Mediterranean, 1991). See also Neville M. Goodman, *International Health Organizations and Their Work* (London: Churchill Livingstone, 1952); Yves Beigbeder, *The World Health Organization* (The Hague: M. Nijhoff, 1998); and Norman Howard-Jones, *International Public Health between the Two World Wars: The Organizational Problems* (Geneva: World Health Organization, 1978).

[5] Randall M. Packard, *A History of Global Health: Interventions into the Lives of Other Peoples* (Baltimore: Johns Hopkins University Press, 2016).

[6] Mark Harrison, *Contagion: How Commerce Has Spread Disease* (New Haven: Yale University Press, 2012).

[7] Paul Weindling (ed.), *International Health Organizations and Movements, 1918–1939* (Cambridge: Cambridge University Press, 1995); Iris Borowy, *Coming to Terms with World Health: The League of Nations Health Organisation, 1921–1946* (Frankfurt am Main: Peter Lang, 2009).

[8] Marcos Cueto, *The Value of Health: A History of the Pan American Health Organization* (Rochester: University of Rochester Press, 2007); Céline Paillette, "Épidémies, Santé et Ordre Mondial: Le Rôle des Organisations Sanitaires Internationales, 1903–1923," *Monde(s): Histoire, Espaces, Relations* 2:2 (2012), 235–256.

[9] Amy L. S. Staples, *The Birth of Development: How the World Bank, Food and Agriculture Organization, and World Health Organization Have Changed the World, 1945–1965* (Kent, Ohio: The Kent State University Press, 2006).

also relied for more recent periods of the agency on Nitsan Chorev's study of the WHO from a sociological perspective.[10]

Our book is a narrative history of the WHO and is organized in ten chapters. The first chapter, "The Making of an International Health Establishment," deals with the formation of an institutionalized international health order in the nineteenth and early twentieth centuries. It first focuses on the multinational sanitary conferences that began in 1851. These conferences were inspired in part by the fear of mid-century cholera pandemics, perceived to be exogenous threats to the West. The chapter also discusses the construction of other "quarantinable" diseases likewise perceived as exogenous threats to the West: yellow fever and bubonic plague. Attention is directed to the organizations that evolved from the sanitary conferences by the early twentieth century – the *Office International d'Hygiène Publique*, the Pan American Sanitary Bureau, and the League of Nations Health Organization (LNHO). The International Health Division of the Rockefeller Foundation and the United Nations Relief and Rehabilitation Administration (UNRRA), a relief organization created by the Allies during the later stages of World War II, are also considered.

The second chapter, "The Birth of the World Health Organization, 1945–1948," analyzes the activities and post–World War II legacies of health agencies, especially the LNHO and UNRRA. Officials of the LNHO played a key role in carrying over social-medicine ideas into the early postwar period and to the new multilateral organization. UNRRA left a residual budget and redeployed personnel who were fundamental in creating the new specialized health agency. The response to a 1947 epidemic of cholera in Egypt and aspects of the First World Health Assembly in 1948 are examined to illustrate how the WHO validated its existence in public health and political circles. In a larger context, the WHO was part of a broader postwar design: the creation by the industrialized Western nations – especially the United States, the United Kingdom, and Western Europe – of a reorganized, stable, international capitalist economy and monetary order with a set of multilateral institutions that facilitated technical cooperation and hegemony of the United States and respected the possessions of European Western colonial powers.

The third chapter, "The Start-Up Years, 1948–1953," describes what happened after the Soviet Union and its allies denounced the WHO's excessive closeness to the United States and walked out from 1949 to 1956. The policies of the first two heads of the organization, Brock Chisholm and Marcolino Candau, are discussed, as are the challenges of organizing regional offices, especially in

---

[10] John Farley, *Brock Chisholm, the World Health Organization and the Cold War* (Vancouver: UBC Press, 2008); Nitsan Chorev, *The World Health Organization between North and South* (Ithaca: Cornell University Press, 2012).

sub-Saharan Africa where European colonialism persisted. Chisholm and Candau both attempted to move the agency from the old idea that infectious diseases were exogenous threats to developed nations to a new one that these diseases were menaces to global health security and that all nations had rights to protection from infectious diseases with the help of improved health systems. The former was also adamant in supporting multilateralism as an alternative in order to resist the Cold War pressures of the superpowers, namely the United States and the Soviet Union.

The fourth chapter, "The Cold War and Eradication," addresses what was the agency's principal modus operandi in the 1950s: vertical intervention. Its design in WHO's headquarters in Geneva and in most countries was a clear case of the technocratic perspective mentioned before. This was an American style of disease control, in large part because the US State Department saw vertical eradication programs as ideal weapons with which to counter communist influence in the developing world, believing that through such programs poor people would be moved out of poverty and thus become resistant to communist "seduction." The influence of this American perspective was particularly evident in the WHO in the mid-1950s when the agency declared its commitment to a vertically structured Malaria Eradication Program (MEP). However, by the late 1960s, it was clear that MEP had failed in both medical and political terms.

The fifth chapter, "Overcoming the Warming of the Cold War: Smallpox Eradication," delves into the Smallpox Eradication Program (SEP), which extended from 1966 to 1980 and, unlike MEP, came to a widely heralded and triumphant conclusion. The chapter analyzes the opportunities offered by a less antagonistic phase of the Cold War known as "Détente" and examines the crucial cooperative roles played by both the Soviet Union and the United States within the framework of the WHO. The chapter also examines the collaboration of the US Centers for Disease Control (CDC) and the leadership provided by D. A. Henderson, assigned by the CDC to Geneva. It demonstrates that the differences between SEP and MEP were fundamental and not merely of degrees of eradication intensity.

Chapter 6, "The Transition from 'Family Planning' to 'Sexual and Reproductive Rights,'" focuses on the specter of overpopulation in the 1950s and 1960s and how that specter affected the WHO. It studies the role played by private entities, such as the Population Council and the Ford Foundation, in convincing first the US government and then multilateral agencies of the urgent need for population control. The chapter also probes how callous family-planning policies influenced the WHO and the changes of population policy during the administration of Ronald Reagan, and, later, during and after the international conferences in Cairo and Beijing in the mid-1990s, which replaced the notion of family planning with that of sexual and reproductive health.

Chapter 7, "The Vicissitudes of Primary Health Care," investigates one of the most rich and complex periods in WHO history. The visionary Halfdan Mahler served as director-general from 1973 to 1988 and his tenure was marked by both highs and lows. The notion of Primary Health Care (PHC) was articulated as one of the central elements of the resounding Alma-Ata Declaration of 1978. The Alma-Ata Declaration also announced the goal of "Health for All by 2000" in response to the demands of developing nations for greater health equity and social justice. It was a case of the socio-medical perspective of the agency. Major donor nations reacted negatively to Mahler's initiatives by promoting an alternative Selective Primary Health Care (SPHC) agenda which undermined the spirit of Alma-Ata. During the 1980s, SPHC led to narrower and more technically focused programs and to a competition from UNICEF.

In the eighth chapter, "The Response to the HIV/AIDS Pandemic," the WHO's responses to AIDS is scrutinized. The initial response, valiantly promoted by the director of the Global AIDS Program at the WHO, Jonathan Mann, opened the way to a new understanding of the link between health and human rights. Mann made clear that global disease outbreaks were not only biological threats but serious challenges to human rights, as health security concerns oftentimes, at least initially, displaced the defense of human dignity and health access as the central foci of global initiatives. Mann found himself at odds with the WHO's new, increasingly unpopular Director-General Hiroshi Nakajima, and as a result by the early 1990s the WHO had lost its leadership position in the response to AIDS. It was displaced by the UN's creation of the Joint United Nations Programme on HIV and AIDS (UNAIDS) and was only able to recover some of the initiative in the early twenty-first century when it launched the "3 by 5" initiative (3 million people receiving antiretrovirals by 2005). This program was inspired by the promotion of the right of universal access to essential medications, a right that was usually challenged by transnational pharmaceutical companies.

Chapter 9, "An Embattled Director-General and the Persistence of the WHO," focuses on one of the most difficult periods in WHO history, the 1990s. The rise to dominance of neoliberal policies under Presidents Ronald Reagan and George H. W. Bush, certain that private-company practices were superior to those of the public sector in efficiency and problem-solving, had a strong negative impact on the WHO and other UN agencies, which were harassed by the US government as part of its general weakening of the public sector and strengthening of private institutions and market capitalism. During this period, the WHO was particularly vulnerable because Director-General Nakajima's poor leadership, management deficiencies, and lack of effective collaboration with other agencies all contributed to a widespread perception of an agency adrift. Yet the WHO somehow survived, and this chapter will discuss the strategies it used to regain credibility and navigate the 1990s.

Chapter 10, "The Competitive World of Global Health," reviews the political, economic, and institutional impacts of globalization on international health. In the 1990s "global health" was defined as different from "international health" in that its focus was transnational factors that affected populations which drew responses from non-state organizations that sometimes acted independently of existing international organizations and nation states. Global health was also related to economic globalization and neoliberalism. Globalization gave particular prominence to the World Bank and the Gates Foundation and explains the programmatic initiatives of Director-General Gro Harlem Bruntland (1998–2003). In contrast to Nakajima who was backed by developing countries, Brundtland was aligned with the new donors and the major industrialized nations. In the period after Brundtland, under director-generals Jong-wook Lee and Margaret Chan, the WHO moved back to some extent to earlier organizational priorities. Most notably, in this period a Commission on the Social Determinants of Health produced a series of publications that, seemingly in the spirit of Alma-Ata, called for the reduction of worldwide health disparities through programs of social reform. This chapter also deals with the global financial crisis of 2008, which led to worsened poverty and health for many poor people around the world and to budget and staff cuts in WHO.

Finally, Chapter 11, "The World Health Organization in the Second Decade of the Twenty-First Century," discusses the role played by the World Health Organization in the Ebola epidemic of 2014 as well as the controversy it generated and situates in historical context the election of an African as director-general by the World Health Assembly of 2017. The chapter discusses the efforts of the WHO to validate itself after several years of criticism from nation states and multilateral agencies. It also describes the persistence of two conflicting perspectives in the history of the WHO – the socio-medical and the biomedical – and summarizes the critical issues that the organization faces today in a political context substantially different from the one in which it first emerged. Finally, the chapter raises some questions about the future of the WHO in a complex political context.

1   The Making of an International Health
Establishment

The WHO's roots can ultimately be traced to the development in the mid-nineteenth century of international health as a systematic area of regulation and action. International health emerged primarily as a response to pandemic threats perceived as coming menacingly from outside Western Europe. Thanks to new steamship and railroad technology, increased and rapid world commerce and travel allowed cholera, and later yellow fever and bubonic plague, to leave their traditional endemic sites in colonies and poor countries and reach the economically advanced nations of "the West." Physicians, merchants, and politicians converged on the need to protect their populations, businesses, and territories from epidemic outbreaks by modernizing and standardizing quarantine and other border health controls. Many Europeans believed that in the mid-nineteenth century they could inaugurate a period of real progress in sanitation. International health would steadily carve out a niche as a specialty of public health, a concern of governments, a tool to ensure safe commerce, and an activity that provided new types of medical and diplomatic careers.

The First Meetings in Europe

In 1851, the French government organized the first International Sanitary Conference in Paris to discuss cholera, a disease marked by the frightening and dramatic onset of cramps, vomiting, convulsions, and diarrhea.[1] Cholera had long been restricted primarily to India, but beginning in 1829 it spread

---

[1] See Neville M. Goodman, *International Health Organizations and Their Work* (London: J. & A. Churchill, 1952); Norman Howard-Jones, *The Scientific Background of the International Sanitary Conferences, 1851–1938* (Geneva: World Health Organization, 1975); Richard J. Evans, "Epidemics and Revolutions: Cholera in Nineteenth Century Europe," *Past and Present* 120 (1988), 123–146; Juan Mateos Jiménez, "Actas de las Conferencias Sanitarias Internacionales (1851–1938)," *Revista Española de Salud Pública* 79 (2005), 339–349; William F. Bynum, "Policing Hearts of Darkness: Aspects of the International Sanitary Conferences," *History and Philosophy of the Life Sciences* 15 (1993), 421–434; B. Hillemand & A. Ségalicine, "Les Six Conférences Sanitaires Internationales de 1851 a 1885 Prémices de l'Organisation Mondiale de la Santé (OMS)," *Histoire des Sciences Médicales* 48 (2014), 131–138; 47 (2013), 37–44.

rapidly throughout the world. Cholera found a home in unsafe domestic water systems in overcrowded European urban centers. The disease caught European medicine unprepared because it was little known on the continent. Traditional land cordons, quarantines, and forced confinements of the sick seemed useless, and traditional treatments did little to preserve or restore health.

The 1851 meeting was attended by representatives of twelve governments – including Austria, Spain, the Papal States, France, and the United Kingdom – and inaugurated a series of meetings where the participants would vary but almost always included France and the United Kingdom. The first six meetings (1851, 1859, 1866, 1874, 1881, and 1885) paid most attention to cholera since several cholera pandemics from Asia reached Western Europe and the Americas during the nineteenth century. But more generally, these meetings concentrated on the construction of a uniform system of maritime quarantine as a line of defense between Western Europe and "the East." They also helped establish a network of medical officers, researchers, and diplomats to debate the methods and materials to be used in the disinfection of vessels and ports. A widely accepted, but not fully implemented general goal of these conferences was to find ways to "destroy the disease at its birth [rather] than to try and stop it on its march."[2]

Only three governments endorsed the 1851 convention, but in 1859 the French government organized a second conference in Paris in the hope of obtaining greater recognition of the need for maritime sanitary agreements. Although the majority of delegates from the 11 attending countries were diplomats, most were unable to secure commitments from their governments. The difficulties in creating a binding system of maritime sanitary regulation resulted from several factors. First, most countries had no uniform public health legislation, and many governmental health agencies were subordinate departments in the ministries of the Interior or Justice. A second major factor in explaining the lack of ratification of proposed sanitary conventions was the system of international law that had prevailed in Europe since the Treaty of Westphalia of the mid-seventeenth century. The "Westphalian system" of international diplomacy was based on the precept of non-intervention in the domestic affairs of individual nation states. There was a fear of the unintended consequences and loss of sovereignty that could come with intergovernmental accords. Even in the late 1880s, some representatives to the international sanitary meetings insisted that conventions should be understood as recommendations but not as obligations to set up strict quarantines.[3] As a result,

---

[2] *Proceedings of the International Sanitary Conference, Fifth Washington, DC, 1881* (Washington, DC: US Government Printing Office, 1881), p. 177.

[3] Patrick Zylberman, "Civilizing the State: Borders, Weak States and International Health in Modern Europe," in Alison Bashford (ed.), *Medicine at the Border: Disease, Globalization and Security, 1850 to the Present* (New York: Palgrave Macmillan, 2006), pp. 21–40, p. 27.

different cross-border rules continued to exist among countries, meaning that a ship with confirmed cases of cholera on board could be treated differently at different ports.

The small number of formalized conventions was also a result of ongoing medical debates about whether cholera was an imported contagion or a locally produced miasmatic illness. Most nineteenth-century physicians believed that cholera originated in foul air particles produced by decomposed organic living matter and general pollution; miasmatic particles flourished in hot and humid climates and especially affected individuals with weak physical constitutions or who had intemperate and "immoral" lifestyles. Miasmatically inclined physicians thus explained epidemic outbreaks as products of precarious sanitation and opposed strict quarantines. Others argued in favor of contagion and believed that cholera was dispersed by the sick arriving from abroad. They favored stringent quarantine regulations and urged the inspection, and isolation if needed, of passengers, sailors, merchandise, cargoes, and even mail. Many British physicians and health authorities had an intermediate position, sometimes enforcing quarantines and sometimes prioritizing local sanitation. Variations in professional opinion also had a relationship with British public opinion that could strongly support quarantines when epidemic outbreaks occurred in major ports. Large commercial firms, especially if they were engaged in the importation and exportation of goods, typically overemphasized cholera's miasmatic origin, resisted maritime quarantines, and, when they were imposed, would try to convince politicians that their imposition would destroy the economy more severely than the epidemics themselves.

These mixed attitudes persisted even after the work of the London physician John Snow (1813–1858), who argued in an 1849 pamphlet that drinking water contaminated by the feces of cholera patients transmitted the disease. Snow's work and the discovery of the cholera bacillus in 1883 by the German physician Robert Koch reinforced the beliefs of the contagionists and eventually led to a general installation of better plumbing and sewage systems to stop the oral-fecal transmission of the disease in cities of developed countries. Snow and Koch's work did not convince all physicians, nor did it diminish the need felt by port authorities to strictly control the arrival of "infected" people and merchandise. The relevance and policy implications of their work were not fully recognized until the twentieth century. Miasmatic theory remained intellectually viable and had many adherents into the early twentieth century. Port authorities were also likely influenced by the widespread stigmatization of the diseased, which meant holding individuals, communities, or nations (usually non-Caucasian) responsible for epidemics, an attitude that reinforced the cultural dimensions of European imperialism.

Arab pilgrims were thus commonly portrayed as vectors of cholera. They were suspected of carrying the disease annually from India to Mecca and

Medina and there infecting other Muslim pilgrims who carried it back to Europe. Fear of infected pilgrims and the Oriental poor persisted in Europe well beyond the end of the nineteenth century. According to a contemporary public health journal, "Fully one-third of the pilgrims are indigent, and beggars furnish the principal food for [the] epidemic."[4] These traveling poor were thought to carry "exotic" infectious diseases rare in industrialized countries but common in less-developed nations. Indians and Arabs carried cholera, and later yellow fever was thought to be carried by immigrants from the Caribbean and bubonic plague by immigrants from China. In the case of plague, Asian immigrants thought to be carrying it became scapegoats of public authorities in developed countries, who actually burned down several Chinatowns. Thus, the new sanitary regime, despite much good that it accomplished, also reinforced the gap between "civilized" Europe and the "backward" regions of the world.

Despite banding together against the uncivilized "other," the European powers also frequently broke into intense and unproductive rivalries. For example, the fourth sanitary conference, held in Vienna in 1874 and attended by 21 nations addressing the sanitary implications of the opening of the Suez Canal five years earlier, saw flare-ups of tension between France and Germany, which had fought the Franco-German war in 1870–1871. Another flare-up occurred during the sixth International Sanitary Conference, held in Rome in 1885, where the competing imperialist interests of France and England in Egypt – and the Middle East more broadly, impeded an agreement.

It was only in 1892, at the Seventh International Health Conference in Venice, that progress was made toward international health regulation. Representatives, and later governments, approved clear and rigorous sanitary protocols for monitoring the Suez Canal. The movement of people through the Canal was a growing concern because between 1868 and 1892 the number of pilgrims taking the sea route to Mecca more than doubled. As a result, Europeans now felt dangerously close to India. The Conference at Venice stipulated that all ships using the Canal should be classified according to whether they had a case of cholera on board or not. On-site medical inspection targeted sailors, passengers, baggage, paper, hides, skins, cotton, linen, and cattle. The Venice meeting also endorsed two other ideas that would receive further support in the future. The first was that every government had to notify others about cholera outbreaks within their borders. The second was the more vigorous assertion of an idea initially proposed at the Vienna Conference of 1874: that there was a need for an office or international clearinghouse for the notification and exchange of information on epidemics.

---

[4] Wallace S. Jones, "Italy, International Sanitary Conference," *Public Health Reports* 12:19 (May 7, 1897), 452–459.

Until the 1890s, demands for information on epidemics were overwhelmingly about cholera. But in the late nineteenth century, when cholera was subsiding in Europe, two other pandemic diseases became urgent concerns: yellow fever and bubonic plague. Initially, yellow fever was thought to be restricted to the Caribbean. But it soon became clear that although they did not reach the global distribution of cholera, yellow fever outbreaks occurred in several European and US cities. Moreover, in 1878, a yellow fever epidemic had devastated Mississippi, Louisiana, and Tennessee, and not long before, in 1871, a tragic epidemic of yellow fever had struck Buenos Aires.

In 1903, the 11th International Sanitary Conference that gathered in Paris confirmed the mode of transmission of yellow fever. This confirmation was based on the work of Carlos Finlay (1833–1915), a Cuban, and of US Major Walter Reed (1851–1902) who worked in Havana in the wake of the Spanish American War (1898). Finlay first, and then Reed, identified the vector of the fever: a mosquito that came to be known as *Aedes aegypti*. Careful field studies showed that the mosquito was never far from human dwellings and bred in artificial water containers. This discovery was followed by a successful program to reduce the *Aedes* larvae in Havana. Public health leaders around the world endorsed and replicated the successful control method.[5] In related actions, the 1903 meeting approved specific periods of quarantine for specific diseases and also removed most merchandise from the quarantine list.

The Paris conference likewise addressed bubonic plague. Epidemics of plague had ravaged Europe during the Middle Ages and Early Modern periods but after the sixteenth century entered a long period of decline with irregular resurgent outbreaks. For much of the nineteenth century, plague was believed to be a disease confined to rural Russia and China, with occasional outbreaks in the Middle East. In 1894, bubonic plague spread from southern China to Hong Kong and then globally, reviving memories of the plague pandemics of the Middle Ages.[6] But bacteriologists now led the responses to plague, an indication that miasmatic ideas had been brushed partly aside. Alexandre Yersin, Shibasaburo Kitasato, and Waldemar Haffkine all played roles in this international effort, and it was the work of a Pasteur Institute bacteriologist working in India, Paul-Louis Simond, which confirmed that the plague bacillus thrives in the stomach of rat fleas (*Xenopsylla cheopis*), suggesting that rodents, hidden in the cargo of ships, were to blame for international epidemics. The discovery oriented sanitary work toward the "de-ratisation" of warehouses, ports, and ships. The specific methods included washing ships down with a

---

[5] Mariola Espinosa, *Epidemic Invasions: Yellow Fever and the Limits of Cuban Independence, 1878–1930* (Chicago: University of Chicago Press, 2009).

[6] See Myron Echenberg, *Plague Ports: The Global Urban Impact of Bubonic Plague, 1894–1901* (New York: New York University Press, 2007).

strong solution of mercuric chloride; using rat poisons, fumigation, regular garbage collection, and disposal in urban areas; and maintaining lazarettos for the isolation of the sick.

The possibility of a permanent specialized agency for international health was also seriously discussed at the 1903 Paris conference. The idea had first come up at Vienna in 1874 and had been broached again in Venice in 1892. But there was a new seriousness in 1903, connected with fresh concerns about cholera. In 1900, a controversial railway line – built by the Ottomans with the help of German engineers – was nearing completion. The railway line was named "Hejaz" after its station in central Damascus. The Hejaz line significantly reduced the time of travel between Istanbul and Mecca, which was especially pertinent because the Berlin to Baghdad Railway was already operational. It was assumed that these two lines would be used by thousands of pilgrims to Mecca from Russia, Central Asia, Iran, Iraq, and other countries close to Western Europe. The prospect of heightened cholera transmission to Europe along these same railway lines provided the incentive European health officials needed to establish a permanent institution for gathering and monitoring global epidemiological data and for supervising quarantine standards. Article 181 of the sanitary convention, approved at Paris in 1903, urged the French government to initiate a process to establish a permanent health office. Four years later, in December 1907, a new agency called the *Office International d'Hygiene Publique* (OIHP) became a reality, thanks to an agreement signed in Rome by representatives of the 12 nations attending the International Sanitary Conference that year.

International Health Agencies and Social Medicine

The principal object of the Paris *Office* was to "collect and bring to the knowledge of the participating States the facts and documents of a general character which relate to public health, and especially as regards to infectious diseases, notably cholera, plague, and yellow fever, as well as the measures taken to combat these diseases."[7] There was no intention to establish an organization with executive powers or to intrude into the public health administrations of the participating countries.[8] The *Office*'s first director was a retired French diplomat, Jacques de Cazotte, who was familiar with international health affairs. He was assisted by a secretary-general and a small technical staff receiving salaries from no other source. The initial budget of the agency was estimated to be 150,000 francs, which was considered sufficient to

[7] Goodman, *International Health Organizations*, p. 97.
[8] Cited in "The International Office of Public Health," *The British Medical Journal* 2:2548 (October 30, 1909), 1297–1298, p. 1298.

accomplish assigned tasks and to promote staff loyalty to the agency in contrast to continuing loyalty to their governments.

However, this latter goal was never fully achieved, despite the fact that, formally, the OIHP was an international agency whose authority resided in an independent "Permanent Committee" composed of representatives designated by member states (usually physicians, often the current or retired director of the national health department, although sometimes diplomats or administrators with expertise in public health). French physicians and diplomats dominated the organization from the start. The headquarters of the agency was located in Paris and the official language was French. The Francophone staff built a clearinghouse for gathering, validating, and disseminating information on outbreaks of cholera, plague, and yellow fever and for compiling the best methods to control these diseases. The governments of participating countries had to inform the agency of "pestilential diseases" and distribute epidemiological information through diplomatic channels. The OIHP had no authority to do field work; yet, over time, the agency conducted limited investigations on diseases, provided some relief in emergencies, and published a monthly *Bulletin*. One of its major assets was the meetings of its Permanent Committee, twice a year for about ten days each session.

The unspoken mission of the OIHP was to protect its predominantly European signatory states from transmissible diseases that threatened to arrive from afar.[9] Its role was to organize surveillance, disseminate useful information, and coordinate preparedness efforts, all these measures being aimed at keeping infectious diseases out, or, if they arrived nevertheless, under tight control. The *Office*'s unspoken goal was *not* the improvement of the health of the world's people but the protection of certain favored nations from the "grande maladies epidemiques" originating primarily in less favored ones. This mission was to be accomplished by the enforcement and, when necessary, the updating of the legally sanctioned international sanitary conventions.

Several basic activities thus preoccupied the staff of the *Office* and its governing committee during the early years.[10] One was collecting all available data on the "reportable" diseases specified in the conventions: cholera, plague, and yellow fever. Another was tinkering with the categories of notification and the rules of quarantine, so that vessels could now be classified as "infected" or "suspect" based on clinical or laboratory criteria rather than the port of

---

[9] This spirit was still evident in the early 1920s; US Representative Rupert Blue, US surgeon general in late 1922, submitted his "Report of the October Meeting of the *Office International d'Hygiene Publique*, October 20th to November 2nd, 1922," assuring: ". . . all nations [represented] were convinced of the necessity of a line of defense between the Orient and Europe," United States National Archives, College Park, Maryland, RG 90, Group 12, Box 1.

[10] G. Abt, *Vingt-Cinq Ans D'Activite de L'Office International d'Hygiene Publique, 1909–1933* (Paris: *Office International d'Hygiene* Publique, 1933).

departure. The application of new bacteriological science also allowed the close examination (including the troublesome practice of rectal swabbing) of seemingly healthy cholera "carriers." The dissemination of science likewise led to an interest in international standard-setting, for both serums and vaccines and for epidemiological reporting. A few other issues also came under the mandate of the *Office* (to collect and transmit "the facts and documents of a general character of interest to public health"), and in this connection some effort was made to gather information about tuberculosis treatment, venereal disease, leprosy, water purification, and a few other issues. The OIHP's procedure was to collect and publish what various countries did while only occasionally urging them to adopt new measures or standards. Overall, the OIHP in its early years was true to its founding mission and served primarily as a forum for discussion and the exchange of information. In modern parlance, it was a "knowledge management" agency, not a field agency, and the knowledge it managed was public health information that was thought useful to help protect member nations from the incursion of infectious diseases. The *Office* worked in this fashion until World War I forced it to suspend operations except for the publication of its *Bulletin*.

Despite the disruptions they caused, World War I and its immediate aftermath provided the setting for several new international health organizations. The first on the scene, actually founded just before the war in 1913, was the International Health Division (IHD) of the Rockefeller Foundation. It was a private health philanthropy and operated in the United States, China, Europe, Latin America, and other regions of the world. The Foundation had its origins in an American family that possessed the world's greatest oil fortune and decided to spread Western medicine with a missionary zeal. In a short time, the IHD was the most powerful unit of the Foundation and an informal ambassador of the United States.[11] The Foundation's main presupposition was that considerable worldwide poverty was due to infectious diseases that undermined productivity. It carried out important campaigns against hookworm, yellow fever, and malaria as well as for the promotion of the American model of medical education. The Foundation's expectation was that if workers could be cured of their ills, they would become productive citizens and allow their societies to progress. A second assumption was that the Foundation's work should be concentrated on those diseases for which a technology of control existed. Finally, there was the assumption that those who designed health programs knew what was best for the recipients of the aid. There was little regard for community participation in decision-making, although in

[11] John Farley, *To Cast Out Disease: A History of the International Health Division of the Rockefeller Foundation, 1913–1951* (New York: Oxford University Press, 2004).

practice local actors sometimes made their voices heard in ways that changed elements in the original program.

An important regional health agency was the Pan American Sanitary Bureau, created as an international office in the Americas in 1902, renamed in the early 1920s as the Pan American Sanitary Organization, and renamed again as the Pan American Health Organization (PAHO) in the late 1950s. It was initially attached to the US surgeon general's office, had a small budget, and its membership was initially limited to certain Latin American countries. It complemented the work of the more powerful Rockefeller Foundation but developed some of its own initiatives such as those against bubonic plague and smallpox.

Another new international health organization came into existence at the end of World War I: the League of Nations Health Organization, or LNHO. Mainly because of the disruptions, troop movements, and social turmoil associated with World War I and its immediate aftermath, fearsome epidemic diseases now loomed again in the "East": typhus in Russia, which threatened to spread through Poland to Western Europe because of the thousands of people fleeing from the epidemic and from famine, and cholera, smallpox, dysentery and typhoid in the Ottoman Empire, which threatened to spread through Greece. The newly created League of Nations was empowered by Article 23f of the Covenant to "take steps in matters of international concern for the prevention and control of disease."[12] A League-sponsored conference in April 1920, attended by France, Great Britain, Italy, Canada, Japan, Poland, and the United States (which not far in the future opted not to become a member of the League of Nations) and representatives of the OIHP and the League of Red Cross Societies (LRCS) with full voting rights, recommended a temporary epidemic commission, established in May 1920, whose task was to help direct work in afflicted countries, primarily Poland, at least initially.

The presence of the OIHP representatives at the London conference was to be expected, but the LRCS's participation needs some explanation. The LRCS was a new player in the world of international public health. It was largely the creation of wealthy and politically well-placed Americans, who wanted to shift the focus of the International Committee of the Red Cross, Swiss-run and based in Geneva since 1863, from only assisting military medical services during wartime to providing public health services in peacetime. The Americans wanted to organize new humanitarian enterprises to engage in the struggle against epidemic disease, destitution, and other causes of ill health, and this led

---

[12] Francis Paul Walters, *A History of the League of Nations* (London: Oxford University Press, 1952), Vol. 1, p. 59; Goodman, *International Health Organizations*, p. 102.

to a "civil war" between what became two rival Red Cross organizations.[13] Because of strong American interest and President Woodrow Wilson's personal support, the LRCS was invited to participate in a series of emergency conferences in 1919 and 1920, including the one planning the epidemic commission. Indeed, encouragement for "duly authorized voluntary national Red Cross Associations" to play a central and official role in international health efforts was written into the Covenant of the League of Nations as Article 25.[14] The LRCS cut a wide swath because of the enthusiasm of its leaders, its diplomatic support by the US government, and, not least, by the expectation that it would help pay the bills for the epidemic commission and similar work without unduly taxing the resources of the countries formally involved.[15]

The man who emerged as the leader of the epidemic commission was Ludwik Rajchman, a talented and cosmopolitan Polish medical scientist and head of the Polish State Institute of Hygiene since its creation in 1918.[16] He was an outstanding young bacteriologist who had worked with Nobel Laureate Elie Metchnikoff at the Pasteur Institute in Paris and then held several concurrent investigation, teaching, and editorial positions in London from 1910 to 1913. Rajchman came into contact with leading British officials and politicians and also had excellent political connections in Poland. In January 1920 he had accompanied the Polish prime minister to the first official session of the League of Nations. By early 1921, he was principally in charge of the work of the Epidemic Commission, which had set up headquarters in Warsaw and borrowed offices and personnel from the State Institute of Hygiene. The Commission assisted existing national health organizations by providing drugs, vaccines, hospital equipment, soap, food, and clothes and established disinfecting sanitary stations on roads near relevant borders. As he oversaw work in the field, Rajchman insisted that participating governments pay their fair share and not allow the largesse of the LRCS and other relief agencies to let them off the hook. He wanted governments to acknowledge that international medical relief was a legitimate and important responsibility and that nongovernmental philanthropic institutions should not be rewarded with perhaps illegitimate authority. Rajchman (see Figure 1.1) was himself rewarded, however, by being named, in August 1921, medical director of the League of Nations' provisional Health Section.

---

[13] John F. Hutchinson, *Champions of Charity: War and the Rise of the Red Cross* (Boulder, CO: Westview Press, 1996), pp. 279–345.

[14] Walters, *A History of the League*, p. 60; Bridget Towers, "Red Cross Organizational Politics, 1918–1922: Relations of Dominance and the Influence of the United States," in Weindling (ed.), *International Health Organizations*, pp. 43, 46, 50–51, Note 26.

[15] Towers, "Red Cross Organizational Politics, 1918–1922," p. 53.

[16] Marta A. Balińska, *For the Good of Humanity: Ludwik Rajchman, Medical Statesman* (Budapest: Central European University Press, 1998).

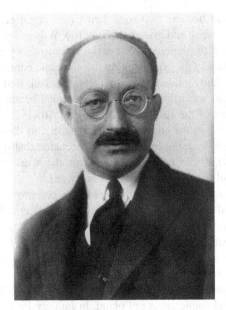

Figure 1.1 Ludwik Rajchman, a Polish physician and bacteriologist who completed post-doctoral studies at the Pasteur Institute in Paris, was medical director of the Health Section of the League of Nations between 1921 and 1939. Among his other accomplishments, he was a respected leader of European social medicine.
Courtesy: United Nations Archives at Geneva.

A provisional Health Committee had already been appointed to oversee Rajchman's work and was one outcome of complex negotiations that had been underway for several years in an attempt to create a single international health agency by including the OIHP under the aegis of the League or, alternatively, by integrating the League's Epidemic Commission into the OIHP. However, political developments made creating a single international agency difficult. During the 1920s, the US Congress declined to join the League of Nations, despite the fact that President Woodrow Wilson had participated in its initial design and actively promoted America's participation. Congressional reaction was a demonstration of the widespread anxiety of US politicians that international organizations and agreements might override American laws and sovereignty. A by-product of American isolationism was the strength it gave to the resistance of some OIHP members, particularly the French, to merge with the League of Nations' Commission. The French felt a proprietary authority over the OIHP and did not want to yield any of it to the British, who strongly supported the League of Nations, supplied its first secretary-general, and wanted to gain recognition in international health via the League's new health activities. For its part, even though the United States chose not to become a member of the League of Nations, many leading American medical experts such as C.-E. A. Winslow of Yale University became advisers to the League while Alice Hamilton of Harvard University and US Surgeon General Hugh Cumming served as members of the League's Health Committee. In 1924, after the possibilities of a merger between the OIHP and the League's health initiatives had disappeared, the League created a Permanent Health Committee to continue and enlarge the work of its Epidemic Commission. This led to the creation of another major health agency, the League of Nations Health Organization (LNHO).

Despite the fact that there were communications, occasional cooperation, and some overlap of personnel between the OIHP and the LNHO, the leaders of both agencies strove to maintain their independence. For leaders of the OIHP, international health work primarily consisted in the collection, validation, and dissemination of epidemiological information. Leaders of the LNHO criticized the absence of executive function in the OIHP and made clear the LNHO was more than a sanitary watchtower.[17] Another difference between the two organizations was that the language used in OIHP communications and publications was almost exclusively French, whereas the LNHO was more diversified in its staff and used both French and English in its publications. (A group portrait of part of the staff of the League of Nations Health Organization appears in Figure 1.2.) For example, of the 66 officers and clerical staff who had appointments in the LNHO's headquarters in Geneva in 1932, the majority were Swiss (17), but there were 8 Brits, 6 Poles, 1 American, and 1 Chinese.[18] A difference between the two agencies was that the focus for the OIHP was the border crossing of infectious disease, whereas the LNHO went well beyond that to the consideration of the health conditions within countries and between regions.

By the mid-1920s, the architecture of the LNHO included a Health Committee and a Health Section that was part of the League of Nations' Secretariat. The Health Committee was composed of 16 senior officials from national public health services or medical experts selected for their technical qualifications and not as representatives of their governments (hence some American membership). The intention was to construct a technical international body of

[17] See Ludwik Rajchman to Wickliffe Rose, RF, (no day) May 1922, Rockefeller Foundation Archives [hereafter RFA], Record Group 1.1, [hereafter RG], Series 100, Box 20, Folder 165, Rockefeller Archive Center [hereafter RAC].

[18] "Health Section-Section D'Hygiene" in *League of Nations, Staff List' of the Secretariat, Showing Nationalities and Salaries for 1932* (Geneva: League of Nations, 1932), pp. 50–53.

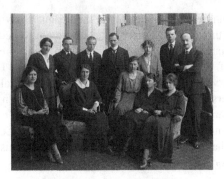

Figure 1.2 Staff: League of Nations Health Organization in the late 1920s. Rajchman is standing on the right. It is interesting to note the number of women in this photograph even though they worked in secretarial and clerical positions.
Courtesy: United Nations Archives at Geneva.

civil servants. The Health Section was the executive organ of the LNHO.[19] By 1933, the LNHO's staff had grown to 18 technical officers. Non-professional personnel numbered 35 individuals, and nearly 100 experts in national health administrations and science research centers collaborated actively with the LNHO.[20] Thanks to a broad and elastic charter, the LNHO undertook a variety of changing tasks, and in the process, helped to define the meaning of international health.

Ludwik Rajchman became the undisputed, if often controversial, leader of the LNHO.[21] The League of Nations' secretary-general, the British Eric Drummond, had appointed Rajchman medical director of the Health Section in August 1921 for a period of seven years (in 1928 he was reappointed for a similar period). Rajchman recruited, as members of the Health Committee, international health experts who served the LNHO without salary. They included Thorvald Madsen, head of the Serum Institute in Copenhagen; George Buchanan, senior medical officer of the British Ministry of Health; and the Croatian Andrija Stampar (see Figure 1.3), who headed the newly

[19] League of Nation Secretariat, Information Section. The Health Organization of the League of Nations (Geneva: n.p., 1923), p. 6.

[20] "Brief Review of the Program Accomplished Since 1 January 1923, LNH" RFA RG 1.1 Series 100, Box 20, Folder 170 and "Development of the Health Organization of the League of Nations, Assistance of the Rockefeller Foundation, 1933" RFA, RG 1.1, Series 100, Box 21, Folder 177, RAC.

[21] Folder "Rajchman, Ludwig" Series Personnel S, Years 1919–1946, Box 861, File 167, [LNA-UNG] and Theodore M. Brown & Elizabeth Fee, "Ludwik Rajchman (1881–1965), World Leader in Social Medicine and Director of the League of Nations Health Organization," American Journal of Public Health 104:9 (2014), 1638–1639.

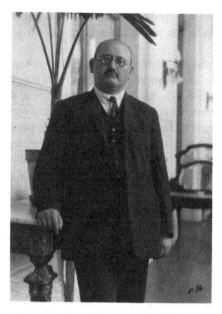

Figure 1.3 Andrija Stampar, the Croatian public health and social medicine leader who worked in China in the mid-thirties for the League of Nations Health Organization. Stampar participated centrally in the creation of the World Health Organization in the 1940s.
Courtesy: United Nations Archives at Geneva.

founded Ministry of Public Health in the Kingdom of Serbs, Croats, and Slovenes (later Yugoslavia).

Rajchman promoted social and medical reforms despite the fact that the LNHO did not have these specific goals in its mandate. Examples of wide-ranging LNHO activities were studies and programs to improve nutrition, child health, rural sanitation, and vital statistics. A number of diseases not prioritized by the OIHP, such as malaria, tuberculosis, sleeping sickness, and cancer became the focus of LNHO commissions populated by international experts. The Commission on Cancer, formed in 1923, compared recovery as the result of the surgical resection of tumors to recovery in patients using radium therapy. The Malaria Commission, created one year later, was one of the most important units of LNHO. Its work was considered urgent because after World War I malaria cases grew in Eastern Europe due to the movement of troops and populations from malarial to non-malarial regions and the disorganization of medical services. The Commission criticized the high cost and insufficient world output of quinine, studied the relationship between poor housing and malaria, and organized international malaria courses in Hamburg, London,

Paris, and Rome.[22] The LNHO also helped create an anti-leprosy center in Rio de Janeiro and studied reforms in the health systems of the Soviet Union, Greece, and Bolivia.

One of Rajchman's goals was to establish in Geneva a global medical library for researchers from all over the world. More urgent was the promotion of exchanges between public health officials from different parts of the world in order to create a global health network.[23] Rajchman hoped to foster "a new spirit of common service" because he believed that international public health work was a transnational duty, shared by professionals beyond borders and in service to people rather than governments. In 1923, 92 public health officers from 18 countries took part in LNHO-sponsored exchanges, and a year later the number grew to 127 from 20 countries.

Rajchman then turned his attention to other areas of interest. One was the laboratory-based standardization of sera, serological tests, and other biological products. International biological standardization was a special priority of Thorvald Madsen, an internationally respected bacteriologist, director of the Danish State Serum Institute in Copenhagen, and chair of the League of Nations' Health Committee. Madsen and Rajchman shared a mutual respect. They began working together to promote a standardization agenda within the LNHO and succeeded in organizing important conferences on therapeutic and diagnostic sera and in creating a network of investigators and laboratories. The issue was urgent because World War I had seriously disrupted communication and created a confusing variety of measurements for the potency of sera used for common infectious diseases such as diphtheria, tetanus, and syphilis. After the War, divergent measurements for antitoxins, sera, vitamins, hormones, and drugs such as digitals, pituitary hormone, and insulin existed among different laboratories. In terms of pharmacopeia, there was great variety in the compositions of medicinal preparations. As a result, many physicians were confused when writing their prescriptions. By 1924 the LNHO created a Permanent Commission on Biological Standardization, chaired by Madsen, which held a series of conferences on the standardization of sera, serological tests, and drugs. Members of the OIHP and of the serological institutes of Austria, Belgium, France, Germany, Great Britain, Italy, Japan, Poland, Switzerland, and the United States participated in these meetings. They established new standards for biological products and a precise relationship between weight and effect for major medications. A decision to centralize this biological information in the Copenhagen Sero-Therapeutic State Institute, which Madsen directed, capped these efforts.

[22] "Health Work of the League," *The British Medical Journal* 2:2826 (July 14, 1934), 72.
[23] Victor G. Heiser, "The Health Work of the League of Nations," *Proceedings of the American Philosophical Society* 65:5, Supplement (1926), 1–9, p. 9.

Rajchman also pushed forward an epidemiological intelligence plan. The LNHO, early on, started compiling and publishing a weekly epidemiological record and a series of epidemiological intelligence reports. But in a January 1922 memo to Drummond, Rajchman referred to the "comparative study" of information contained in the individual annual health reports published by various countries and to "a comprehensive survey of the epidemiological situation of the world." These ambitions intruded into the territory of the OIHP, as Rajchman was told in no uncertain terms by Dr. George Buchanan, a senior medical officer in Great Britain's Ministry of Health and England's representative to the OIHP and the LNHO's Health Committee. Because Rajchman was courting the Rockefeller Foundation as a possible funder for his epidemiology projects, Buchanan wrote to Wickliffe Rose of the Foundation, complaining that Rajchman's plan pushed intrusively into the sphere of the OIHP and would be tantamount to creating a "superepidemiologist at Geneva" as the pivot of the work.

The Foundation held firm and, in fact, worked closely with Rajchman in the latter part of 1922 to recruit an outstanding individual to head the LNHO's new and comprehensive "international service of epidemiological intelligence and public health statistics."[24] That individual was the American epidemiologist, economist, and statistician Edgar Sydenstricker, who was employed by the United States Public Health Service.[25] He had also pioneered in the development of statistical methods for determining patterns of morbidity in communities. Yet despite Sydenstricker's importance in the United States, US Surgeon General Hugh Cumming was willing to let him go to Geneva to work with Rajchman for a year. Cumming made it clear to Rajchman that he was willing to support the LNHO's epidemiological and biostatistical ambitions even if it meant distancing himself from the OIHP on whose Permanent Committee he sat.[26] More immediately, Cumming's acquiescence brought Sydenstricker and his talent to Geneva, where in January 1923 he quickly set to work to transform Rajchman's aspirations into tangible research methods, data sets, and publications. The LNHO's epidemiological publications now became more sophisticated, reliable, and wide-ranging and were greatly enhanced by a Sydenstricker innovation: graphs and maps used to present comparative national data in visually compelling ways.[27]

If the enthusiasm and ambition of the LNHO were great, its budget was precarious. Initially, the LNHO was dependent on the financial largesse of

---

[24] Borowy, *Coming to Terms*, pp. 103–105.
[25] Harry M. Marks, "Epidemiologists Explain Pellagra: Gender, Race, and Political Economy in the Work of Edgar Sydenstricker," *Journal of the History of Medicine* 58 (2003), 34–55.
[26] Wickliffe Rose to Ludwik Rajchman, July 21, 1922, LNA-UNG, Class 12B, Box 839.
[27] Frank G. Boudreau, "Health Work of the League of Nations," *The Milbank Memorial Fund Quarterly* 13:1 (1935), 3–7.

some European governments, mostly Britain. Decisive help came from Selskar M. Gunn of the Paris Office of the Rockefeller Foundation and from the Foundation itself.[28] Beginning in 1922, the Foundation made several grants to support the LNHO's publications, meetings, data collection and analytical activities, fellowships for public health interchanges, and the general budget.[29] Between 1922 and 1934, the Foundation contributed between USD 1,700,000 and 2,000,000 to the operating budget of the LNHO, and by 1933 it was paying the salaries of 25 of the 53 LNHO staff members. The Foundation continued its support almost until the end of the interwar period, granting USD 200,000 for the years 1936 and 1937.[30] This help was crucial during a period when Europe was passing through severe financial crisis and political turmoil.

Rockefeller aid included substantial support for the LNHO's principal extra-European undertaking: its "International Epidemiological Intelligence Bureau for the Far East," inaugurated in the British possession of Singapore in March, 1925.[31] In a part of the world from which epidemiological data had previously been obtainable only with difficulty, the Far Eastern Bureau became a reliable clearinghouse of information on disease outbreaks. The Bureau ultimately surveyed the health conditions of 140 ports and served as a major node in a communication network that included Pretoria, Karachi, Madras, Saigon, Hong Kong, Shanghai, Tokyo, Wellington, Honolulu, and ports in India and China. It drew data from 40 different national or colonial administrations and sent monthly, weekly, and daily cables and radio transmissions to Geneva reporting on epidemic outbreaks. Because the area surveyed included China and several European colonial dependencies, such as French Indochina and the Dutch West Indies, the Far Eastern Bureau became a priority for both the European powers and the Rockefeller. Over time, the Bureau widened its general mission to include "earnest studies of the great public health problems of the East" and promoted specific inquiries into pneumonia and plague, the value of oral vaccination against cholera, and the efficacy of dried smallpox

---

[28] Socrates Litsios, "Selskar Gunn and China: The Rockefeller Foundation's 'Other' Approach to Public Health," *Bulletin for the History of Medicine* 79:2 (2005), 295–318.

[29] George K. Strode, Memorandum on the Health Organization of the League of Nations and the Relationship thereto of the International Health Division of the Rockefeller Foundation [1925] RFA, RG 1.1, Series 1.1, Box 22, Folder 184, RAC.

[30] "Request from the Health Organization of the League of Nations, 12 July 22," "League of Nations – Consolidation of Pledges, 18 March 1928," and "League of Nations Health Section, 21 December 1934," the three documents at RFA, RG 1.1, Series 100, Box 20, Folder 164, RAC.

[31] Lenore Manderson, "Wireless Wars in the Eastern Area: Epidemiological Surveillance, Disease Prevention and the Work of the Eastern Bureau of the League of Nations Health Organization, 1925–1942," in Weindling (ed.), *International Health Organizations*, p. 109. Rockefeller's grants to the Bureau appear in "League of Nations Health Section, Appropriations and Budgets, 1929," RFA, RG 1.1, Series 100, Box 20, Folder 164, RAC.

vaccine. The Far Eastern Bureau was the only solid and long-lasting extension of the LNHO outside Europe.[32]

The League did, however, make sporadic efforts to extend its work into Africa. In May 1922, the Health Committee appointed a subcommittee of experts from Belgium, France, and Great Britain (which all now held mandatory authority over formerly German African colonies) to study sleeping sickness and tuberculosis in central Africa. The subcommittee produced a lengthy report by mid-1923 which confirmed that both diseases were clearly on the rise. It took another nine years before Rajchman was able to follow up, by working with the government of the Union of South Africa to organize a public health meeting of delegates from neighboring countries. That meeting took place in November 1932 in Cape Town and discussed yellow fever, plague, and smallpox. In 1935, a second conference was held in South Africa, this one in Johannesburg.[33] The European powers viewed the LNHO's efforts with some suspicion because they perceived those efforts as potential threats to their colonial authority in the region. When it became clear that the LNHO would not publicly question colonial control, tensions abated, but the LNHO's efforts to establish a solid presence in Africa remained rather limited.

But another late 1930s extra-European LNHO initiative was bolder. That initiative was the "Intergovernmental Conference of Far-Eastern Countries on Rural Hygiene," held in August 1937 in Bandoeng, Java, then part of Dutch Indonesia.[34] During the 1930s, "rural hygiene" had become a major LNHO focus that drew attention to the overwhelming needs of rural populations. These populations bore an enormous burden of disease and mortality, had limited access to modern medical providers or the benefits of scientific public health practices, and struggled with the devastating consequences of the worldwide economic depression – not least, massive nutritional deficiencies. The LNHO approached these problems from an intersectoral perspective and focused not only on the access to medicine but also on the fundamental challenges of educational uplift, economic development, and social advancement. Throughout the thirties, in a series of conferences and reports focused on rural hygiene in Europe, LNHO concentrated on three basic issues: how to ensure effective medical care in rural communities, how best to organize public health services in rural districts, and how to raise the overall environmental, social, and economic status of rural areas.

---

[32] Frank G. Boudreau, "International Health," *American Journal of Public Health* 19 (1929), 863–878.

[33] League of Nations, *Pan-African Health Conference, 1935 Johannesburg* (Geneva: League of Nations, 1936).

[34] Socrates Litsios, "Revisiting Bandoeng," *Social Medicine* 8:3 (2014), 113–128.

In 1932, the League of Nations delegate from India, with the support of the Chinese delegate, proposed a conference on rural hygiene in Eastern countries. It took a few years for a formal response, but in May 1936 LNHO officially accepted an invitation from the Dutch government to host a conference at Bandoeng. This rural hygiene conference was to be different in several ways from the European conferences. For one thing, several of the countries represented were only ambiguously sovereign nations and others were colonial states. Moreover, it was understood that, compared to Europe, the depth of poverty was greater and the level of education lower in much of the vast Asian rural population. Andrija Stampar, the Croatian public health leader who had participated in several of the European "rural hygiene" conferences, spent considerable time in China in the mid-thirties on special missions for the LNHO. There, amid China's revolutionary turmoil, Stampar viewed health problems through a wide lens. In 1936, his detailed report to LNHO stated: "After working nearly three years in China ... successful health work is not possible where the standard of living falls below the level of tolerable existence. ... It follows that the best health programme is to raise the standard of living of the people ... Of perhaps even greater importance is the removal of social grievances, such as the sense of exploitation by the landlord."[35] In seeming synchrony with Stampar, Rajchman insisted that his handpicked staff attendees at Bandoeng include individuals with a "thoroughly sympathetic attitude toward the native populations."[36]

These "Eastern" specifics were reflected in the final recommendations of the Bandoeng meeting. Some repeated the themes of intersectoral collaboration and basic health education familiar from the European rural hygiene conferences. But there were also open references to "land reform," emphasis on honoring indigenous languages, insistence on the populace's "free will" in adopting plans for "betterment," and a clearly stated understanding that public health work would be an "entering wedge" for economic development and self-governance. Although action subsequent to the Bandoeng conference fell far short of conference rhetoric, several of the recommendations not only showed glimpses of the priorities of nationalist independence movements such as that led by Gandhi in India but also of a commitment to the broad principles of "social medicine."[37]

---

[35] Stampar is cited in *Quarterly Bulletin of the Health Organisation of the League of Nations* 5 (1936), 1090–1126. This report is reprinted as "Health and Social Conditions in China" in Mirko Drazen Grmek (ed.), *Serving the Cause of Public Health: Selected Papers of Andrija Stampar* (Zagreb: University of Zagreb, 1966), pp. 123–151, quotations pp. 149–160.

[36] Theodore M. Brown & Elizabeth Fee, "The Bandoeng Conference of 1937: A Milestone of Health and Development," *American Journal of Public Health* 98:1 (2008), 42–43.

[37] Amrith, *Decolonizing International Health: India and Southeast Asia, 1930–65*.

The LNHO under Rajchman had, in fact, been moving strongly toward social medicine principles, that is, to approaches to public health problems that emphasized social and economic as opposed to biomedical factors. This perspective was present to some extent in the twenties, as in the epidemiological studies relating typhus to famine, the Malaria Commission's insistence that malaria was a "social disease," and the attention devoted to the connection between medical insurance and public health.[38] But the social medicine focus emerged far more clearly in the thirties, for a variety of reasons. The state of the world, especially the worldwide economic depression and the social and political disruptions that followed from it, was of major significance. These trends may in some sense have allowed Rajchman to follow more consistently interests in social medicine for which his socialist political proclivities prepared him. The shift was signaled in new studies on tuberculosis, which the LNHO had approached largely from technical perspectives in the twenties but considered in the broader context of income, working hours, diet, and living conditions in the thirties. A memorandum prepared by the Health Section in August 1932, "Economic Depression and Public Health," stated its new orientation with particular clarity:

Although the mortality and morbidity statistics of the various countries have not hitherto supplied any indication that the crisis is now exercising an influence on the state of health of the populations which can be measured statistically, warning signals have nevertheless multiplied in the last few months, especially in Germany. ... Many facts have already been quoted in medical literature pointing to an increase in the number of cases of open tuberculosis among adults, and also ... among children; an increase in the number of cases of rickets is also reported ... In a working-class quarter of Berlin, the children of the unemployed were definitely backward from the point of view of weight and growth. Another symptom of the economic depression is the increase in tuberculosis morbidity, skin diseases and nervous affections and in the number of difficult or morally neglected children.[39]

Studies from the social medicine perspective developed more fully in the thirties, with three areas having particular importance: nutrition, housing, and

---

[38] For the LNHO's movement toward social medicine, see Weindling, "Social Medicine at the League of Nations Health Organization and the International Labour Office Compared," in Weindling (ed.), *International Health Organizations*, pp. 141–146. On typhus, see Weindling, *Epidemics and Genocide* (Oxford: Oxford University Press, 2000). On malaria, see Hughes Evans, "European Malaria Policy in the 1920s and 1930s: The Epidemiology of Minutiae," *Isis* 80 (1989), 45–49; on social insurance, see Lion Murard, "Health Policy between the International and the Local: Jacques Parisot in Nancy and Geneva," in Iris Borowy & Wolf Gruner (eds.), *Facing Illness in Troubled Times, 1918–1939*, (Frankfurt am Main: Peter Lang, 2005), p. 226.

[39] "Economic Depression and Public Health," Geneva, August 20, 1932, LNA-UNG, Class 8A, Box 5866, Series 1409, Dossier 37494. See Theodore M. Brown & Elizabeth Fee, "Cognitive Dissonance in the Early Thirties: The League of Nations Health Organization Confronts the Worldwide Economic Depression," *American Journal of Public Health* 105 (2015), 65.

the public health effects of the economic depression. Expert committees pursued these lines of work, and the LNHO's newest periodical, the *Quarterly Bulletin of the Health Organisation*, regularly published impressive and often quite lengthy papers and reports on this fresh range of topics.[40] A notable author was Jacques Parisot, chair of hygiene and social medicine at Nancy and a founding editor of *Revue d'Hygiene et Medecine Sociales*.[41] When Parisot joined the League's Health Committee in 1934 and then replaced Thorvald Madsen as chair in 1937, the LNHO's shift from biomedicine to social medicine would seem to have gained even further momentum. There was more to Parisot's election as Health Committee chair than met the eye, however. Balińska sees it, in fact, as part of a plot against Rajchman and his allies in the LNHO, a judgment which is consistent with scholarly accounts of the League's history in the later thirties.[42] The reality was that Rajchman had been in political difficulty for some time, and many in powerful positions both within the League and beyond wanted him out. A problem derived from his strong defense of China against Japan's aggression in the 1930s and the suspicion that he stepped beyond his League-sanctioned technical role. The Japanese government requested the League to curtail Rajchman's activities in China, and he was not, in fact, allowed by the League's authorities to remain in the country. With the rapid rise of European fascism in the thirties, Rajchman was not secure in Europe, either, as his left-leaning politics were increasingly labeled "communist," "pro-Soviet," or even "Jewish-Masonic." After Italy's annexation of Ethiopia in 1936 and during the Spanish Civil War, his sympathies were firmly with the left while the League sputtered in neutral, capitulated to the right, or allowed itself to become captive to British-French foreign policy priorities in support of Munich appeasement. Rajchman even lost the backing of his "home" country as the Polish government became increasingly

---

[40] S. R. Christophers & A. Missiroli, "Report on Housing and Malaria," *Quarterly Bulletin of the Health Organisation of the League of Nations* 2 (1933), 357–482; "Rapport de la Commission de l'Habitation," *Quarterly Bulletin of the Health Organisation of the League of Nations* 6 (1937), 543–592; M. Vignerot, "La Maison et l'Amenagement Ruraux," *Quarterly Bulletin of the Health Organisation of the League of Nations* 8 (1939), 92–151; "Rapport de la Commission de l'Habitation," *Quarterly Bulletin of the Health Organisation of the League of Nations* 8 (1939), 789–858; A. Goetzi, W. Kornfeld, & E. Nobel, "The Effects of the Economic Depression on the Population of Vienna," *Quarterly Bulletin of the Health Organisation of the League of Nations* 3 (1934), 461–522; "Report on the Best Methods of Safeguarding the Public Health During the Depression," *Quarterly Bulletin of the Health Organisation of the League of Nations* 2 (1933), 286–332; "The Most Suitable Methods of Detecting Malnutrition Due to the Economic Depression," *Quarterly Bulletin of the Health Organisation of the League of Nations* 2 (1933), 116–129; W. R. Aykroyd, "Diet in Relation to Small Incomes," *Quarterly Bulletin of the Health Organisation of the League of Nations*, 2 (1933), 130–153; E. Burnet & W. R. Aykroyd, "Nutrition and Public Health," *Quarterly Bulletin of the Health Organisation of the League of Nations* 4 (1935), 232–474.
[41] Murard, "Health Policy between the International and the Local," pp. 207–245.
[42] Balińska, *For the Good of Humanity*, pp. 112–113.

right-wing. Thus, despite his clear support of the LNHO's change of focus to social medicine, Rajchman felt no joy in Parisot's election and less than two years later was himself, like Madsen, compelled to resign. His elimination as head of the Health Section was part of a general "purge" of perceived left-wing elements in the League Secretariat conducted by Joseph Avenol, Drummond's successor as secretary-general. Avenol rationalized Rajchman's dismissal as an economy-based decision, telling him in a letter of January 4, 1939, that "restructuring entails the disappearance of the directorate of the Health Section."[43]

The polarization of European politics and ideology, along with major changes in the internal workings of the disintegrating League, was primarily responsible for this turn of events. Indeed, much that happened to Rajchman is explained by the title of Barros' history of Avenol's tenure as secretary-general: "Betrayal From Within."[44] But it was also true that Rajchman's old Health Committee enemies, such as England's George Buchanan, had never relented in their attacks and assaulted him with more powerful ammunition after his shift to social medicine.[45] Even if he still had support in the leadership of the Rockefeller Foundation, after 1938 there were no more Rockefeller funds at his disposal to administer. Rajchman had no option remaining but to leave, and he chose to leave with grace. In his resignation letter of January 29, 1939, he wrote: "I am leaving without bitterness, conscious and happy to have been able to glimpse that international collaboration is possible, that it can be disinterested."[46]

The Final Years of the League of Nations Health Organization

The world of international health – like the world at large – was dramatically disrupted by the coming of World War II. In September 1939, when Germany invaded Poland, the LNHO sent a message to world health authorities explaining that communications would be "delayed." In fact, they were soon so compromised that only in late 1941 was it possible to publish the annual epidemiological report for 1938.[47] The League of Nations had to trim its

---

[43] Balińska, *For the Good of Humanity*, p. 121.

[44] James Barros, *Betrayal from Within: Joseph Avenol, Secretary-General of the League of Nations, 1933–1940* (New Haven: Yale University Press, 1969), pp. 185–188.

[45] See, for example, George Buchanan to Ludwik Rajchman, May 1933, LNA-UNG, Class 8A, Box 549.

[46] Balińska, *For the Good of Humanity*, p. 123.

[47] League of Nations, Radiotelegraphic information concerning the sanitary situation in Eastern port, Geneva, September 1, 1939, RFA, RG 6.1, Series 1.1, Box 38, Folder 465, RAC; "Activities of the Health Organization of the League of Nations during the War," *Chronicle of the World Health Organization*, Special Number, No Volume, (1945), 2–16, p. 15, World Health Organization Library.

operations and reorganize its structure. The Secretariat of the League merged several units into three new departments, one of which was the Department of Health, Drug Control, and Social and Cultural Questions that absorbed the LNHO.

During the war, the LNHO could not count on many of its most important former officers and advisors. Rajchman spent most of World War II in Washington, DC, New York, and London, initially as a representative of the Polish government-in-exile and later working on the organization of health services for areas of Europe liberated by the Allies. Stampar returned to Yugoslavia in 1939 as professor of hygiene and social medicine at the Zagreb School of Medicine. But when the German army occupied Yugoslavia in 1941, Stampar was sent to a jail in Austria where he remained until the end of the War. LNHO advisor René Sand was sent from Belgium to Germany and was not released until the liberation of Belgium by the Allies. After serving in the French Army, Jacques Parisot was captured by the Germans in June of 1940 and sent first to a concentration camp and later to a Czech prison. After release from prison, Parisot stayed in occupied France. Thorvald Madsen worked in German-occupied Copenhagen, seemed sympathetic to the Nazis, kept a low profile, and stayed away from Geneva.

The outbreak of World War II also brought changes to the OIHP, which made the controversial decision to work under Nazi supervision and relocated from Paris to Royat, a town in Vichy France.[48] During the war, leaders of the LNHO regarded the OIHP as a "German-controlled agency located in an enemy-occupied territory."[49] When in 1940 several units of the League of Nations moved to Princeton, New Jersey in the United States and others to London, the leaders of the LNHO considered moving outside of continental Europe but decided to stay in Geneva. The Far Eastern Bureau in Singapore lost its links with Geneva after the Japanese occupation of February 1942, and the LNHO staff of the Bureau moved to Canberra, Australia, but then had to suspend their activities.

A small LNHO contingent remained in Geneva and bravely soldiered on: the French Yves Biraud and the Swiss Raymond Gautier, the latter an LNHO officer since 1924 and director of the Far Eastern Bureau from 1924 to 1930. Biraud and Gautier worked together with a small clerical staff, and in 1939 Gautier officially replaced Rajchman as medical director, a position he would retain until the end of the war. This small Geneva group somehow kept

---

[48] "Annexe II Au Procès-Verbal de la 10e Séance-Jeudi 31 October 1946," in *Office International d'Hygiene Publique, Session Ordinaire du Comité Permanent* (Paris: *Office International d'Hygiene Publique*, 1947), 153.

[49] Raymond Gautier, "The Future Health Organization," May 31, 1943, Series Health 8A, Years 1939–1942, Box 6150, File 41755 League of Nations Archives, United Nations Archives, Geneva [hereafter LNA-UN].

up the irregular publication of the *Weekly Epidemiological Record*, and even managed to publish several numbers of the *Bulletin of the Health Organization*. The LNHO was officially "neutral" by virtue of being in internationally neutral Switzerland, but in reality, established close ties with the Allies. Starting in 1942, LNHO representatives attended meetings in London and Washington to examine, with public health experts from the United States and the United Kingdom, the postwar nutritional and health requirements of the countries occupied by the Nazis, Fascists, and Japanese. During 1942 and 1943, Gautier moved to London to work on postwar planning, formally "on loan" from the League.

In March of 1943, Gautier wrote an 11-page confidential report entitled "International Health in the Future."[50] This report contained an outline of a future "supranational" health agency, meaning that the projected agency would take the initiative of intervening in emergencies "without waiting for a governmental request." Gautier considered the OIHP an unworthy German-controlled organization that should not be revitalized after the war. He also recognized that the LNHO would not survive in its present form but could, he hoped, be the basis for a new agency independent of the "interference" of diplomats. Gautier's document contained a sentence that in a more refined form would later be incorporated in the Preamble to the WHO Constitution: "For health is more than the absence of illness; the word health implies something positive, namely physical, mental, and moral fitness. This is the goal to be reached."[51] It was a clear statement of the socio-medical perspective that would later inspire and identify some members of the WHO. The Constitution stipulated a function that would be a matter of discussion for years: The WHO was to be the directing and coordinating leader on international health.

In 1944, the LNHO made a comprehensive study of health conditions in Europe that was turned over to UNRRA. In October 1944, Gautier, US Surgeon General Thomas Parran, Frank Boudreau (an American who had been executive director of the Milbank Foundation and executive secretary of the Health Organization of the League of Nations), and Rockefeller IHD Associate Director George K. Strode, along with other medical leaders, met and agreed on two principles: the need to build an international health organization for the postwar period and the importance of the United States taking the initiative to convene "as soon as possible" a conference on world health.[52] It was out of this conference that the World Health Organization would emerge.

---

[50] Raymond Gautier, "Confidential-International Health in the Future, 1943," Series Health 8A, Years 1939–1942, Box 6150, File 41755 [LNA-UNG].

[51] Gautier, Confidential-International Health in the Future, 1943, p. 1.

[52] Raymond Gautier, "From Atlantic City to Montreal and Further," October 25, 1944, Series Health 8A, Years 1939–1942, Box 6150, File 4127 [LNA-UNG].

2 The Birth of the World Health Organization, 1945–1948

During World War II, the most destructive war in history, Europe, Asia, and other areas of the world suffered devastating human carnage, widespread material destruction, terrifying food scarcity, shattered public health and medical care systems, and massive waves of displaced persons. Intense fears of epidemic outbreaks that would rapidly spread worldwide were understandably pervasive, and many thought that for pragmatic reasons a new international health organization had to be created because they believed that the health institutions of the interwar period would prove woefully inadequate to meet massive postwar challenges. That new organization, the World Health Organization, would in fact be formally launched in 1948, and included in its foundation idealistic as well as practical considerations. The purpose of this chapter is to examine the early institution-building process. The key focus during the immediate postwar period was an "Interim Commission" of the projected WHO. The roots of this new commission can be traced, to some extent, to idealistic visions of a new world order in health that carried over from the prewar period, but more directly, to pragmatic relief operations that were organized during the latter years of the war.

Legacies of World War II

Early in 1942 the Allied powers began to call themselves the "United Nations," that term first making an appearance in a January 1942 declaration in which 26 nations pledged to employ their "full resources, military or economic" in their unified fight against the Axis nations. The same term was applied a year later to a relief organization, the United Nations Relief and Rehabilitation Administration (UNRRA), which was established in 1943 when 44 nations signed an agreement to coordinate their relief activities, initially targeting primarily European civilian victims of the war.[1] The UNRRA would

---

[1] Jessica Reinisch, "Internationalism in Relief: The Birth (and Death) of UNRRA," in Mark Mazower, Jessica Reinisch, & David Feldman (eds.), *Past and Present Supplements, Supplement Post-War Reconstruction in Europe: International Perspectives, 1945–1949* 6 (2011), 258–289.

ultimately provide relief in more than 30 countries overrun by the Axis powers in Europe, northern Africa, and Asia. At its peak, it had a budget of USD 3.7 billion, $2.7 billion of which came from the United States. No other relief organization at that time had anything remotely approaching this level of financial clout.

Initially, the UNRRA concentrated on the provision of food, fuel, clothing, shelter, and other basic and urgent necessities, but soon its work expanded to include medical and health services. The enlargement of the UNRRA's medical and health operations led to the creation of a health division. Wilbur Sawyer, who had been the director of the International Health Division of the Rockefeller Foundation before the war, became director of the UNRRA's Health Division soon after his retirement from the IHD in 1944. Under Sawyer, the goals of the UNRRA's Division were the rehabilitation and restoration of hospitals, medical clinics, and laboratories; the prevention of epidemics by the distribution of drugs and the insecticide dichlorodiphenyltrichloroethane, known as DDT (initially to control typhus); and the administration of the International Sanitary Conventions (the latest one had been approved in Paris in 1926 and modified in 1938, and it had been complemented by agreements on aerial navigation in 1933). A 1944 agreement authorized the UNRRA to assume this former responsibility of the OIHP, with the expectation that at the end of the War a decision would be made about the continuity or termination of that organization. Thanks to the UNRRA, postwar European epidemic outbreaks did not get out of control (unlike in other wars, where the number of victims of epidemics was frequently greater than the number of soldiers who died in battle), encouraging the optimistic belief that this achievement could be extended on an international scale with modern medical science and technology. DDT would be used in other places in the early post–World War II period (see Figure 2.1, depicting a health worker from India writing the date of insecticide spraying on a poster featuring the WHO emblem).

The UNRRA's health staff included professionals of many different nationalities, but they were primarily US and British citizens. Some would continue working in international health beyond the UNRRA's lifespan. The American Henry van Zile Hyde, for example, worked with the health committee of the UNRRA, later at the State Department's Division of International Labor and Health Affairs, and eventually represented the United States in the organizing meetings of the WHO and in early World Health Assemblies. In many settings, the UNRRA replaced broken national health systems, thus going beyond its formal mandate as a relief agency and becoming a reconstruction agency instead. This dual approach created mixed feelings among the leaders of the UNRRA, some of whom liked the idea of being in control of health system reconstruction, especially when it happened in Western European countries

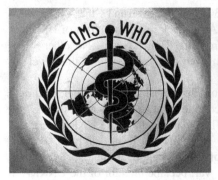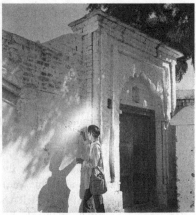

Figure 2.1 In this 1949 photograph, a health worker from India writes the word DDT and the date of spraying on a poster with the emblem of the WHO on a treated house in Uttar Pradesh. The emblem of the World Health Organization consists of the UN symbol on which is superimposed a staff with a snake coiling around it, the traditional symbol of medicine.
Courtesy: World Health Organization Photo Library.

closely allied to the United States. Nevertheless, most US diplomats understood that reconstruction would be a heavy burden and set as their highest priority the creation of a new multilateral agency.

The first step in creating this agency was deciding on the fate of the existing agencies, the OIHP and the LNHO. The OIHP was not taken seriously because the organization had been compromised by its collaboration with the Nazis.[2] There was also little possibility of restoring the LNHO because the United States did not want to continue the League of Nations. There was, instead, a strong push to create a new set of international institutions and to locate a new health organization within it. At a meeting in London in April 1944, a glimpse of the future appeared when Allied representatives from ministries of education proposed the establishment of a "United Nations Organization for Educational and Cultural Reconstruction" that would later become the basis for UNESCO. According to Raymond Gautier, the best the

[2] Despite being accused of collaborating with the Nazis, Pierret, the director of the OIHP, managed ephemeral support from the new government of France. But the insistence of the United States on dissolving the OIHP as soon as possible prevailed. See Howard B. Calderwood, "France and Pierret," in Department of State, "Memorandum of Conversation, Subject Position of the International Office of Public Health, 15 January 1946," Howard B. Calderwood World Health Organization development collection Years 1945–1963, MS C 171, Box 1. Folder "1946 Items 47–59," History of Medicine Division, National Library of Medicine [NLM].

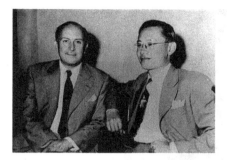

Figure 2.2 Geraldo de Paula Souza from Brazil (left) and Szeming Sze from China. Both participated in founding the United Nations San Francisco Conference in 1945, and with Karl Evang of Norway, advocated for the inclusion of a health agency in the Constitution of the UN.
Courtesy: World Health Organization Photo Library.

surviving staff of the LNHO could hope for was to place a new health agency under the authority of the "United Nations" and empower it to continue the LNHO's work.[3]

Many of the early staff of the new World Health Organization would thus be drawn from active and retired LHNO personnel. The UNRRA also provided staff for the new multilateral agency. This was the case for Neville Goodman of Great Britain, who after a career in international health became director of the Health Division in the UNRRA's European Office and later moved to the WHO as director of the Field Services Division. The UNRRA was also instrumental in rescuing the Far Eastern Bureau in Singapore, which, thanks to new funds, reopened in 1946. In part due to pressure by Biraud, in March 1947 the Bureau became a responsibility of the organizers of the World Health Organization. The technical commissions of the LNHO, such as the biological standardization commission, were also preserved and assigned to the WHO.

The UNRRA had among its officers prominent young health workers from all over the world. These included Simon Sze, a Chinese national who had studied medicine at Cambridge, and the Brazilian Geraldo de Paula Souza from the school of hygiene in Sao Paulo (Souza and Sze appear in Figure 2.2). Unlike Goodman, Sze and de Paula Souza were new to international health. Both attended the United Nations Conference on International Organization that took place in San Francisco from April to June 1945, where 50 countries ultimately signed the United Nations Charter. As UNRRA staff members, Sze and Souza could not present proposals, so they arranged to be members of the

[3] Raymond Gautier, "For Whom the Bell Tolls," August 15, 1944, Series Health 8A, Years 1939–1942, Box 6150, File 4274 [LNA-UNG].

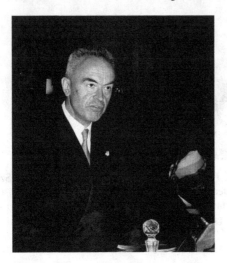

Figure 2.3 Karl Evang, director-general, Public Health Service, Norway. Evang played an important role in the early years of the WHO. This photograph shows him speaking at the World Health Assembly in 1956. Courtesy World Health Organization Photo Library.

delegations of their home countries.[4] De Paula Souza and Sze succeeded in inserting the concept of a health agency into the constitution of the UN (previously they had coordinated with Karl Evang from Norway (see Figure 2.3) and even with some members of the United States and Great Britain). The declaration submitted by the delegations of Brazil and China on May 28, 1945, asserted that the creation of that health agency "cannot be dodged at this Conference. International health security, now more than ever, is becoming a matter of immediate and urgent concern." The Brazil-China declaration asserted that the proposed international health organization be part of the responsibility of the Economic and Social Council, which would be in charge of defining the role of the specialized UN agencies.[5]

---

[4] In 1944, Simon Sze was the general secretary of the Chinese Medical Association and later wrote *The Origins of the World Health Organization: A Personal Memoir 1945–1948* (Boca Raton: L.I.S.Z. Publications, 1982). In 1948, Sze joined the Secretariat of the UN in New York, where after a few years he became medical director. On Souza, see Cristina Campos, *São Paulo pela Lente da Higiene: as Propostas de Geraldo Horácio de Paula Souza para a Cidade (1925–1945)* (São Paulo: Rima, 2000). Following the war, Evang became Norway's director-general of Health. See K. Ringen, "Karl Evang: A Giant in Public Health," *Journal of Public Health Policy* 11:3 (1990), 360–367.

[5] "Joint Declaration by the Delegations of Brazil and China Regarding International Health Cooperation," July 9, 1948, Howard B. Calderwood World Health Organization Development Collection MS C 171, Years 1945–1963, Box 1. Folder "items 1–10," NLM.

According to other accounts, however, the British and Americans were already thinking about the possibility of an international health agency before the San Francisco meeting and wanted to design the institution themselves. They believed that a general international organization, that is, the UN, should be set up first and that technical organizations should follow under the UN's aegis. The US Department of State made sure to have the Charter of the emerging UN amended to facilitate the handover of the UNRRA's funds and health functions to the UN Economic and Social Council as a preparatory step toward the new health agency.[6] The resolution proposed by Sze and Souza was approved unanimously, and the San Francisco meeting also approved a UN constitution, which in articles 55, 57, and 59 formally provided for the organization of specialized agencies, including one having worldwide responsibilities in health.

The declaration approved in San Francisco called for a general conference to "be convened within the next few months for ... establishing an international health organization ... to which each of the governments here represented will be invited to send representatives." In February 1946, the UN Economic and Social Council designated a group of medical leaders as a "Technical Preparatory Committee" (TPC), which by June of that year would call a meeting formally to organize an "international," "global," or "United Nations" health organization (the name of the new organization was not yet settled). The TPC was composed of 16 experts (a number similar to the one used by the LNHO Health Committee) officially selected for their technical competence and not as representatives of their respective countries. Eight were from Europe, five from the Americas, and three were from Asia.[7] None came from Africa. The TPC's mandate also included the preparation of a draft charter for the new health organization and the setting of an agenda for its founding World Health Assembly.

The first meeting of the TPC took place on March 18, 1946, in Paris. There was an attempt by diplomatic officials of the United States and the United Kingdom to limit the membership of the TPC to a small group of technical experts because they feared that large meetings would become politicized and might interfere with foreign policy goals. However, it was impossible to keep the TPC's work completely apolitical because several of its members came from the social medicine perspective. For example, the TPC's chairman was

---

[6] George Woodbridge, *UNRRA: The History of the United Nations Relief and Rehabilitation Administration Vol. 1* (New York: Columbia University Press, 1950), p. 303.

[7] They were: Gregorio Bermann from Argentina, René Sand from Belgium, Manuel Martínez Báez from Mexico, Karl Evang from Norway, A. Cavaillon from France, D. Knoparris from Greece, Brock Chisholm, Josek Cancik from Czechoslovakia, Wilson Jameson from the UK, C. Mani from India, Parran from the United States, Aly Twefik Shousa Pasha from Egypt, Geraldo H. de Paula Souza from Brasil, and P. Z. Kin from China.

the respected social medicine leader René Sand. The TPC could agree, however, on certain basic organizing principles.[8] The most important of these was
to build a health organization with a high degree of independence from the UN
since the lack of autonomy of the LNHO in relationship to the League of
Nations was then considered to have been an impediment to its success. Other
principles included reinforcing the links between new medical discoveries and
public health initiatives and involving as many member states as possible in
the work of the TPC. The latter principle meant that countries could be
members of the emerging health agency without yet being official members
of the UN.

It is interesting to note that Rajchman, the forceful leader of the LNHO
during the interwar period, was not part of the TPC. An American official
explained that Rajchman was "pushed aside" despite his credentials because he
was considered "too forceful" by organizers of the new health agency.[9] He had
made bold proposals during the war for a new international health agency that
would include a unit as some "sort of control in colonial empires," a plan that
was considered "wild" by British authorities.[10] By contrast, the international
health newcomer Thomas Parran, the US surgeon general, played an influential
role in the TPC. He had a reputation for being an able medical politician and
had a broad commitment to socio-medical principles. In the late 1940s he was
serving his third term as surgeon general (1945–1948), and the USPHS which
he oversaw had 14,187 civil service personnel and a professional staff of 2,152
in the commissioned corps. His budget and staff were much larger than those
of any other national or international health organization. Many medical
experts believed Parran would become director of the new international health
organization. Yet his advocacy of national health insurance drew strong
opposition from the American Medical Association and other conservative
political forces in the United States, and President Truman made the strategic
decision not to reappoint him after 1948.[11]

---

[8] These principles are discussed in World Health Organization, Official Records, Number 1,
Minutes of the Technical Preparatory Committee for the International Health Conference held
in Paris, March 18 to April 5, 1946 (Geneva: United Nations World Health Organization,
Interim Commission, 1946).

[9] Transcript of an oral interview with Professor Milton P. Siegel by Mr. Gino Levy with the
participation of Norman Howard-Jones, Tape One, November 15, 1982, p. 15, World Health
Organization Archives, Geneva [hereafter WHO], www.who.int/archives/fonds_collections/
special/milton_siegel_tapes.pdf.

[10] Gautier, "For Whom the Bell Tolls." One of Rajchman's proposals during the War, "United
Nations Health Organization," The Lancet 1 (6399), 584. He also previously published "A
United Nations Health Service, Why Not?" Free World (1943), p. 3, newspaper clipping Series
Health 8A, Years 1939–1942, Box 6150, File 41755 [LNA-UN].

[11] "World Health Job Posed for Parran," The New York Times, July 14, 1946, p. 4. See also Lynne
Page Zinder, "New York, the Nation, the World, the Career of Surgeon General Thomas
J. Parran Jr., MD (1892–1968)," Public Health Reports 110 (1995), 630–632, and Jeanne

Before being dismissed, Parran had helped build US support for a new international health agency. In 1944, the State Department sponsored a "Commission to Study the Organization of the Peace," which included Parran and medical experts such as C.-E. A. Winslow, a professor at Yale and occasional advisor to the LNHO who advocated for a postwar international health agency. Later, the Department convened a more formal Advisory Health Group, consisting of 47 American health leaders that met in Washington, DC, in October 1945. It was chaired by Parran and included E. I. Bishop, director of health in the New Deal's Tennessee Valley Authority; Frank G. Boudreau, a former LNHO officer; Martha M. Eliot, associate chief of the Children's Bureau and occasional advisor to the LNHO and the UNRRA; James Doull, director of the Office of International Health Relations of the US Public Health Service; Hugh S. Cumming, director of the Pan American Sanitary Bureau; Morris Fishbein, editor of the Journal of the American Medical Association; Raymond B. Fosdick, president of the Rockefeller Foundation; General James S. Simmons, chief of preventive medicine services of the US Army; George Strode of the International Health Division of the Rockefeller Foundation; and Winslow. The Advisory Health Group strongly urged the federal government and Congress to move quickly to establish a new international health agency. The group argued that the health systems of many countries had been destroyed during the war and those countries were now experiencing outbreaks of diseases that, because of new means of rapid transportation, represented a menace to the rest of the world. There was thus a need to maintain the continuity of health agencies, such as the UNRRA, that existed before or during the war.[12] The group found that some officers of the Department, such as Undersecretary of State Dean Acheson, were already convinced of the need for an international health organization. American health leaders knew that they had to advance these arguments of self-interested pragmatism because they had to fight for a new multilateral health agency against a US Congress committed to a tradition of isolationism, a tradition which intensified after the election of November 1946 when conservative Republicans took control of both the House and Senate.

During the initial postwar years, foreign policy leaders in the US and UK governments maintained a wary but overall cordial working relationship with the Soviet Union. This period of cordiality can be traced to 1942 and became

---

L. Brand, "The United States Public Health Service and International Health, 1945–1950," *The Bulletin of the History of Medicine* 63 (1989), 579–598, p. 579.

[12] "Annex 7, A Resolution, Department of State Advisory Health Group, 12 October 1945, Washington, DC," in *International Health Conference, New York, June 19 to July 22, 1946, Report of the United States Delegation, Including the Final Acts and Related Documents* (Washington, DC: US Government Printing Office, 1947), pp. 90–91, National Library of Medicine.

more pronounced in 1944, when ideological differences between the United States and the Soviet Union were temporarily put aside for the sake of achieving the common goals of defeating the Nazis and establishing a basis for a new world order. An illustration of the cordial relations between the two sides in this period was Parran's friendly relationship with medical leaders of the Soviet Union and his willingness to recognize Soviet achievements in public health. Many politicians and diplomats in the United States, the United Kingdom, and the Soviet Union believed that cordial relations were ephemeral and that open military conflict would ensue after World War II. Nonetheless, these suspicions did not dominate diplomatic circles until the late 1940s and early 1950s.

The participation of the US government in the creation of multilateral organizations despite deep wells of congressional suspicion that derived from traditional isolationist foreign policy was possible thanks in part to a more professional and specialized Department of State with energetic new leaders. These included the secretaries Edward R. Stettinius, Dean G. Acheson, and George C. Marshall. George Kennan, the force behind the United States policy of "containment" of communist influence, became director of the Department's powerful Bureau of Policy Planning in 1947. Kennan's containment policy held that competition between capitalism and communism was inevitable but that direct, armed confrontation should be avoided because of the risk of mutual annihilation through nuclear warfare if open conflict began and escalated.

The application of Kennan's ideas by President Harry Truman in the late 1940s indicated a change in the political atmosphere and the beginning of the Cold War. The principal factors in the background to this change were the United States' and the Soviet Union's efforts to expand their areas of influence, most immediately in the supervised reconstruction of devastated Europe (the West by the United States, and the East by the USSR). In May 1947, the US Congress responded to a direct appeal by President Truman by voting USD 400 million in military and economic aid to Greece and Turkey to keep them from "falling" to communism. Truman's "Doctrine" was thus to "contain" communism and not allow it to spread in order to avoid "domino"-like regional and ultimately wider geopolitical shifts in the US-USSR balance of forces.

According to the new policy, the US government sent financial aid, expert personnel, and military forces to provide active aid to countries threatened by "communist takeover." Truman's announcement formally ended the friendly relations between the Soviet Union and the United States and began an American "get tough" policy. Leaders of the United States and the United Kingdom also spoke openly of their disapproval of the violent Soviet takeover in Czechoslovakia in 1948, a move justified by the USSR because the eastern European country had a communist leader with a pro-Western orientation.

The Soviets were also moving in a similar confrontational direction. In October of 1947, they had taken a step toward confrontation with their former allies by forming the Cominform (Communist Information Bureau) to coordinate the activities of Europe's communist parties. It was a step toward relaunching the global ambitions of the Soviet Union as in the Comintern, created in 1919 as the "Third International," which Stalin had dissolved in 1943 to calm his World War II allies. By late June 1948, tension escalated significantly when the Soviets began the Berlin Blockade, attempting to shut down all East German contact with the West. They also pursued a general policy of building up nuclear arms. From the Soviet Union's perspective, it made perfect sense to establish a ring of satellite states as a buffer between them and Germany, which had invaded it twice in three decades. Soviet authorities also pointed out that the territory they annexed, such as the Baltic States and Eastern Poland, had belonged to Russia before World War I. The British, who like the French were still trying to recover full control over their colonial empires, decided to combine their interests with US Cold War policy and in 1949 joined with the United States in the formation of the North Atlantic Treaty Alliance (NATO), a full-fledged military alliance aimed at defense against prospective Soviet aggression in Europe.

Planning for the Future

The planning and early implementation phases of the WHO encompassed the brief postwar euphoria and the coming of the Cold War. Work formally began in March and April of 1946 when the TPC met in Paris. In addition to the 16 designated experts, representatives of four organizations attended the meeting: the Pan American Sanitary Bureau, the OIHP, the LNHO, and the UNRRA. The delicate issue of the absorption of some or all of these was initially deferred. The immediate task was to prepare a draft constitution on the basis of four documents submitted respectively by Cavaillon and Leclainche from France, Jameson from the United Kingdom, Parran from the United States, and Stampar from Yugoslavia (who basically used the draft prepared by LNHO's officers Gautier and Biraud toward the end of the War). All the drafts focused on matters of organizational structure but also aimed for a wider political base than that of the LNHO. Because Parran's proposal, modeled on the US Public Health Service, was considered the most comprehensive and complete, it became the basis for the final document.

A substantial feature of the final document, its well-known preamble, did not exist in Parran's draft. According to some sources, Stampar was responsible for this inspiring section, called by many the *"magnacarta* for health."[13] However, as noted in Chapter 1, the basic ideas and wording of the preamble can be found in documents drafted by Gautier and Biraud of the LNHO that circulated among international health experts during the War. "Health is a state of complete physical, mental, and social well-being and not merely the absence of disease or infirmity", is the most often quoted language, but the full preamble contained nine principles, including the responsibility of governments to provide health, the primacy of the healthy development of children, and the need for the extension to all nations of the benefits of medical science without distinction of "race, religion, political belief, economic or social condition."[14] Health was a fundamental right of all citizens in all countries of the world. This idealism was also foundational for other UN agencies, and in December 1948 the UN General Assembly approved a landmark Universal Declaration of Human Rights. The socio-medical perspective of the agency would identify with this section Preamble and this Declaration.

An unresolved issue was the name of the new organization. The first name suggested was "International Health Organization." Some strongly believed that the term "United Nations Health Organization" was more appropriate because, unlike the first option, it did not evoke the International Health Division of the Rockefeller Foundation. The Chinese delegation made a strong case for "World Health Organization" as the best title to convey the global character of the agency and the growing spirit of internationalism that was evident at the San Francisco meeting. According to one of those present, the decision to adopt the term "world" as part of the title of the organization served to emphasize the notion that international health included colonial and developing countries and that "peoples of the world cannot exist half sick and half well, any more [than] they can exist half slave and half free."[15] He concluded that many health problems could only be solved on a worldwide basis.[16] This idea resonated with the long-standing belief in international health that "disease has no borders."

---

[13] "60 Delegates Sign Health Charter," *The New York Times*, July 23, 1946, p. 9.

[14] Brock Chisholm, "A New Look at Child Health," reprint from the May 1948 issue of *The Child*, p. 2, Brock Chisholm papers [WHO].

[15] "Annex 7, A Resolution, Department of State Advisory Health Group, 12 October 1945, Washington, DC," in *International Health Conference, New York, June 19 to July 22, 1946, Report of the United States Delegation, Including the Final Acts and Related Documents* (Washington, DC: US Government Printing Office, 1947), p. 9, National Library of Medicine.

[16] Brock Chisholm, "The World Health Organization," *International Conciliation* 437 (1947), 111–116, p. 111.

The TPC's "Conference for the Establishment of an International Health Organization" began on June 19, 1946, in New York City, and lasted five weeks.[17] The Indian lawyer Ramaswami Mudaliar, first president of the UN Economic and Social Council, chaired the opening session. Norwegian diplomat and politician Trygve Lie, first secretary-general of the UN, welcomed participants. Parran, chairman of the US delegation, was unanimously elected president of the Conference. Delegates of 51 nations and non-voting observers attended as well as representatives from 13 organizations. Spain's Franco regime was initially excluded due to its wartime alliances with Nazi Germany and Fascist Italy. After difficult negotiations led by a few Latin American countries, Spain was allowed to participate in spite of not yet being a member of the UN. In contrast to the LNHO, the WHO allowed full membership to states as long as they accepted its Constitution and their applications for membership were approved by a majority vote of the World Health Assembly. Although the decision about Spain was framed as a "technical" issue, political considerations played a role because Franco's right-wing regime became an ally of the United States during the Cold War. A generally less intensely political agenda item was dealing with the OIHP, the LNHO, and the UNRRA and deciding whether or not to modify, absorb, or terminate them. The decision was to dissolve all of them and to entrust their former functions, such as maintaining epidemiological surveillance and the sanitary conventions, to the organizing committee of the new health agency. This decision was justified with arguments about the need to avoid chaotic duplication of effort or rivalry between several new multilateral health agencies. It is important to mention that the WHO was not intended to perform every function of international health. For example, the new multilateral agency was not intended to be a funding organization or a medical research center (but could help to network with these kinds of institutions). Other matters were part of a negotiation between the emerging superpowers. For example, initially the Soviet Union was unwilling to accept the proposal of the United States that resolutions could have binding power and negotiated that most decisions would be reached by consensus and occasionally by majority vote (needing two-thirds in important issues). The United States and the Soviet Union agreed to keep out of the functions of the agency an important issue that would reappear many years later with anti-AIDS drugs: the power to regulate the importation of pharmaceuticals – especially substandard pharmaceuticals.[18]

---

[17] *International Health Conference: New York, NY, June 19 to July 22, 1946: Report of the United States Delegation, Including the Final Acts and Related Documents* (Washington, DC: Government Printing Office, 1947).

[18] "Russians Accept UN Health Rule," *The New York Times,* September 16, 1946.

The Conference approved the WHO's Constitution and created an Interim Commission (IC) to oversee international health work until the First World Health Assembly. The IC was able to operate thanks to a loan of USD 1.3 million from the UN and grants from the UNRRA for a total of USD 2.7 million. It had a staff of 15 individuals, with the Swiss Gautier serving as counselor and later director of its Geneva office.[19] The Conference also decided additional details of the IC's absorption of the OIHP (which included taking over its library and archives) and the LNHO (taking over the collection and dissemination of epidemic disease information and annexing the Singapore Bureau of Epidemiological Intelligence). The IC also absorbed the health work of the UNRRA in China, Greece, Ethiopia, Italy, and Poland. In 1947, the UNRRA had completely transferred its health functions to the IC, but contrary to expectations, its residual funds went to UNICEF instead of the WHO. Rajchman, Poland's representative to the committee for the liquidation of the UNRRA, convinced other members of the committee that a children's fund should be established to succeed UNRAA and started with leftover funds.[20]

At the end of July 1946, the Peruvian Carlos Enrique Paz Soldán, who was then presiding over the meeting, nominated Parran as chairman of the Commission. But Parran withdrew his name and proposed the Soviet Fedor G. Krotov, a lieutenant general in the Red Army and deputy health minister. The Russian was unable to occupy the post for any extended time because of health reasons, and Stampar was elected chairman. With a solid reputation in international health, Stampar then became the leading candidate to head the WHO. However, his support by the USSR undermined his position in the West as the Cold War intensified. In an internal memorandum written by a US State Department officer, Stampar was designated as a "problem" with a "good many views of his own" and as "one of the obstacles to be hurdled rather than a definitive ally."[21] Brock Chisholm (see Figure 2.4), a Canadian psychiatrist with experience in the military and as deputy minister of health, seconded Stampar. The Canadian, who began to stand out as a leader accepted by most countries, mentioned in his speech the universalistic justification that would

[19] The World Health Organization, "Report of the Interim Commission to the First World Health Assembly, 1948," Part 1 Activities, Official Records, Number 9 (Geneva: United Nations World Health Organization Interim Commission, 1948), p. 69.

[20] Interview with Martha A. Eliot, November 1973–May 1974, p. 188, Family Planning Oral History Project, Cartoon 2, Schlesinger Library, The Arthur and Elizabeth Schlesinger Library on the History of Women in America, Radcliffe Institute for Advanced Study at Harvard University, Cambridge, Massachusetts [hereafter AESL].

[21] Otis E. Mulliken to Louis Williams, February 2, 1946, Howard B. Calderwood World Health Organization Development Collection, Years 1945–1963, MS C 171, Box 1, Folder "1946 items 82–90," NLM.

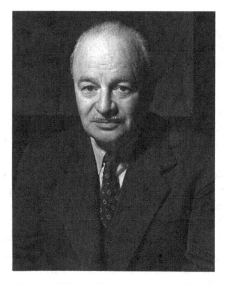

Figure 2.4 Brock Chisholm, a Canadian psychiatrist served as the first director-general of the World Health Organization from 1948 to 1953. Courtesy: Smithsonian Institution Archives.

drive some officers of the agency: "The environment of every person in the world now is the whole world."[22]

Most participants in the New York meeting of the IC left with the impression that the definitive creation of the agency would not take long. The decision had been to convoke the first session of the WHO as soon as "practicable" but no later than six months after the date the Constitution came into force, namely when it was ratified. Sixty national representatives signed the Constitution of the WHO (including the Soviet Union, who for the first time signed a document of a specialized agency of the UN). Yet, the formal establishment of the WHO depended on the acceptance of its Constitution by at least 26 members of the UN, and at the New York meeting only the delegates of China and the United Kingdom had the power to commit their governments. All the other delegates had to await ratification of the Constitution by their parliaments or other legislative bodies, a procedure initially thought of as a formality. It was not, and the ratification of the Constitution took longer than expected. The Interim Commission asked the UN General Assembly of 1947 to impress upon delegates the importance of

---

[22] Candau's intervention in "From Verbatim Minutes of Eight Plenary Session of International Health Conference, 2 July 1946," Folder 736, Box 54, Martha A. Eliot Papers [AESL].

early ratification since "essential progress in international health" was being seriously hindered by the long delay in establishing the WHO.[23]

In the case of the United States, the delay lasted about 18 months and was due partly to politics and partly to cumbersome procedures in Congress. The Senate accepted the WHO Constitution unanimously and rather quickly, but five of the seven members of the House Committee on Foreign Affairs voted to table the resolution and entrap it because it could not come to the floor of the House unless passed by this Committee. It did not help that the Republicans, more prone than Democrats to isolationism in foreign affairs, were then in control of Congress. An officer of the Rockefeller Foundation wrote in disbelief, "It seems to me incredible that the US ... will be on the outside looking in" in the formation of international health policies.[24] The WHO's supporters were worried because other multilateral organizations, such as the Food and Agriculture Organization (FAO), created in 1943, and the United Nations Educational, Scientific and Cultural Organization (UNESCO), founded in 1946, were making rapid progress. Moreover, FAO leaders seemed eager to encroach on the health field and a similar tendency existed with other multilateral agencies. But the IC could not spend time focused only on these matters because the emergent health agency soon had a real health challenge to deal with.

An Epidemic in Egypt

In September 1947 a cholera outbreak in Egypt – then a country of about twenty million people – captured worldwide attention. The outbreak stirred dreadful memories of devastating cholera epidemics and pandemics in the nineteenth century. Postwar circumstances were such that when the IC responded it in effect became, at least in part, a field agency and not merely an information management agency, and these events accelerated and shaped the institution-building process of the WHO. According to an American WHO officer, the work in Egypt was the most dramatic episode in the history of the Interim Commission.[25]

The first site of cholera in Egypt was El Korein, a village of 15,000 inhabitants on the eastern side of the Nile Delta. Three days later the epidemic reached Cairo, and in three weeks all provinces of lower Egypt reported cases

---

[23] Cited in "Hopes and Fears of International Health," *The Lancet* 253:2 (September 27, 1947), 474–475, p. 474.

[24] Paul F. Russell to Harold Hilman, April 7, 1948. Folder 28, Box 60, American Society of Tropical Medicine and Hygiene, Records. Center for the History of Medicine (Francis A. Countway Library of Medicine).

[25] Frank A. Calderone, "WHO: Activities and Prospects," *United Nations Bulletin* 4:1 (1948), 28–29, p. 28.

of cholera. By mid-October the disease affected Upper Egypt with more than 8,300 cases and 3,200 deaths having been reported.[26] The peak of the epidemic came in late October with 900 new cases and 500 deaths per day. There was fear and anxiety in Europe because several of the cholera epidemics that hit the continent during the nineteenth century had first reached Egypt and were then introduced to Europe by sea travel. The flight of frightened people contributed to the rapid diffusion of the epidemic. Its spread was also due to the basic lack of proper sanitation. Although cholera most likely ultimately came from the Bengal province in India where the disease was endemic, it found propitious conditions in Egypt.[27] The fear about its spread and expansion quickly became a matter of urgent concern in Europe and the rest of the world.

King H. M. Farouk I, who had ruled since 1936, was the titular leader of Egypt. But the British Empire was really in control because Egypt until recently had been a British Protectorate and the British still controlled the Suez Canal and the country's main agricultural product, cotton. Nevertheless, Egyptian doctors promptly reported and spoke openly about the epidemic outbreak, none more effectively than Aly Tewfik Shousha.[28] Shousha had trained in medicine and bacteriology at Berlin and Zurich and served for a time as the head of the bacteriologic Institute of Cairo. He had become under-secretary of state for health in 1940 and was the second in command in the Egyptian Ministry of Health when the epidemic hit. Later, he was one of three vice-chairmen of the IC and the first director of the Eastern Mediterranean Regional Office (EMRO) of the WHO. The IC and European health authorities counted on Shousha to control the epidemic.

The first responses to cholera in Egypt were tinged with panic and hysteria. Neighboring countries closed their borders to passengers, goods, and mail from Egypt. The Greek government canceled all flights to Cairo and used small planes to spray its own cities with DDT in an irrational "anti-fly campaign." The Italian government decided that passengers arriving from Egypt by air should be kept under observation, the French government forbade admission of passengers and even mail from Egypt, and several countries prohibited the import of foodstuffs and cotton from Egypt. Other examples of desperate measures were land quarantines; prohibition of public markets, public gatherings, and the sale of ice-cream; and suppression of the movement of pilgrims from Egypt to India that was about to start in October. For *The*

---

[26] "Cholera in Egypt," *The Lancet* 253:2 (November 1, 1947), 657–658, p. 657.

[27] See Robert Pollitzer, *Cholera* (Geneva: World Health Organization, 1959), p. 48, and Ministry of Public Health, *Egypt Annual Report of the Department of Laboratories for the Year 1947*, (Cairo: Government Press, 1950), p. 65.

[28] Rene Francis, *Public Health in Egypt*, (Cairo: n.p., 1951).

Lancet, these responses were a reminder that cholera was a "disease of fear" which could lead too readily to a return to the "quarantine of the jungle."[29]

The IC helped fight the cholera epidemic in Egypt by supporting the health measures commanded by Shousha, such as house-to-house search and isolation of the sick, but especially by coordinating and becoming the clearing-house of the supply of tons of vaccine and medical equipment from all over the world (such as syringes, hypodermic needles, blood plasma, sodium chloride and glucose for rehydration, and sulfonamides). By early November, the quantity of vaccine was sufficient to inoculate one out of every six persons in the country, and later in the month enough vaccine was available to immunize more than half of the inhabitants of Egypt. In addition, other countries in the region, such as Syria and Saudi Arabia, received vaccine supplies as a precaution. In terms of the rapidity of response, supplies sent from the United States reached Egypt in fewer than three days, a remarkable achievement at the time.[30]

The epidemic was brought under control within six weeks and no country west of the Persian Gulf was affected. In 1902 an epidemic of cholera had a case fatality rate of 85 percent. In 1947, the total number of cases was 20,804 with 10,277 deaths for a case fatality rate of 50 percent.[31] Other health improvements were linked to the campaign, such as better water systems, chlorination, and the construction of new sanitary infrastructure. Cholera vaccination was employed on a large scale during the last months of 1947. Related to this campaign was the reorganization and expansion of the Vaccine and Serum Laboratory in Cairo. A second campaign of cholera vaccination was undertaken in February 1948. An illustration of the campaign's dimension is that during 1948, 161,015 stools were examined and all "suspicious" cases of diarrhea or vomiting were treated and the patients examined bacteriologically.[32]

Autumn, sanitation, education, and vaccination seem to have ended the epidemic. Only ten cases were reported in early 1948, and later that year the country was declared "clean" or free from the disease. There were no cholera cases the next year. Although the safety and cost-effectiveness of the vaccine later became controversial issues, a contemporary study in Egyptian hospitals showed that the fatality rate among the inoculated was lower than among the non-inoculated, and only in 1973 did the WHO remove cholera vaccination

[29] "Cholera and Hysteria," *The Lancet* 253:2 (November 29, 1947), 797–798, p. 798.

[30] Folder "International Health, Cholera Epidemic, Egypt, 21 October–5 November 1947," Series 0544, Box 3, United Nations Archives, New York [hereafter UN-NY].

[31] Aly Tewfik Shousha, "Cholera Epidemic in Egypt (1947), a Preliminary Report," *United Nations Bulletin* 1:2 (1948), 353–381.

[32] Egypt, Ministry of Public Health, *Annual Report of the Department of Laboratories for the Year 1948* (Cairo: Gov. Printing Press, 1951), p. 2, National Library of Medicine.

from international travel requirements. Early in 1949, the Interim Commission received an Anti-Cholera Memorial Medal from the Egyptian government, and Shousha was lavishly praised for his leadership in controlling the epidemic.

The Egyptian epidemic was a learning experience for the IC on how to react to an emergency and yet keep up long-term planning. The IC's response became a form of validation of the WHO's institutional worth, as it was tangible evidence that the new international health organization would not be merely a debating society or a forum for empty and repetitive speeches. The epidemic seemed to be a well-timed, practical demonstration that world health was indivisible and that no nation could consider itself safe while epidemic disease existed in any part of the globe.[33] The phrases frequently repeated since the nineteenth century – "disease has no frontiers" and "microbes need no passports" – acquired new meaning.

Another by-product of the WHO's intervention in the epidemic was that it facilitated public health work between 1948 and 1951 among the approximately one million Palestinian refugees in Lebanon, Syria, and other countries of the region during a very tense and volatile political period. In 1948, the WHO collaborated with the ephemeral United Nations Relief and Works Agency for Palestine Refugees in the Near East on a series of health programs, including an antimalaria program. The UN had begun work in the region a year before, just after the proposed partition of what had been Mandatory Palestine into a Jewish state, a Palestinian state, and an internationally administered zone – an arrangement that failed, as have so many subsequent proposed "solutions" to Israel/Palestine problems.[34]

The First World Health Assembly

As the IC approached its second year without having yet received ratifications of the WHO Constitution from the United States, the Soviet Union, or France, its leaders decided to call an international meeting in the hope of pressuring foot-dragging countries.[35] The pressure worked, and the first World Health Assembly was finally convened between June 24 and July 24, 1948, in the *Palais de Nations* Assembly Hall in Geneva. Delegates and observers from 70 countries and organizations attended the meeting, and Stampar was elected

---

[33] Yves Biraud & P. M. Kaul, "World Distribution and Prevalence of Cholera in Recent Years," *Epidemiological and Vital Statistics Report, Monthly Supplement to the Weekly Epidemiological Records* 1:7 (1947), 141–152.

[34] World Health Organization, *The First Ten Years of the World Health Organization* (Geneva: World Health Organization, 1958), p. 144.

[35] Henry van Zile Hyde, *World Health Organization – Progress and Plans* (Washington, DC: US Government Printing Office, 1948), p. 1.

president of the Assembly. The first session of the Assembly received con-
firmation of ratification from its 26th member, the Byelorussian Soviet
Republic. But a peculiar US ratification notice that had arrived a few days
before the opening of the meeting had to be discussed. The US Congress
insisted that the United States be allowed to withdraw unilaterally from the
WHO with a year's notification, something that no other country requested.
This congressional action reflected the persistence of American isolationism.
The peculiar form of United States ratification was criticized by the New York
Academy of Medicine, the American Public Health Association, and a variety
of other American medical spokesmen.[36] Trygve Lie, the UN secretary-
general, asked the Health Assembly to interpret the US position and make a
final decision.

The day before the issue was brought to the attention of the first World
Health Assembly there was a dinner involving Parran and Nicolas Vinogradov,
the head of the delegation of the Soviet Union, plus a few members of their
respective delegations. There was until then no inkling of the attitude that
would be taken by the Soviet delegation with regard to the atypical United
States conditional confirmation of the WHO's Constitution. Parran showed
Vinogradov the draft of the speech he was going to deliver at the plenary
session and made clear that the United States wanted its acceptance of the
Constitution to be approved unanimously by the Assembly. According to an
account of the conversation: "The Soviet group did not commit itself, taking the
attitude that the Constitution was a sacred instrument and that the US committed a crime against the Constitution by its reservation." The Americans, worried
that the approval might fail in the Assembly, called Stampar after dinner, and
the Croatian calmed them by saying that it was characteristic of the Soviets not
to give an immediate decision in such circumstances.[37] Trying to convince the
Soviet Union and a number of European delegates who believed that the
United States should have a provisional membership pending an amendment
of the WHO's Constitution, Parran, as leader of the United States delegation,
assured the Assembly that the United States' stipulation was merely a formality and that the US federal government's true support of the WHO was
exhibited in its payment of more than 35 percent of the Organization's

[36] "Doctors Hit Delay on UN Health Unit," *The New York Times*, March 22, 1948, p. 15; United
States, Committee on Foreign Affairs House of Representatives, *Eightieth Congress, First
Session, Hearings before Subcommittee No.5 – National and International Movements:
A Joint Resolution Providing for Membership and Participation by the United States in the
World Health Organization and Authorizing an Appropriation therefore, 13, 17 June and 3 July
1947* (Washington, DC: US Government Printing Office, 1947).

[37] The dinner is described in "Confidential, United States Delegation, First Session of the World
Health Organization, 2 July 1948," Folder 743, Box 55, Marta M. Eliot Papers [AESL].

expenses.[38] Yet Parran had only limited credibility because he was no longer US surgeon general. Parran's position was supported by Stampar and by delegates from the United Kingdom and India, who saw the action of the US Congress as a mere legal technicality.[39] Yet the tension surrounding debate on this issue is illustrated in the retrospective account by an American delegate of the speech given by the representative of the Soviet Union:

He [Vinogradov] started blasting the US ... [Stampar] understood Russian; you could see his face falling and looking grimmer and grimmer ... it was obvious that ... [Vinogradov] was just giving us the works. Then [we] ... saw the big grin on Stampar's face and knew we were in. But that was a very tense situation, because just the opposition of the USSR could have kept us out of the World Health Organization. Well, of course, with the financing of it and everything else, they would have been really politically stupid to have thrown us out of it; they had nothing to gain.[40]

In another anecdote Stampar told Martha M. Eliot during the meeting that he had learned before the meeting that the Russians had "talked to Moscow ... with the result that the outcome was what it was." An American who was also at the meeting retorted to Eliot: "Maybe Stampar knew, but the rest of us sure sweated it out!"[41] Eliot later became an important officer at the WHO (see Figure 2.5).

The World Health Assembly then got down to business. The Executive Board held its first session during the closing days of the World Health Assembly and a second and more extended one in October 1948. The EB fully restored epidemiological intelligence as an international health activity and assembled a staff of epidemiologists in Geneva to collect reports from all parts of the world, validate their data, and transmit it widely to health and port sanitary authorities. Journals that frequently used the same titles as former publications of the LNHO and the OIHP – such as the *International Digest of Health Legislation*, *The Weekly Epidemiological Record*, and *Epidemiological and Vital Statistics Report* – were restarted and these were followed by a series of new publications such as *The Bulletin of WHO*, *The Chronicle of the World Health Organization*, and the *Official Records of the World Health Organization*.[42] Some of these publications, such as the *Chronicle*,

---

[38] According to a newspaper article, the Soviet Union paid only 6 percent, the UK almost 12 percent, and France and China 6 percent each. Howard A. Rusk, "World Health Organization Needs Active Help of US," *The New York Times*, April 4, 1948, p. 42.

[39] Norman Howard-Jones, "The World Health Organization in Historical Perspective, *Perspectives in Biology and Medicine* 24:3 (1981), 467–482.

[40] Oral History Interview with Henry Van Zile Hyde, July 14 and 16, 1975, Harry S. Truman Presidential Library and Museum, n.p.

[41] Marta M. Eliot to Henry Van Zile Hyde, February 17, 1959 and Van Zile to Eliot, March 6, 1959, Folder 759, Box 56, Martha M. Eliot Papers [AESL].

[42] World Health Organization, Publishing for a Purpose: Fifty Years of Publishing by the World Health Organization (Geneva: World Health Organization, 1998).

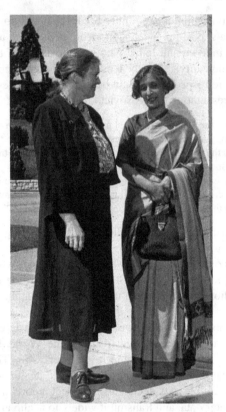

Figure 2.5 Martha M. Eliot (left), a noted American pediatrician and child health advocate, was assistant director-general of the WHO from 1949 to 1951. Here she appears with Rajkumari Amrit Kaur, India's health minister and president of the Third World Health Assembly that took place in Geneva in May of 1950. Credit the WHO/J. Kernen.
Courtesy: World Health Organization Photo Library.

soon appeared in the five official languages of the UN (Chinese, English, French, Russian, and Spanish). In January 1949, when the fastest means of communication was radio, the WHO began transmitting daily epidemiological radio broadcasts with network nodes in Washington, DC, Geneva, Singapore, and Alexandria.[43]

The World Health Assembly put into practice the organizational scheme specified in the WHO constitution: a World Health Assembly, a Secretariat,

[43] Brock Chisholm, "Achievements of First World Health Assembly," *United Nations Bulletin* 5 (1948), 636–637.

and an Executive Board. The Assembly would be made up of delegates appointed by each member state, three per country (countries could send to the Assembly alternates and advisers, but they had no vote). Representatives of philanthropic foundations, of other multilateral or bilateral agencies, and of medical associations could be observers at the Assembly. The Assembly would meet once a year to vote on policy proposals, review the activities of the Executive Board and the Secretariat, adopt or change international regulations, approve the WHO's budget, elect the director-general and the Executive Board, and consider applications for membership which were sent to the director-general. Every nation was equal in the Assembly since it worked on a "one state, one vote" principle regardless of economic or political power. The mode of operation was mainly consensus; decisions had to be accepted by all member states. In addition, the WHO was not to function as a supranational organization in a regulatory sense. It could not impose sanctions or enforce rules on its members (as Gautier had envisioned in 1943). Moreover, the WHO's help to a given country could only be provided in response to a specific request from its national health administration. Initially, this help concentrated in two areas that reflected the two perspectives of the agency: either strengthening health administration, education and training, maternal and child health, or environmental sanitation, which were all suffused with a social medicine perspective, or controlling communicable diseases as the prime example of the technocratic perspective.

The WHO's budget was based on assessed contributions, that is, dues paid by governments according to their country's wealth and population. The WHO's Secretariat, which runs day-to-day operations, was headed by a director-general and three assistant director-generals appointed by the director-general. The director-general, proposed by the Executive Board and formally elected by the Assembly for a five-year term (until 2017, the assembly confirmed the candidate proposed by the Board), enjoyed considerable power. He prepared the budget and oversaw all technical and administrative services. Finally, the Executive Board, composed initially of eighteen "technically qualified" individuals to serve for three years (each year one-third of the Board members will change), met twice a year to implement policies and carry out the decisions of the Assembly (the number added two to the LNHO Health Committee and the TPC). During the WHO's initial years there was some tension between the Secretariat and Executive Board as they sorted out what their respective functions were.

The election of the Executive Board and the appointment of the assistant director-generals carried a challenge for the superpowers that continued through the history of the WHO: to ensure a geographical balance. It was not easy to achieve this goal. The first Executive Board had a disproportionate number of representatives from powerful countries in the Western Hemisphere, including the United States, and nine from Europe, including the Soviet Union. Although this changed a little in the 1950s as citizens from Australia, Ceylon, China, Egypt, India, Iran, and South Africa became members of the EB, the hegemony of the United States, the United Kingdom, and their allies persisted.[44]

The WHO had other components that gave the organization an aura of technocracy and maintained continuity with the past. Like the LNHO, the WHO established internal and external expert committees. These advisory panels produced reports that after an Executive Board's authorization were published in the *Technical Report Series*. These publications even continued to be numbered as if they were a continuation of the reports published during the interwar years by advisory panels of the LNHO. The expert committees, which included many of the world's leaders in their respective fields, could organize meetings and provide technical guidance in the formulation and execution of policy. They could also promote research and facilitate networks of investigators.

A far-reaching decision of the first World Health Assembly was to establish the WHO's permanent headquarters in Geneva. The United States and many Latin American countries favored a city in the Western Hemisphere where some of the meetings of the Interim Commission had taken place. The United Kingdom supported for some time the idea of London as the base for the agency (a proposal that was withdrawn) but finally supported Geneva. The Soviet Union, India, Brazil, and France favored Geneva on the grounds of its excellent work facilities and continuity with the LNHO. Another unspoken and quite Eurocentric reason for preferring Geneva was that continental proximity would make it easier for the WHO to help European countries devastated by World War II. Favoring Geneva also reflected aspirations that the WHO's main office be located near European centers of medical excellence. Generous Swiss contributions – in currency and land – facilitated the decision. WHO headquarters would initially occupy an enlarged section of *the Palais de Nations* the former headquarters of the League of Nations.

The First World Assembly also worked out agreements with other agencies such as the United Nations, the UN Food and Agricultural Organization, the International Civil Aviation Organization, the UN International Labor Organization (ILO), and UNESCO. Two nongovernmental organizations with which the WHO was associated in its early years were the International Committee of the Red Cross and the League of Red Cross Societies, both with headquarters in Geneva. Working out a relationship with UNICEF was complicated. UNICEF was created in 1946 as the United Nations International Children's Emergency Fund ("International" was later dropped but

---

[44] Van Zile Hyde, *Challenges and Opportunities in World Health: The First World Health Assembly* (Washington, DC: Government Printing Office, 1948), p. 6.

the acronym stuck) to provide emergency food and health care to children in countries devastated by World War II. UNICEF later enlarged its remit to the entire globe and in 1953 became a permanent part of the UN system. UNICEF's initial chairman of the board was the former head of the LNHO, Ludwik Rajchman, who – as described before – did not participate in the organization or early work of the WHO.

During its first years, UNICEF developed a number of health programs related to maternal and child care. The WHO's officers believed that UNICEF was stepping into WHO territory, recruiting top medical staff and dealing with the health of older people and not only children. Discussions were carried out between the WHO and UNICEF in the attempt to avoid unnecessary overlap and to coordinate work. In 1948, these discussions arrived at a slowed down with the creation of the Joint Committee on Health Policy UNICEF-WHO that would meet at least once per year and report to the executive boards of the WHO and UNICEF. The Joint Committee stipulated that all medical programs undertaken by UNICEF would proceed only on the recommendation of the Joint Committee with the concordance of the WHO. The latter agency was recognized as the "the highest international authority in the [health] field."[45] UNICEF carved out a niche as a "supply" organization, in charge of fundraising and the procurement of vehicles, drugs, and other medical materials, but not administering programs directly. The "technical direction" of health programs was always to be a primary responsibility of the WHO.

One of the tasks of the First World Assembly was the election of the director-general. Almost by consensus, Brock Chisholm became the first DG of the WHO on a 46 to 2 vote. The other members of the first WHO Secretariat, appointed shortly after Chisholm, were three assistant director-generals: the Swiss Gautier in charge of Technical Services, the British William P. Forrest in charge of Advisory Services, and the American Milton P. Siegel in charge of Administration and Finance. In addition, other positions were filled by former staff members of the LNHO and the UNRRA: the French Biraud became director of the Division of Epidemiology, the American Frank Calderone was confirmed as director of the Liaison Office with the UN in New York, the British Neville Goodman was appointed director of the Division of Field Operations, and the British Norman Howard Jones was appointed director of the Division of Editorial and Reference Services. In this initial group, no Soviet or citizen of a developing country was appointed. Only at the end of 1948 would the Secretariat include four members from communist countries – two from Czechoslovakia, one from Poland, and one from Romania.

---

[45] UNICEF/WHO Joint Committee on Health Policy, 1st session, 1st meeting, Geneva, July 23, 1948, JC.1-UNICEF/WHO/Min/1, Folder 961–4-1, First Generation of Files [WHO].

Chisholm and the Executive Board also oversaw the recruitment of the WHO rank-and-file staff. By 1949 the WHO's staff came to a total of 254, of whom 194 worked at Geneva, 29 at the New York Office, and 32 were "in the field." An enthusiastic American officer who had worked for a year at the agency described his experience in 1949 as "everything is in the formative and exciting stage of development."[46] The work of the Geneva officers included considerable travel and their identity became that of "international" civil servants with loyalty to a multilateral agency rather than to the governments of their home countries. For Chisholm, the staff had to work with no prejudice as "world citizens" and develop empathy with all sorts of people.[47] The first WHO officers signed a statement which read: "I solemnly swear to exercise in all loyalty, discretion and conscience the functions entrusted to me as a member of the international service of the World Health Organization . . . and not to seek or accept instructions in regard to the performance of my duties from any government or other authority external to the Organization."[48] These oaths posed problems for American employees because they set off alarms with United States "security" agencies and complicated Chisholm's relationship with the US government, as we will see.

Chisholm's opinions increasingly implied a questioning of the Cold War. As a supporter of multilateralism, he called for all governments to support the UN and advocated the idea that world health and "world peace" – a code term during the Cold War – were indivisible and closely interrelated. He also condemned the world's division between the superpowers as a threat to peace and as the "most serious obstacle to economic and social progress." He also subscribed to a trope that was common at the end of the Second World War and would last for decades: All medical knowledge needed to control and eliminate the major disease scourges was in place, but physicians and health workers had to convince governments to invest in the health of people.[49]

Although many expected that Chisholm would have an easy time with the Americans, that was not often the case and intrusive security investigations of the WHO staff were only part of the problem. Chisholm also disliked the vertical style of public health campaigns that marked many United States and Rockefeller Foundation programs and which Americans now suggested for the

[46] Marta M. Eliot to Hugh Lavell, July 20, 1949, Folder 753, Box 229, Martha M. Eliot papers [AESL].

[47] Chisholm, "The World Health Organization," *International Conciliation*, p. 115.

[48] The oath appears in "United Nations, World Health Organization, 22 Nov 1948," Frank A. Calderone Papers, Series World Health Organization, Box 6, Folder 5, Archives and Special Collections, Columbia University Health Sciences Libraries, New York.

[49] Brock Chisholm, "Address by the Director General of the World Health Organization," in World Health Organization Third World Assembly, First Plenary Meeting, Geneva, May 8, 1950, Provisional Verbatim Record, p. 24, http://apps.who.int/iris/bitstream/10665/100446/1/WHA3_VR-1_eng.pdf, last accessed March 1, 2018.

WHO. He believed that the WHO should have a broad agenda and concentrate on several health problems at once. He wanted programs addressing malaria, tuberculosis, sexually transmitted diseases, maternal and child care, and mental health. After a trip to Pakistan, India, Ceylon, Singapore, Thailand, the Philippines, Hong Kong, and Japan, he stated his conviction on a different meaning of "technical assistance." For the Canadian, it was the challenge of adapting a technique to a culture and not "fitting a culture to a technique overnight."[50] Chisholm was able to make mental health a priority in the first years of the WHO, an innovation in international health because traditionally mental health was not given much importance. He believed that the worst enemy of peace was the uncontrolled destructive force of the human personality. Chisholm launched an ambitious and wrongfully optimistic program against tuberculosis. The misplaced optimism was related to cost-effective biomedical agents that had become widely available – tuberculin tests, BCG vaccine, and the antibiotic streptomycin. With the help of UNICEF, the Scandinavian Red Cross, and the Danish National Health Service, the WHO created a Tuberculosis Office in Copenhagen in 1948 that launched an impressive anti-TB campaign that reached millions in more than 30 countries on all continents (a year later the agency also established an important anesthesiology training center in the same city). According to the *WHO Newsletter*, it was the largest health campaign against tuberculosis ever undertaken.[51] Some years later, the WHO reported a 50 percent drop in respiratory tuberculosis between 1938 and 1950 in 21 countries, most of them in Europe (in India, another country where an important campaign was implemented, mass vaccination encountered the mistrust of many people who saw it as an imposition of outsiders).[52] The scope and intensity of the anti-tuberculosis campaign in South Asia is suggested in Figure 2.6. As McMillen has shown, the campaign faced many scientific and political uncertainties. Resistance to TB drugs emerged quickly and BCG was never definitively proven to be an effective vaccination. Also, McMillen demonstrates that the campaign followed a pattern, that can be traced back to the Rockefeller Foundation campaigns of the early twentieth century, of promoting global solutions to local problems by relying on technological fixes rather than the improvement of social and economic conditions. Despite the many technological breakthroughs in TB control, the disease persisted.[53]

---

[50] "Chisholm," April 3, 1952. Folder 757, Box 56, Martha M. Eliot Papers [AESL].

[51] World Health Organization, "Progress in the Fight against the 'White Plague,' *WHO Newsletter* 1 (September 1947), 7, *WHO Newsletter* 1948–1956, WHO Library.

[52] The information in this paragraph is from J. B. McDougall, "Editorial: The World Health Organization and Tuberculosis, Aims, Objects and Accomplishments," *The American Review of Tuberculosis* 64:2 (1951), 218–222.

[53] Christian W. McMillen, *Discovering Tuberculosis: A Global History, 1900 to the Present* (New Haven: Yale University Press, 2015).

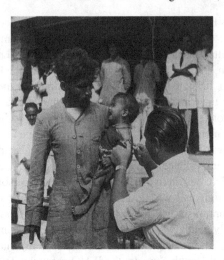

Figure 2.6 An infant girl receives BCG vaccination against tuberculosis at a
United Nations-funded clinic in Pakistan, circa 1950.
Photo by Unations/FPG/Hulton Archive/Getty Image.

Despite this success, Chisholm faced criticism. According to a Rockefeller
officer, he had to field questions from the WHO's Executive Board about
whether the budget had expanded too quickly on personnel and administration and not enough on "operations." The first World Health Assembly
had approved a relatively small budget of 4.8 million, of which more than
half went to repay expenses incurred by the Interim Commission. Some
representatives saw this budget as insufficient and called for a budget of
USD 8 million. As a benchmark, the New York City health budget for
1948 was USD 13 million a year. In comparison with other UN agencies,
especially the wealthier UNICEF, the WHO was a "relatively poverty-
stricken organization."[54]

Chisholm also faced opposition because of his attempt to establish a
population-control program at the WHO. Despite the fact that the WHO had
no official population policy until early 1952, Chisholm managed to send one
expert to India responding to the government's request to receive assistance for
its population problem, help six different Indian centers devoted to population
control, and advise on the methods of controlling overpopulation. Chisholm's
ideas on overpopulation as a menace to global health followed the lead of
Julian Huxley, the first director-general of UNESCO, who believed in the need

---

[54] Excerpt from Robert Struthers Diary. Paris, January 16, 1950, RFA, RG 2, Series 100, Box 495,
Folder 388, RAC.

of population control programs for India and other developing countries. Like Huxley, Chisholm considered family planning "essential" and confronted the opposition of several delegates at the 1952 World Health Assembly. Chisholm was also opposed by the Vatican and Catholic countries such as Ireland, Italy, Belgium, and France that did not consider population growth a health problem.[55] In addition, many European government officials did not regard population control as a priority because in the wake of World War II, Europe seemed, if anything, to be underpopulated. Despite these tensions, Chisholm persisted in his efforts to validate the WHO in a challenging political climate.

---

[55] The Vatican and World Population Policy: An Interview with Milton P. Siegel by Stephen D. Mumford, www.population-security.org/29-APP3.html, last accessed January 11, 2018.

3   The Start-Up Years, 1948–1955

By the mid-1950s, the WHO found a place among a growing network of multilateral agencies, secured the contributions of member countries to its budget, and conducted a remarkable but problematic campaign against tuberculosis. At the same time, it faced significant challenges. The agency had to come to terms with the escalating Cold War and the consolidation of a bipolar world and needed to deal with the anxieties of British, French, Dutch, Belgian, and Portuguese governments trying to hold on to or rebuild their colonial empires as these began to crumble. It also had to respond to the growing demands and expectations of developing countries. The WHO's technical priorities, programs, and decisions were never divorced from the political context or politics, inside and outside the agency. Like other UN agencies, the WHO abandoned dreams of a collaborative community of nations and began coming to terms with new international political realities, including revived imperial goals, decolonization, and assistance to newly independent developing countries. The agency also moved closer to US foreign policy and became partially captive to US resources and priorities. The WHO wound up pursuing a pragmatic course of limited objectives, settled upon an institutional structure incorporating compromises over decolonization and regionalization, and undertook a select number of programs.

The Political Context and Institutional Developments

A direct result of Cold War tensions at the WHO was the withdrawal of the Soviet Union along with the Ukrainian and Byelorussian Soviet Republics (which had independent seats in the World Health Assembly) in 1949. The Geneva Secretariat was informed of these decisions by telegram in February 1949, a few months before the Second World Health Assembly was to meet in Rome. Before and shortly after that Assembly, Bulgaria, Romania, Albania, Poland, Czechoslovakia, and Hungary also sent notifications of withdrawal. The formal reason given was dissatisfaction with the work carried out by the multilateral agency, but underneath this public rebuke was anger aimed at the WHO and the United States for withholding medical resources from Eastern

Europe. The Soviets felt that although they had paid a very high price in human and material terms during the Second World War, they received little help after the war from the Marshall Plan, United States bilateral agencies, or multilateral organizations. Believing for good reason that the Americans dominated the WHO and the UN, the Soviets decided to boycott these agencies.

Contributing to the boycott decision was a growing conviction on the part of the Soviets and their allies that there were two dramatically opposing views about public health, that of capitalism and that of communism. The Soviets argued that the United States did not recognize the inseparable connections between social, economic, and health problems. They denounced poor working conditions and exploitation under capitalism as the roots of disease and held the conviction that the United States would never do the same. The Soviet Union also declared the need for nationalizing medical services. In 1949 a communist delegate to the World Health Assembly denounced the agency as the battleground of "two opposing points of views ... [that of the Soviet Union] standing for the interest of humanity, which demands that the attainment of medical science should serve the whole human race ... while the capitalist camp represents the interest of a minority who consider science as a source of income and as a weapon of war."[1] Later, the Polish minister of health used similarly harsh words: The WHO had "surrendered to the imperialistic States and in particular to the United States."[2]

Despite this increasingly tense political and ideological atmosphere, Stampar and Chisholm hoped that social medicine principles would still be among the priorities of the WHO. Stampar argued that the WHO should concentrate on four principles: "social and economic security, education, nutrition, and housing."[3] However, as Amrith has suggested, a social medicine perspective, if taken seriously, implied questioning the inequality of land ownership in rural areas and the multitude of inequities that produce poor housing, misery, and illness in urban areas. To avoid these sensitive positions and the displeasure of the United States in response to them, the WHO began to embrace a framework of "technical assistance," based on an ideology that can be traced to US governmental discourses at the end of World War II. "Technical assistance" was instrumental in conveying the idea

[1] "Statement of the Delegate from Poland Irène Domanska," Official Records of the World Health Organization, No. 21, Second World Health Assembly, Rome, June 13 to July 2, 1949, Decisions and Resolutions, Plenary Meetings Verbatim Records, Committees Minutes and Reports: Annexes (Geneva: World Health Organization, 1949), pp. 105–106.

[2] Cited in "Poland Decides to Withdraw from WHO," Chronicle of the World Health Organization 4:10 (1950), 324–325, p. 324.

[3] Cited in "Dr. Stampar Yugoslavia, Points from Speeches," Chronicle of the World Health Organization 3:8–10 (1949), 217–224, p. 221.

that development was primarily a matter of transferring knowledge of science and technology, thus avoiding the need to address the economic interests and social realities that led to underdevelopment.[4] The Second World Health Assembly voted to provide funds and design technical health programs for developing countries, making the WHO one of the first UN agencies to offer specific assistance to these countries but also reinforcing the impression of heavy United States influence. In response, the US surgeon general made a strong statement (in the Third World Health Assembly of 1950) to underline the commitment of his country to health multilateralism:

We believe in the open forum of discussion at these Assemblies. We believe in resolution of honest differences of opinion by discussion and we trust the judgment of sincere people. This means we subscribe to the concept of constructive debate and decent restraint. We respect the outcome of ballots – which need not be reassured by suggestions of sinister political motives to gain power. . . . I hope you will believe me – my Government – [and] the people of the United States of America stand squarely behind the ideals of WHO.[5]

On a practical level, the decision by the Soviet Union and its allies to leave the WHO had an impact on the finances of the organization. Obviously, the absent countries (and several others) did not pay their assessed contributions, so in 1949 it was necessary to defer settlement of an outstanding loan from the United States and to keep to the same budget level as that approved at the First World Health Assembly.[6] Some delegates tried to minimize the reality of financial troubles and the walkout of the Soviet Union and maintain their optimism about the future. During and after the Assembly, Chisholm insisted that the WHO was the international health organization of all nations. Knowing that there were Russian physicians and health officials who did not want the USSR to pull out of the WHO, he offered to visit the Soviet Union to dispel any "misunderstandings." His request was turned down by the Soviets. But Chisholm pointed out that the WHO's Constitution made no provision for withdrawal from membership. He therefore claimed the nine communist countries were "inactive" rather than "withdrawn" and announced that he would wait for their return (a decision that later created a path for their smooth reentry). C.-E. A. Winslow, in an *American Journal of Public Health* article, endorsed Chisholm's conciliatory stance: "The erring brothers have their seats waiting for them when they desire to mend their ways."[7] Some with

---

[4] Amrith, *Decolonizing International Health*, p. 122.

[5] "Address by Surgeon General Leonard A. Scheele, Third World Health Assembly," Geneva, May 27, 1950, Folder 755, Box 56 Martha M. Eliot Papers [AESL].

[6] "The World's Health," *The Lancet* 258:1 (May 13, 1950), 920.

[7] Charles-Edward Amory Winslow, "International Health," *American Journal of Public Health* 41:12 (1951), 1455–1482, p. 1458.

high-status positions in the WHO also tried to help. For example, Rajkumari Amrit Kaur, a minister of health from India and president of the World Health Assembly, attempted privately to persuade Vyacheslav Molotov, the Soviet foreign minister, that the United States was "not running WHO."[8]

Shortly after the Rome Assembly, however, an international conflict erupted that reinforced Soviet perceptions: the Korean War (1950–1953). This war between South and North Korea was also a proxy conflict between the United States and its allies, on the one hand, and the People's Republic of China and the Soviet Union, on the other. A simmering civil war erupted into open warfare on June 25, 1950, when North Korean forces supported by the Soviet Union and China invaded the south in an attempt to "unite the country." That same day, the UN Security Council declared the North Korean advance an "invasion" and called for an immediate ceasefire. Two days later, the Council, with the Soviet Union absent because it was boycotting the UN, decided to send forces to "defend" South Korea, with the United States providing the vast majority of the military personnel. This "police action," formally on behalf of the UN, allowed the Truman administration to avoid asking Congress for a declaration of war and to frame the whole episode as a search for peace within the UN-overseen international order. The WHO became involved in the conflict when UN Secretary-General Trygve Lie requested assistance for victims of epidemics in South Korea. The WHO argued that an even-handed offer of medical assistance was rejected by North Korea.[9] Nevertheless, it was difficult to avoid the perception that the UN and the WHO were implicated in the Cold War and on the US side. In the following years, some WHO officers would try to distance their agency from this perception, but others would tolerate or even embrace it.

For its part, the US State Department, in a May 1953 memorandum to the White House, had bluntly stated that "In the Cold War the UN has become a major means for diplomacy and propaganda in combating the political warfare of the Soviet Union and in rallying the strength of the free world through a wide variety of measures."[10] Moreover, Willard L. Thorp, assistant secretary of state for Economic Affairs, had emphasized at the 1950 annual meeting of

---

[8] US Resident Delegation, Geneva to Department of State, July 24, 1953 [the comment appears in a report of an interview with Chisholm where a US diplomat refers to the meeting between Molotov and Rajkumari Amrit Kaur], US Department of State Records, Record Group 59, Decimal File 398.55, Years, 1950–1954, Box 1634, Folder 5, National Archives and Records Administration (hereafter RG 59 & NARA).

[9] "WHO's Offer of Assistance to Korean Epidemic Victims," *The Department of State Bulletin* 27:699 (November 17, 1952), 495.

[10] Memorandum prepared in the Department of State for the White House, May 29, 1953, in William Z. Slany & Ralph R. Goodwin (eds.), *Foreign Relations of the United States, 1952–1954, vol. III United Nations Affairs* (Washington, DC: US Government Printing Office, 1979), pp. 70–73, p. 70.

the American Public Health Association that a clear relationship existed between national security and the worldwide struggle against disease and poverty. Disease and poverty must be fought, he suggested, because they "feed communism" and thus threaten the "very survival of our democracy."[11] Congressman Frances P. Bolton would explain the US government support for the WHO as follows: "In our global struggle against communism, one of our principal endeavors is to keep the free world strong. Disease breeds poverty and poverty breeds further disease. International communism thrives on both."[12] US foreign policy thus clearly conceived of multilateralism and international health as useful tools in the struggle to halt the spread of communism.

The tension between the superpowers and the relationship of the Soviet Union with the UN and WHO changed thanks to an unexpected event in March 1953: the death of Joseph Stalin, the hard-line communist leader. For three years, it was not clear who would lead the Soviet Union. An incipient de-Stalinization came with the rise of Nikita Khrushchev, who emphasized "peaceful coexistence" and "friendly" competition with the United States, both inside and outside the UN system. In July 1955 the Soviet Union formally stated its intention to rejoin the WHO and fully participate in the UN. The WHO accepted the reentry of the USSR and Soviet-allied countries and requested payment of only a small percentage of their back dues. The financial side of the decision was further eased because Soviet payments were allowed in nonconvertible rubles and were used mainly for the purchase of Soviet supplies and services. All communist countries – with the notable exceptions of China and North Korea – returned to the WHO in 1956.[13]

The presence of the Soviet Union within the WHO now became more visible. Even when it was in "inactive" status in the early 1950s, the USSR always had a few staff members in the WHO. In 1958, two years after returning to "active" status, their number had grown to 22. Soviet scientists were also well-represented on the 40-expert committees of the agency, and a Soviet physician, Nicolay I. Grashchenkov, served as WHO's assistant

[11] A summary of the speech in "Defense and World Health," *Public Health Reports* 65:49 (1950), 1611–1613.

[12] "Honorable Frances P. Bolton of Ohio in the House of Representatives, Extension of Remarks on World Health Day," April 7, 1954, in United States, Congressional Record, Proceeding and Debates of the 83rd Congress, Second Session Volume 100-Part 4, April 1, 1954 to April 28, 1954 (Washington, DC: US Government Printing Office, 1954), p. 4844.

[13] James Frederick Green & Howard B. Calderwood, "Notification by the USSR Concerning Participation in the World Health Organization," February 14, 1956, R.G. 59, Decimal File 398.55, Years 1946–1962, Box 330, Folder WHO membership, NARA. On the Soviet Union during the mid-1950s, see Vladislav Zubok and Constantine Pleshavok, *Inside the Kremlin's Cold War, from Stalin to Khrushev* (Cambridge: Harvard University Press, 1996).

director-general (succeeded in 1961 by another Russian, Oganes V. Baroyan).[14] In 1962, the World Health Assembly's president was S. C. Kuraŝov of the USSR, the first time a physician from a communist party was elected to that position.

In these circumstances, the US Department of State argued that the United States had to win the competition with the Soviets in the international health arena. For the Department's assistant secretary for International Organization Affairs, the Soviet leaders "realized that the economic and social services performed, largely under US leadership, by the United Nations and the specialized agencies, threatened communist plans in the world. They were frightened by the impact made upon the underdeveloped countries by free-world aid."[15] US State Department officials suspected that the Soviets would seek to frustrate the activities of the WHO and the UN.[16] According to these officers, Soviet obstructionism would attempt to undermine efforts to "modernize" underdeveloped countries. This expectation did not lead solely to a reinforcement of American influence in multilateral agencies such as the WHO but to the stepping up of US bilateral aid.

The national-security dimension of American domestic and foreign policy had an impact on the WHO. From the beginning of UN multilateralism, US security agencies investigated Americans who participated in the conferences they organized – and even more intensely, those who worked in them. A member of the United States delegation to the First World Health Assembly revealed:

It seems that when one represents this great country in an international congress, the Federal Bureau of Investigations is deeply concerned and some of my friends informed me that I have been investigated. In fact, on my return I received a copy of the letter which the Assistant Deputy Commissioner of the Federal Security Administration sent to the Secretary of State. It was a great comfort to know that I had been certified as a loyal and trustworthy citizen.[17]

Regulation became stricter in the following years. In 1950, US Senator Joseph McCarthy accused the US federal government and the UN of being infiltrated by communists. One result was that the US State Department and the FBI strengthened their already rigorous "clearance" regulations for Americans

---

[14] Maureen Gallagher, "The World Health Organization: Promotion of US and Soviet Foreign Policy Goals," *Journal of the American Medical Association* 186:1 (1963), 29–34, p. 34.

[15] Francis O. Wilcox, "International Organizations: Aid to World Trade and Prosperity," *The Department of State Bulletin* 37 (1957), 749–754.

[16] David McKey, "Advancing US Economic Policies through the United Nations," *The Department of State Bulletin* 30:779 (1954), 826–830, p. 828.

[17] James Raglan Miller, "World Health Assembly Geneva, 1948, Notes by an Amateur in Public Health," *Connecticut State Medical Journal*, newspaper clipping, Folder 744, Box 55, Marta A. Eliot Papers [AESL].

working at the UN and its agencies. One notable early WHO staff member who had a difficult time with these regulations was the physician and sociologist Milton I. Roemer, who worked as an officer in social and occupational health between 1950 and 1951. Roemer admired Soviet public health and believed that the United States needed a national health insurance system. In Geneva, the US Consulate seized his passport and informed him that it could only be used to return to the United States.[18] The incident was not an isolated event. The relationship between the US government and the first director, the Canadian Brock Chisholm, was considered "unsatisfactory" by Secretary of State John Dulles because when he asked the Canadian to suspend hiring US nationals pending receipt of the McCarthyite US clearance forms in 1952, the Canadian strongly objected, stating he would discuss the matter with his Executive Board. The United States delivered a formal request for full cooperation, and forms were distributed directly to Americans working in WHO headquarters by the US representative in Geneva. Later, the second director-general, Marcolino Candau, was more lenient with these forms. Previously, Trygve Lie, the first secretary-general of the UN, who occupied the position between 1946 and 1952, allowed the FBI, for a few years, to set up an office within the New York headquarters of the organization to vet all Americans on the staff.[19]

Other, less left-leaning Americans, such as Milton Siegel and Martha M. Eliot, had less trouble. Eliot served as assistant director-general from 1949 to 1951 (previously, she was alternate to Parran on the Standing Technical Committee on Health of UNRRA and was the only woman attending the International Health Conference of New York of 1946 that approved WHO's Constitution).[20] Eliot was also chair of WHO's Expert Committee on Maternal and Child Welfare, which held its first session in Geneva in 1949, but, most relevantly, she maintained close ties with the US State Department and left Geneva in 1951 to become chief of the US Children's Bureau (where previously she had been associate chief).

The Cold-War alliance of the US State Department with governments of Western Europeans, many of them experienced in colonial medicine, explains why initially many tropical medical doctors formed the bulk of WHO's staff. An example was the Frenchman Pierre Dorolle, who was appointed WHO's

[18] Henry F. Nichol, US Resident Delegation, Geneva, July 31, 1953, "Interview with Dr. Candau, Director General, WHO," R. G. 59, Decimal File 398.55, Years, 1950–1954, Box 1634, Folder 6, NARA. See also Emily K. Abel, Elizabeth Fee, & Theodore M. Brown, "Milton I. Roemer: Advocate of Social Medicine, International Health, and National Health Insurance," *American Journal of Public Health* 98:9 (2008), 1596–1597.

[19] WHO Library, RC2/AFR/9, Summary of Statement made by Brock Chisholm, July 31, 1952, Regional Committee for Africa, Second Session Monrovia.

[20] "Obituary: Dr. Martha M. Eliot," *Chronicle of the World Health Organization* 32:6 (1978), 249.

deputy director-general in 1950. He had been trained in tropical medicine in France, and had been a former *Directeur du Service de la Santé Publique* in French Indochina. He had also served as a public health officer in the French colonies in Saigon and Hanoi.[21] Like other European physicians sympathetic to social medicine, he saw no contradiction between defense of European imperial prerogatives and the support of social medicine.

By the early 1950s the WHO had developed and approved a four-year plan for fellowships and by 1956 had provided more than 5,000 of them to health professionals from 149 countries, thus helping to build or reconstruct public health systems.[22] It had also completed work in standardization, such as in the Sixth Revised List of Diseases, Injuries, and Causes of Death; the International Pharmacopoeia that was instrumental in making drugs and medical substances used in different countries of identical strength and purity; the list of biological standards for drugs; and International Sanitary Regulations (1951). More than 130 countries adhered to the sanitary regulations, thus enabling the WHO to replace earlier and less comprehensive conventions (that standardized control of smallpox, plague, cholera, yellow fever, louse-borne typhus, and other diseases).

Not all went smoothly for the WHO in terms of finances. The Second World Health Assembly approved a budget for 1950 of USD 7.5 million but owing to several countries not paying their contributions it had to be reduced to USD 6.3 million. The Third World Health Assembly passed a budget for 1951 which, owing to the same circumstances as in 1950, was reduced to USD 6.15 million. In 1954, the World Health Assembly rejected a US proposal for a more limited budget and approved a total assessment of more than USD 10 million for the 1955 calendar year. The American delegation made a strong case to cut the budget to 9 million and objected to any increase that would entail a rise in the American assessment.[23] The US contribution amounted to 33.3 percent of the total budget of the WHO. American officials were worried that this figure was in excess of the cap of 30 percent that Congress had set for contributions to multilateral agencies.[24] WHO officials thought that exceeding the 30 percent limit was reasonable because the United States had the highest per capita income in the world. The final budget for 1955, which was approved by a

---

[21] "Pierre Dorolle," *Chronicle of the World Health Organization* 4:10 (1950), 323–324.
[22] H. S. Gear, "Ten Years of Growth of the World Health Organization," *The Lancet Special Articles* (12 July 1958), 85–88, p. 86.
[23] "Budget (1955) of the World Health Organization and the United States Assessment," *The Department of State Bulletin* 30 (1954), 964.
[24] "Additional Assessment for World Health Organization," United States, Congressional Record, *Proceedings and Debates of the 83rd Congress Second Session, Vol. 100 – Part 5, 29 April 1954 to 25 May 1954* (Washington, DC: US Government Printing Office, 1954), 7047–7048, p. 7047.

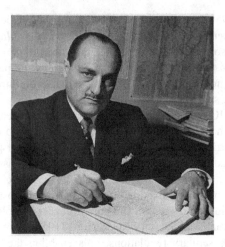

Figure 3.1 Marcolino Candau, a Brazilian physician who had worked with the Rockefeller Foundation and the Pan American Sanitary Bureau. Candau became the second director-general of the World Health Organization in 1953. He was reelected in 1958, 1963, and 1968.
Courtesy: Smithsonian Institution Archives.

28 to 24 vote of the World Health Assembly, was halfway between the US proposal and the initial figure proposed by the Executive Board of more than USD 11 million. The Board argued that it had exercised restraint for the previous three years, partly because it took into consideration American concerns over the growing budget. It was now imperative for the agency's expenditures to increase if its programs were to be developed and the organizational structure sustained. The US Congress eventually agreed to maintain its financial support for the WHO, at least for the time being. The trade-off was that the United States, as the main fiscal underwriter of the WHO, bought a considerable amount of influence with its financial support.

Meanwhile, Chisholm decided not to renew his appointment as director-general, which the Executive Board offered him in late 1952. In January 1953 he formally announced that he was uninterested in a second term, declaring that the WHO should regularly renew its leadership during the early years of its history. Very likely contributing to his decision were his objections to the United States' heavy hand in the organization and his conflict with the Catholic Church over family planning. Chisholm was probably also sensitive to the political reality that a conservative US government was unsupportive of the socio-medical orientation he preferred. The Brazilian Marcolino Candau (see Figure 3.1) became the second director-general of the WHO at the age of 42. He received the nomination of the WHO's Executive Board after defeating candidates from Pakistan and Italy that had been supported by the British and the Italians, respectively, and was elected at the 1953 Sixth World Health Assembly. The candidacy of the Brazilian was enthusiastically supported by Chisholm and the American health leader Fred Soper. Candau's election was the first instance of a procedure which would be followed by the EB until the early twentieth century: to hold a series of secret ballots in which the candidate receiving the least number of votes would be dropped until only two names remained. (Chisholm campaigned "hard" for Candau.)[25] The EB proposal of Candau to the Assembly was endorsed by the US delegation as well as by a bloc of Latin American countries and some European nations.

Candau was a graduate of Rio de Janeiro's Medical School and held a master's degree in public health from Johns Hopkins University. He had worked under Fred Soper's supervision during Rockefeller IHD's fight against *Anopheles Gambiae* in the Brazilian northeast and, later, in programs sponsored by US bilateral assistance. His WHO career began when he joined the Geneva headquarters' staff in 1950 as director of the Division of Organization of Health Services. Within a year he became assistant director-general in charge of Advisory Services. In 1952 he moved to Washington as the Pan-American Sanitary Bureau's assistant director, to work briefly under Soper again. In Geneva, Candau proved to be the WHO's longest-serving director-general, being reelected three times and directing the agency from 1953 to 1973. The US government supported Candau not least because its Department of State believed that with Candau it would be possible to negotiate a reasonable WHO scale of assessments and raise the "minuscule" contribution paid by the USSR. He was also perceived as a supporter of the vertical and technocratic perspective described at the beginning of this book.

Under Candau, who served as director-general for 20 years (1953–1973), the WHO increased its visibility, financial stability, and administrative coherence. He worked closely with the staff in Geneva and developed a reputation for his diplomatic skills, which he used to rally the World Bank, the FAO, the US State Department, and even the US Congress. By the mid-1950s, the WHO administered 120 projects, employed more than 1,000 staff, and included 88 countries, several of which were not UN members. Candau was also responsible for securing a new glass-and-steel building in Geneva and reinforcing the resources and staff of the regional offices. Regional directors came to be elected by the member countries of each region rather than being appointed by the director-general and acquired considerable control over their region's programmatic activities.[26]

---

[25] Farley, *Brock Chisholm*, p. 191.
[26] John Sibley, "UN Health Unit Marks a Decade," *The New York Times*, April 6, 1958, p. 13.

The Challenges of Regionalization

The development of regional offices was, in fact, one of the most notable features of the WHO's organizational evolution in the late forties and early fifties. Plans for regionalization can be traced to the 1946 New York meeting where initially five regions were envisioned: the Americas, South-East Asia, Europe, the Eastern Mediterranean, and the Western Pacific, respectively known as AMRO, SEARO, EURO, EMRO, and the WHO-Western Pacific (no acronym initially used).[27] The creation of the sixth regional office, for Africa, was accomplished only after complex negotiations with European imperial powers and will be discussed in the final section of this chapter. Each regional office was overseen by a committee consisting of representatives of "full members" (independent countries) and "associate members" (usually European colonies). All regions were meant, at least initially, to aggregate countries sharing commonalities such as geographic proximity and similarity of epidemiological profile. The regional offices were responsible for setting regional policies, hiring staff, supervising and carrying out WHO policies in the regions, and organizing meetings with representatives of the governments of each member country. In the late 1940s and early 1950s, these meetings moved from city to city within the regions until a regional "capital" was agreed upon.

Many of the European officers of the WHO initially resisted the idea of regionalization and insisted that countries join the agency individually, each in a direct relationship with Geneva (as countries did in the League of Nations Health Organization). But the adamant insistence by the United States and the Latin American bloc that the Pan American Sanitary Bureau (PASB) continue its existence forced regionalization to prevail. An agreement was signed between the WHO and PASB in 1949 whereby the latter would serve as the regional office of the WHO in the Americas and at the same time continue as a specialized agency of the Organization of American States. PASB would have the authority to elect its own director (in loose consultation with the DG) and the liberty to promote and finance almost all of its own programs. However, Caribbean colonies could join the WHO and PASB if represented by the European power that controlled them. PASB was an important instrument of US foreign policy in Latin America, and it was no doubt for this reason that the US delegation played a heavy-handed role in

---

[27] See Howard B. Calderwood, "The World Health Organization and Its Regional Organizations," *Temple Law Quarterly* 37:1 (1963), 15–27, and Robert Berkov, *The World Health Organization: A Study in Decentralized International Administration* (Geneva: Droz, 1957).

the WHA regionalization debate.[28] The US State Department had also recently established regional bureaus that coincided, approximately, with the geographical areas covered by the regional offices of the WHO, and having multilateral agencies tuned in closely to this American Cold War vision of the world was considered essential to US foreign policy.

Outside of the Americas and Europe, the organization of the WHO's regional offices confronted the political challenges posed by a fraying European imperialism and the tensions of the early postwar period. Imperial powers argued that they would take care of the health needs of the populations in their colonies, but they also allowed colonial nations to become associate members of the WHO regions. Yet in some instances, the so-called administering states or "full members" of the WHO removed colonial dependencies from regional offices almost unilaterally. In other cases, changes were initiated in regional configurations to avoid regional political tensions. One example was Israel, which was a member of the WHO since the Second World Health Assembly and was originally placed, seemingly naturally, in EMRO. But because of its conflict with Arab nations in the Middle East, it was moved to the European regional office. Another example was Pakistan, which joined the Eastern Mediterranean region and not its geographically "natural" area of SEARO because the regional office for South-East Asia was located in New Delhi and there was an enduring conflict between Pakistan and India. The tension of the early Cold War also intruded. In 1949, the Chinese Communists drove the Nationalists onto the island of Taiwan and proclaimed the People's Republic of China on the mainland with a population of several hundreds of millions. Nevertheless, Taiwan, with a much smaller population, was included in the WHO as the representative of China in the Western Pacific region, while mainland communist China was denied a place in the WHO or a seat at the UN.

The location of SEARO's headquarters in New Delhi was justified by the fact that it had the full support of the prime minister of India, was at the hub of a good railway and communications network, and was already the site of regional headquarters for other UN offices such as ILO, FAO, and UNESCO. Beginning in early 1949, the head of SEARO was the physician Chandra Mani, a founding member of the WHO and the deputy director of Health Services in India. He recruited a core staff of 20 from nine different countries to work on health policy and administration while six additional experts were recruited to work on malaria, venereal disease, tuberculosis, environmental sanitation, maternal and child health, and nursing. Mani was aggressive in

---

[28] Javed Siddiqi, *World Health and World Politics: The World Health Organization and the UN System* (Columbia: University of South Carolina Press, 1995).

enlarging the prerogatives of his regional office. In one of his first annual reports, he complained to Geneva that it retained essential functions such as general planning, technical guidance, and budgetary control while leaving responsibility for operating programs to the region.[29]

SEARO initially included the by-then independent countries Afghanistan, Burma, Ceylon, India, and Thailand. After its second regional meeting, SEARO also included Nepal, French India, Portuguese Goa, and the British Maldives Islands.[30] By the early 1950s, the region comprised a combined population of more than 490 million, of whom a very large percentage was poor, malnourished, illiterate, and victim to a number of diseases such as smallpox, malaria, and tuberculosis. The region also suffered from a high infant mortality rate, and life expectancy was between 25 and 35 years. Scarcity of health personnel was dramatic. The doctor to population ratio in the region could be as high as 1 to 120,000, there was only one midwife for as many as 100,000 people and one public health officer for every million. SEARO provided a forum to denounce the difficult working conditions of health workers in the region, including insecurity of tenure, little opportunity for promotion, and low salaries. At the second regional meeting, the director complained: "In India ... the emoluments are so low as to attract only the poorest material into [public health]."[31]

The EMRO office began operations in July 1949 using the resources of the former Alexandria Sanitary Bureau that dated back to the nineteenth century. The site was selected because it received support from the Egyptian government in the form of nominal rent for use of a fine building formerly occupied by the Alexandria Bureau and because of its proximity to Cairo where various UN specialized agencies were already in operation. EMRO's first director was Aly Tewfik Shousha, the leader of the 1947 anti-cholera campaign. He would continue to head the regional office until 1957, when A. H. Taba of Iran succeeded him. The Regional Office included 11 countries with a total population of about two hundred million people. One of EMRO's first preoccupations was an old international health concern: the possible spread of cholera with annual pilgrimages to Mecca. At EMRO's first session in Cairo, Shousha focused on a broader goal: promoting community participation, as health was not something "which cannot be

[29] World Health Organization, Regional Office for South-East Asia, *Report of the Regional Director, 17 August 1950* (New Delhi, Third Session, Regional Committee), p. 12.

[30] World Health Organization, Regional Office for South-East Asia, *Twenty Years in South-East Asia, 1948–1967* (New Delhi: World Health Organization, 1967).

[31] World Health Organization, Regional Office for South-East Asia, "Conditions of Service of Public Health Personnel," August 4, 1949, New Delhi, Second Session, Regional Committee, n.p.

done to people; it must be done for themselves by themselves."[32] In the second session, held in Cairo in 1949, the membership of the regional office became clearer: Egypt, Ethiopia, Iran, Iraq, Lebanon, Pakistan, Saudi Arabia, Syria, and Turkey. In addition, delegates from France, the United Kingdom, and Anglo-Egyptian Sudan (administered by the UK and Egypt until 1956 when Sudan became an independent sovereign state) participated as full members.

The Western Pacific Regional Office included Australia, Cambodia, China, South Korea, Laos, New Zealand, the Philippines, Vietnam, and provisionally the Malay Peninsula. In 1951, Japan was assigned to this region, having entered the WHO that very same year with the daunting task of reconstructing its health institutions. This Regional Office got entangled politically with the Cold War and new forms of imperialism. The beginnings of the regional office were troubled because of the Korean War and its immediate aftermath, and after the war representation of Korea was given to South Korea while communist North Korea was only fully recognized as a WHO member in 1973. Another political problem derived from the demand of European powers to recover authority over territories and colonies occupied by Japan during World War II. Australia and New Zealand, with New Guinea and Western Samoa as colonies, sided with the European powers. The governments of Australia and New Zealand were initially opposed to the creation of one regional office and suggested, unsuccessfully, the formation of two regions: one for the north, with the less-developed countries and colonies, and one for the south, including Australia, New Zealand, New Guinea, and the South Pacific Islands.[33] When the proposal failed, an Australia representative attended the first session of the regional committee but only as an "observer," and in the first years New Zealand did not attend at all.[34] The Cold War would endure in this region with the Vietnam War. In 1956, a WHO Office was established in Saigon to coordinate work in Cambodia, the Laos People's Democratic Republic, and Viet Nam. Between the early and the late 1960s it survived but relieved its duties over Cambodia and Laos. After the end of the war in 1975, the Office was closed but the WHO managed to do some important humanitarian work in the new communist country, and the

---

[32] Cited in World Health Organization, Regional Office for the Eastern Mediterranean, Summary minutes, February 7, 1949, Cairo, First Session, Regional Committee, n.p.

[33] "Position Paper, Western Pacific Regional Organization," May 7, 1951, R.G. 59, Decimal file 398.55, Years 1950–1954, Box 1632, Folder Fourth World Health Assembly, NARA.

[34] An official historical account of the regional agency is: World Health Organization, Regional Office for the Western Pacific Region, *Fifty Years of the World Health Organization in the Western Pacific Region* (Manila: World Health Organization Regional Committee for the Western Pacific, 1988).

Western Pacific Region praised the new government. Only in 1977, after the United Nations Security Council advised the approval of Vietnam to the multilateral agency, was a WHO Office in Hanoi established.

The Philippine government led the opposition to European imperialism and Australia-New Zealand's aggressive position in the late 1940s, insisting that the region should be autonomous and defined as broadly as possible. They succeeded in making Manila the headquarters of the regional office, bypassing Australian cities. This city in the Philippines was a cosmopolitan center and the capital of a country with a tradition in tropical medicine connected to the United States. Besides, Manila was the site of fine medical and nursing schools and urban hospitals, and its epidemiological officers were in communication with hundreds of islands of the archipelago. The first regional director was the Chinese physician I. C. Fang, who had previously served on the WHO Interim Commission under Calderone in New York. Trained at the Peking Union Medical College, he later received a master's degree in public health from the London School of Hygiene and Tropical Medicine. In 1966, Fang was succeeded by Philippine physician Francisco J. Dy, a public-health graduate of Johns Hopkins University.

The European regional office was promoted by Eastern European countries and the Soviet Union, which urged the creation of a regional agency whilst Western European countries generally did not see the pressing need for it. The Eastern European countries argued that the office would help them overcome the legacies of World War II, such as destroyed hospitals, non-operating medical schools, and insufficient medical personnel. But the British, for example, were not convinced of the need to establish a regional office on the continent that already hosted the general headquarters of the WHO. Despite these misgivings, in 1951 a European regional office was established in Geneva and, ironically, Great Britain's Norman D. Begg was appointed the first director of EURO and remained in the post until 1957.

It took five more years to move the EURO office to Copenhagen, the city that won the competition with Nice, Florence, The Hague, Vienna, and Frankfurt. According to EURO's organizers, the boundaries of the region would encompass all of Europe. As in other regional offices, Cold War and colonial politics intervened in various ways. The Federal Republic of Germany (West Germany, supported by the United States and its European allies) requested and was granted membership in 1951, although it was formally still under occupation. The decision created a problem with the German Democratic Republic (East Germany, supported by the Soviet Union and its allies), which was denied membership in the WHO despite several requests. Only in 1973 was a concession made and the GDR allowed to send observers to the World Health Assembly.

The Quivers of AFRO

Of all the WHO regions, the last to be formed was the one for Africa, a continent that had formerly received scant attention from international health agencies but was, not accidentally, the leading site of European colonization and colonial medicine. The delay in creating a regional office was the direct result of the postwar politics of revived colonialism. The excuse frequently offered in WHO circles was that Africa had no convenient and outstanding medical center and most African countries lacked the potential for collaboration because they were still largely controlled by their colonial overseers. Indeed, after World War II all African countries were colonies except Liberia, South Africa, Egypt, and Ethiopia, and the last two were early members of the WHO's Eastern Mediterranean Region. The rest of Africa fell into the UN category of "non-self-governing territories" under the UN "trusteeship" system that had superseded the League of Nations' "mandates" system. The debate on trusteeship was one of the most vigorous at the UN Conference in San Francisco.[35] The outcome was that European governments were not forced to give up their colonies but had to report annually to a UN Trusteeship Division on the living conditions of the colonized people under their jurisdiction. European countries accepted this system because it had become clear that the UN would seek to *improve* colonial conditions rather than question the legality of colonies. In reality there was much to improve, as the colonial powers did little to develop the health, educational, or economic infrastructures of their possessions. Colonial powers, the "administering states," were full members of the WHO, whereas the colonies, known as "non-self-governing territories," could only aspire to become "associate members" with the permission of the administering states.[36]

Several countries and colonial possessions in northern and central Africa, such as Spanish Morocco and British Zanzibar, were assigned to EURO on the basis of the claim that their participation in European commerce was more relevant than their geographic location in Africa. The former Italian colony and newly independent north African country, Libya, requested to be part of the Eastern Mediterranean Region for political and religious reasons and was allowed to join EMRO. The UN trusteeship system explains why many in the WHO did not believe that Africa, more precisely sub-Saharan Africa, should have a regional office: The European powers did not relish the prospect of additional supervision of their colonial activities in the region. It is telling

---

[35] Michael D. Callahan, *A Sacred Trust: The League of Nations and Africa, 1929–1946* (Brighton Portland: Academic Press, 2004).

[36] Annette Baker Fox, "The United Nations and Colonial Development," *International Organization* 4:2 (1950), 199–218.

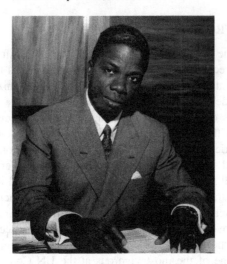

Figure 3.2 Joseph N. Togba, from Liberia, strongly supported the creation and development of a WHO regional office in Africa in the late 1940s and early 1950s.
Courtesy: World Health Organization Photo Library.

that the members of the African working party at the First World Health Assembly were Belgium, France, Portugal, South Africa, and Liberia; with the exception of the last two, all are colonial European empires. Representatives of France and South Africa argued that there should be no rush to create a WHO office in Africa because coming up with the resources for a regional budget was "unrealistic." The leading proponent for the creation of a regional office was a Liberian physician trained in the United States, Joseph Nagbe Togba (see Figure 3.2), but his motives were somewhat suspect, as was Liberia's position in the UN. Liberia was closely and even quasi-colonially connected to the United States, strongly supported the US war effort against Germany in World War II, and had been rewarded with major American investments in Liberian technological development in the postwar period. Togba's proposal was adamantly opposed by South Africa, and less vehemently by France and the United Kingdom, in the First World Health Assembly.

Colonial considerations in partial disguise also dictated the definition of geographic boundaries for the African regional office: "a primary region is suggested for all Africa south of the 20 degree North parallel of latitude to the western border of the Anglo-Egyptian Sudan, to its junction with the northern border of Belgian Congo, thence eastwards along the northern borders of Belgian Congo, thence eastwards along the northern borders of Uganda and

Kenya; and thence southwards along the eastern border of Kenya to the Indian Ocean."[37] As a result of these boundaries, AFRO, with a few exceptions, embraced countries and territories south of the Sahara in an area of about 7,850,000 square miles inhabited by approximately 150 million people. As a region, it was one of the poorest on the globe, in dramatic need of help, and portrayed as incapable of rising out of poverty by itself, thus reinforcing the need for dependence on Europe and the United States in order to achieve "development."

The first AFRO committee meeting took place in Geneva in late 1951. It was attended by representatives of the "full" member countries – Belgium, France, Liberia, Portugal, Spain, South Africa, and the UK – and by a representative of its first associate member: Rhodesia. The Dutch physician François Daubenton, who had worked for UNRRA during World War II and then for the Netherlands Red Cross, had joined the WHO in 1948 as chief of its mission to Ethiopia and a bit later as consultant to EMRO. In 1952 he was chosen to lead the African Regional Office, which was initially administered from Geneva. Daubenton had studied at the London School of Hygiene and Tropical Medicine and at the University of Johannesburg and had considerable experience as a medical consultant to various mining companies in South Africa.[38] His career and the first meeting of AFRO had the odor of colonial medicine. That odor still clung to the second meeting, which took place in Monrovia, Liberia in 1952. Among the participants at that meeting was WHO Director-General Brock Chisholm, who warned against a too-rapid transfer of modern western techniques to Africa and advised AFRO to emphasize "a series of orderly steps requiring direction, control, and constant thought." For his part, Daubenton urged the WHO to promote the participation of "enlightened Africans" capable of winning the understanding and cooperation of the people.[39] The statements of Chisholm and Daubenton suggest that they believed in a version of decolonization that entailed progressive and orderly changes led by enlightened elites. These beliefs also explain why Daubenton was careful to maintain close communication with European colonial medical officers working in London, Paris, Lisbon, and Brussels.

---

[37] A definition consecrated in World Health Organization, First World Assembly, Provisional Verbatim Records of the Eleventh Plenary Meeting, July 10, 1948, A/VR/11. Corr.1, p. 4, apps.who.int/iris/bitstream/10665/98641/1/WHA1_VR-11_eng.pdf.

[38] "General François Daubenton (Obituary)," Chronicle of the World Health Organization 19:10 (1965), 419.

[39] World Health Organization, Regional Committee for Africa, Summary of Statement made by Brock Chisholm, July 31, 1952, p. 21, Second Session, Monrovia, Regional Committee & Report of the Regional Director, August 4, 1952, Third Session, Kampala, Regional Committee, August 13, 1953, p. 24.

In 1953, the regional meeting that took place in Kampala, Uganda resulted in the decision, despite the doubts of some European representatives who considered the step "premature," to move AFRO headquarters to African soil. Daubenton visited Paris with the WHO's legal advisor to negotiate with the French government for the creation of a headquarters office in a French colonial territory. The location selected was Brazzaville, in French Equatorial Africa (later the Republic of Congo), which during World War II had rejected the Vichy regime and worked with the Allied forces. It had also been the site of a 1944 meeting with General Charles De Gaulle, who acknowledged the need for democratic and social reforms in the French colonies. The merits of Brazzaville were used to override Togba's aspiration to house the regional office in Liberia's capital of Monrovia as well as Belgium and Portugal's desire to have it in Leopoldville, the capital of the Belgian colony of Congo. Initially, a small staff of five people moved to the French African city but in a few years they relocated to new and larger quarters in Cité du D'Joué, located 10 kilometers from Brazzaville. The new location included the houses of officers and had the appearance of an enclave or an island of modernity in a sea of poverty that surrounded the compound. These physical arrangements reinforced the view that progress out of colonialism could only be achieved in Africa by the external guidance of European elites and that native societies had to be shepherded into development.

Daubenton announced his retirement in late 1953 and was succeeded by the Portuguese physician Francisco J. Cambournac, who was formally appointed AFRO regional director in January 1954. Cambournac remained head of AFRO until 1964, inspiring confidence during his tenure among the regional committee's members because he came from a tropical medicine tradition and because he was acquainted with the methods of modern international health.[40] Cambournac had studied at Lisbon's *Escola de Medicina Tropical* and pursued a specialization in malariology in Paris and Rome. Cambournac appears in Figure 3.3 at his desk in a typical pose for an officer of the WHO in the 1950s. His work experience included leading a Rockefeller-funded malaria control program in rural Portugal and working in the colonial medical services of Portugal. He was appointed professor of hygiene at the Tropical Medicine Institute in Lisbon in 1946, attended the First World Health Assembly in 1948, and worked as a WHO advisor for Africa. He built a reputation as a skilled public health officer and appeared to be a living example of how colonial medicine and international health could coexist.

---

[40] World Health Organization, Regional Committee for Africa, Annual Report of the Regional Director, July 1, 1956–June 30, 1957 15, Seventh Session, Brazzaville, Regional Committee, p. 15.

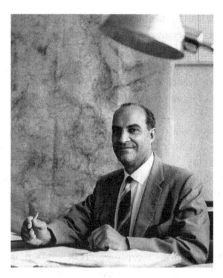

Figure 3.3 Francisco J. Cambournac, the Portuguese director of WHO's Regional Office for Africa, in his office in Brazzaville during the 1950s. He had previously worked in tropical medicine in Portuguese colonies in Africa and in the Rockefeller Foundation's antimalaria programs in Portugal. Credit WHO/Paul Almasy.
Courtesy: World Health Organization Photo Library.

Cambournac never questioned the idea that Europeans had a "civilizing mission" in post–World War II Africa and followed the second technocratic perspective of the agency. Although he did not directly participate in the debates between those who urged independence for Europe's colonies and those who wished to postpone it by offering expanded services and political concessions to decolonizing nations, his writings indicate that he was on the side of the latter. This implied that he favored improvements in public health systems negotiated within the UN system with the participation of colonial administrations. That position was popular at the WHO's Geneva headquarters and in other UN agencies. Yet Cambournac's quest for a place for AFRO within international health would not have been possible without changes in international affairs, most notably those affecting European imperialism. The British, for example, increased their service commitments and recognition of local rights in the colonies because of their fears about their crumbling empire. The British Colonial Development and Welfare Act of 1945, renewed in 1950 and 1955, meant an increase in health expenditures in the UK's African possessions. But the British failed in Egypt, where President Nasser national-ized the Suez Canal in 1956. Thus, in the mid and late 1950s the British began more vigorously to favor indirect rule and the organization of a titular "Commonwealth" under their hegemony because maintaining colonies was getting too expensive and too politically fraught. They accepted the independence of additional African colonies, as in 1956 when British Sudan became an independent nation. The following year, the British colony known as the Gold Coast became independent Ghana under the revolutionary leadership of Kwame Nkrumah.

Conflicting prospects for colonialism also beset the French government. Most French politicians believed it necessary to grant some power to native elites in order to retain their loyalty, while others wanted to resort to authoritarian control over the colonies. In 1946, French colonies started to receive economic development funds from the *Fonds d'investissement pour le développement économique et social des territoires d'outre-mer* (FIDES), and before long France had changed its Constitution to incorporate within it the concept of a "French Union." But calls for a French Union comparable to the British Commonwealth of Nations were greeted in some places with revolts and rebellions. Social unrest in Morocco, Tunisia, Algeria, and Madagascar – which the French government could not subdue – ultimately led to independence. Elsewhere in the French empire, the war in Indochina begun in 1946 ended in France's humiliating defeat in 1954. Pierre Mendès, France's president of the Council of Ministers in the mid-fifties, accelerated the withdrawal of French soldiers from Indochina and agreed with Tunisian nationalist leaders to establish independence in 1956. Charles de Gaulle, France's Fifth Republic president, inaugurated in 1958, was supported initially by conservatives hoping to regain full control by offering rebellious African colonies to be part of a French Union. But by the early 1960s, several former French colonies had become independent. Thus, the political situation favored AFRO's development into an Africa-focused multilateral regional agency.

While these political events played out, AFRO tried to get on with its work with surveys, medical personnel training programs, sanitary engineering projects, and the study of infectious diseases, in particular yellow fever, which was considered a local but not a global threat. Before World War II, yellow fever was known to be endemic in West Africa, from Senegal to Congo, but its spread inland was unknown. With the help of the Rockefeller Foundation, AFRO carried out yellow fever surveys between 1951 and 1953 to determine the southern limit of the infection, hoping to confirm the suspicion that the disease extended far beyond the area where clinical yellow fever was traditionally observed. These studies enlarged the findings of a Rockefeller commission in the late 1920s that the illness was essentially a disease of animals, especially monkeys, introduced into areas inhabited by man. Contrary to some skeptics,

AFRO believed that complete eradication of yellow fever was possible in all African urban communities.

By 1954, AFRO divided its work into four geographical areas: the Central Area (mainly occupied by the Belgian Congo and Angola), the Western Area (with Liberia, Nigeria, and Gambia, among other countries and colonies), the Eastern Area (with Kenya, Uganda, and Zanzibar, among others), and the Southern Area (with South Africa, Rhodesia, and Mozambique, among others). Cambournac also had an interest in developing public health programs that were not common in other regional offices – such as mental health, community development, and medical anthropology (the latter was called applied anthropology in the United States and was then indistinguishable from medical sociology). His predecessor had also supported medical sociology by hiring the French ethnologist Jean Paul Lebeuf. Cambournac renewed Lebeuf's appointment, made him chief of a new section in the regional office, and asked him to comment on all projects from a sociological perspective. For Cambournac, Lebeuf's work was critical and instrumental because learning "the habits and reactions of human beings" was as important as learning the "habits and reactions of insects."[41] The social scientist would help to establish a useful contact between those "who represent progress and those who should receive the maximum benefit from it."[42]

The chief items on the agenda for the 1955 AFRO meeting were the annual report of the regional director and the program and budget for 1956 and 1957. The budget for 1956, including funds from UN technical assistance and the United Nations Children's Fund, was more than USD 3 million; the budget for 1957 was estimated at USD 4.7 million. Although these budgets were smaller than those of other WHO regional offices, they indicate that funding was available and growing. The committee decided to hold its sixth session in September of 1956 in Luanda, Angola, then part of the Portuguese empire. The chairman of the Luanda meeting was a physician from Portugal, demonstrating that imperialism and colonial medicine were alive and well at AFRO. Yet according to Cambournac, the WHO was helping developing independent governments help themselves in their efforts to improve health conditions in Africa.[43]

[41] World Health Organization, Regional Committee for Africa, Annual Report of the Regional Director, August 13, 1952, Third Session, Kampala, Regional Committee, n.p.

[42] "Sociology as the Basis of Health," by J. P. Lebeuf, chief of the sociology section of the WHO Regional Office for Africa, December 1953, in World Health Organization, Division of Public Information, *WHO Special Features* (Geneva: World Health Organization, 1953), 1–3, p. 3. The study later appeared in a journal: Jean Paul Lebeuf, "Sociology as the Basis of Health Education," *Health Education Journal* 13 (1955), 232–238.

[43] Francisco J. Cambournac, "Health in Africa," *American Journal of Public Health and the Nation's Health*, June 1960; 50:6 (1960), 13–19.

Cambournac noted that Africa had never before been a priority for the WHO. Perhaps most strikingly, the 1955 World Health Assembly in Mexico justified the exclusion of Africa from the "global" malaria eradication program by claiming it was "premature" to carry out operations in locations with bad roads, large rural populations, and precarious health systems. Although in sub-Saharan Africa, with few exceptions, all territories were malarious, it was accepted that most adult Africans had a considerable, but not absolute, degree of tolerance for the malaria parasite. Children underwent a severe selection by the disease accounting for high mortality and morbidity, but the fact that malaria was an ever-present problem in sub-Saharan Africa and not a spectacular epidemic allowed non-AFRO WHO experts to believe that there was no urgency about including the subcontinent in malaria eradication.

Some AFRO officers and European medical researchers were very much interested in developing pilot programs, especially in rural areas such as those discussed at a conference in Kampala in 1950, to determine the feasibility of malaria eradication, to create and enlarge malaria-free areas, to identify the most cost-effective interventions, and later to scale-up these programs.[44] These pilot programs – intended to achieve the greatest possible reduction of malaria mortality and morbidity but not eradication – supported by the WHO, especially in Liberia and some British and French African possessions, achieved a temporary decline of malaria morbidity and mortality and turned out to be opportunities to train personnel and develop rural health infrastructures. Yet the combination of medical activities promoted by an international health agency and colonialism was difficult to sustain, and cases of biological resistance both to insecticides and drugs appeared. According to Webb, the antimalarial program encountered local cultural resistance because many Africans believed it was not a priority since they had survived childhood malarial infections and acquired immunity and perceived the disease as a problem of white colonizers.[45] The sustainability of the pilot programs was difficult during a period in which African colonies were rapidly obtaining independence and receiving bilateral aid. Between 1960 and 1964 independence was granted to all the remaining British possessions in East Africa. The Belgian Congo became independent Zaire in 1960, and Rwanda and Burundi were partitioned off from it, becoming separate states a year later. Most of these countries combined control of malaria and eradication and tried to construct basic health

[44] M. Dobson, M. Malowany, & Robert W. Snow, "Malaria Control in East Africa: The Kampala Conference and the Pare-Taveta Scheme: A Meeting of Common and High Ground," *Parassitologia* 42 (2000), 149–166.
[45] James L. Webb, "The Long Shadow of Malaria Interventions in Tropical Africa," *The Lancet* 374:9705 (2009), 1883–1884.

infrastructure instead on emphasizing specific disease-eradication programs. In 1960, the conservative and pragmatic British Prime Minister Harold Macmillan made a famous "wind of change" speech in South Africa, acknowledging the irreversible growth of African independence.

These changes had an impact on the UN, WHO, and AFRO. In October of 1960, 16 new African countries entered the UN. Between 1960 and 1965, 24 new independent African countries joined the UN and the WHO. Since the 10th session of the African regional committee held in Acra, the chairman or vice-chairman of the meeting was a black African. In the early 1960s, after violent confrontations in South Africa where police killed Pan-African Congress demonstrators against apartheid, representatives of former colonies announced that they would not attend AFRO meetings if they were held in the presence of South African delegates (and at the 1963 meeting, when South Africa's representative was called to speak, the rest of African representatives left the room).

The dramatic change in the African region was reflected in the growth and change of its membership. In 1957, there were only three member states and the same number of associate members. Ten years later, the regional office recognized 29 members and only two associate members. In 1965, Alfred Comlan Quenum from Benin became the first African regional director, with the support of the new independent African countries, who was closer to the first socio-medical perspective of the WHO. The year before, the World Health Assembly followed a UN resolution in condemning South Africa's apartheid and deprived it of its voting privileges. South Africa reacted furiously and withdrew from the WHO (remaining an inactive member until 1994 when President Nelson Mandela was elected).

4 The Cold War and Eradication

During the 1950s, the WHO was characterized by confidence in the power of medical science to eliminate or substantially reduce the worldwide burden of disease and, at the same time, by the clear imprint of US foreign policy. In this Cold War era, tension between the Soviet Union and the United States became increasingly palpable. The Soviets now possessed the atomic bomb and had developed a small but significant nuclear arsenal, which shattered American confidence by challenging the US monopoly of these destructive weapons. The United States responded with foreign policy initiatives, military build-up, and bilateral technical aid meant to secure its preeminent place in the Western Hemisphere and in other parts of the world. During this period there was also a studied interaction between American foreign policy and multilateral health organizations.

The growing disintegration of European colonial empires and the consolidation of Nikita Khrushchev's leadership in the mid-1950s opened the way for the Soviet Union's intense worldwide competition with the United States in matters of science, technology, and international health. Indeed, health and development work became a major international arena in which American and Soviet leaders sought to enlarge their spheres of influence. Prophesying the worldwide emergence of socialism, Khrushchev supported national liberation movements in developing "third world" countries and offered to help by providing Soviet technical assistance.[1]

US foreign policy also emphasized non-military aid as crucial in building a developing nation's economic strength and national security. In particular, the US State Department regarded medical and economic assistance for developing countries as tools to repel "enslaving" Soviet influence by contributing to "liberating wars" or "crusades" against disease.[2] This aid strategy

---

[1] See Peter W. Rodman, *More Precious than Peace, the Cold War and the Struggle for the Third World* (New York: Charles Scribner's Son, 1994).

[2] The pairing of the terms "communism" and "slavery" appears in a 1950 report prepared by the Departments of State and Defense and cited by Sergio Aguayo, *Myths and [mis]Perceptions: Changing US Elite Visions of Mexico* (San Diego: Center for US-Mexican Studies at the

was the basis for master health metaphors, for example, between malaria and communism (both were "enslaving" conditions for developing countries). Likewise, "eradication" (of disease and communism) through strenuous, military-like efforts would lead to "modernization." These metaphors reflected the assumption that developing nations should follow the lead and the path of industrialized nations. They were also instrumental in legitimizing self-contained technological solutions that constituted the primarily techno-cratic pattern of initiatives by the world health agency. This pattern was premised on the notion that it was possible to contain diseases at their source with modern technology alone and without significant changes in socio-economic or political conditions.

The Cold War and International Health

The leading American Cold War figure of the 1950s was John Foster Dulles, the US secretary of state from 1953 to 1959 during the two administrations of President Dwight Eisenhower. The grandson of a former secretary of state, Dulles strove to undermine the Soviet's global standing. Although Eisenhower in his 1952 electoral campaign had criticized the "futile" policy of containment practiced by President Truman, once in power both Eisenhower and Dulles followed an expanded version of containment. Eisenhower and Dulles pursued a "rhetorical" diplomacy of belligerent speeches against Communism but limited real confrontation.[3] As they dealt with the Cold War issues of the early 1950s (Korea, Berlin, Iran, and Guatemala), their guiding principle was to stop or "contain" the spread of Soviet ideology and influence.

Under Dulles, the State Department energized its regional branches and reinforced the Bureau of International Organization Affairs (originally created in 1949 to coordinate work with the UN and its specialized agencies such as the WHO). Dulles also contributed to the campaigns of the World Health Organization and the Pan American Health Organization, as depicted in Figure 4.1. There were several reasons for State Department support of international agencies. First, the United States sought to increase its image of humanitarianism and thereby to heighten its global moral reputation. It could accomplish this – and simultaneously reduce the suspicion that its aid was meant to buy a reputation of benevolence – by finding less direct ways to help Western Europe and defeated countries such as Japan to recover. For US United Nations ambassador Henry Cabot Lodge in 1957, "To carry out our

University of California, 1998), p. 42. The phrase "the war on malaria is a race against time" appears in "Report on the War against Malaria," *New York Times*, January 24, 1960, p. 15.

[3] On Dulles, see Richard H. Immerman (ed.), *John Foster Dulles and the Diplomacy of the Cold War* (Princeton: Princeton University Press, 1990).

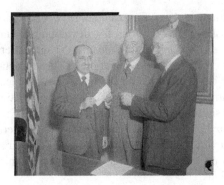

Figure 4.1 US Secretary of State John Foster Dulles, center, presents two checks totaling USD 7,000,000 to two international health agencies in 1957 as part of the US contribution to the malaria eradication program. Marcolino Candau, left, received a check for USD 5,000,000 and the balance went to Fred Soper, director of the Pan American Sanitary Organization.
Credit: Bettmann/Contributor. Source: Getty Images.

own foreign policies under the aegis of the United Nations helps America directly, as we then get credit for practicing altruism instead of power politics."[4] Francis O. Wilcox, the Department of State's assistant secretary for International Organization Affairs, revealed another motive behind overt altruism: to create new markets by increasing the purchasing power of people in areas where per capita income was low and raising their standards of living so that they would be able to buy American goods.[5]

A second reason for active US participation in UN programs was to share the cost of American "humanitarian" activities and thus leverage its investments. Although the budget for US bilateral assistance was always larger than the budget allocated for multilateral assistance, by 1956 the United States had contributed more than USD 23 million to the UN and its ten specialized agencies, thus accounting for 31 percent of the total assessments of these agencies.[6] The UN's pool of manpower and training resources was greater than what the United States could provide alone, and US governmental officials had good reason to believe that international technical experts would

[4] Henry Cabot Lodge, "12th Anniversary of United Nations," *The Department of State Bulletin* 37 (1957), 768.
[5] Francis O. Wilcox, "International Organizations: Aid to World Trade and Prosperity," *The Department of State Bulletin* 37 (1957), 749–754.
[6] United States, Department of State. "Table I United States Contributions to International Organizations from Fiscal Year 1956 Funds," in United States, Department of State, American Foreign Policy, Current Document, 1956 (Washington, DC: US Government Printing Office, 1959), pp. 1432–1433.

carry on projects initiated by the United States. Finally, the State Department was convinced that US aid given through UN agencies would be more acceptable overseas. Many developing countries were protective of their newly won sovereignty and preferred to receive aid from multilateral agencies rather than from one of the Cold War superpowers.

A third reason why the United States promoted international health in the form of direct bilateral assistance and general support for the WHO was that improved health was part of a framework of technical "development" for poor nations. This framework included the notion that progress in developing nations should be orderly, gradual, and controlled by an educated elite of politicians, engineers, and physicians. Such progress would be supported by American professionals who would help by transferring Western technology and by reforming local universities to educate the next indigenous generation. These interventions would create the conditions for an economic and political "take-off" of poor nations, which would then follow an alternative American path rather than the path of socialism promoted by the Soviet Union.

Frequently, modernization within an "underdeveloped" country was understood in terms of a tension between that country's "modern" pole (usually urban, educated, and semi-industrial) and its "traditional" pole (usually rural, illiterate, and subsistence-based). The idea that modernization would come from the urban pole was consistent with health campaigns undertaken by the WHO in the 1950s that were launched by city-based medical elites trained in western medical science. Modernization theory in the 1950s thus considered public health programs as "capital investments," rather than as charitable ventures because healthier and more vigorous people were better for the local and world economies than were those suffering from disease. Modernization and Cold War motives also influenced health agencies by linking health and national security. Improved health was usually portrayed in official US publications as a tool for achieving not only physical well-being but for reducing the vicious cycle of poor health and poverty that could explode into war. Modernization as an ideological basis for US foreign policy received a boost from President Kennedy when he appointed MIT professor Walt W. Rostow to the post of deputy national security Advisor. Rostow had written the definitive works on modernization as a capitalist strategy for development and served as the head of the State Department's Policy Planning Council beginning in 1961.

A fourth reason why international health programs became a priority for the United States was that the government had to convince the world that America was the true defender of "a lasting peace" in a world on the verge of war. For a *New York Times* article, international health was useful for "building strong allies and true friends ... [who] ultimately will make the choice between totalitarianism and democracy ... Peace is never a product of military force alone."[7]

After reorganization within the State Department in 1955, the International Cooperation Agency (ICA) was created as the main non-military bilateral agency. In 1961 it was replaced by the US Agency of International Development (USAID). ICA was a semi-autonomous agency with its own budget and personnel that coordinated all non-military, technical, bilateral programs and was linked with American work at the UN specialized agencies. Dulles provided policy guidance to ICA's director, who reported directly to the secretary of state on all operating programs. John B. Hollister, a former law partner of Robert A. Taft, the noted conservative Republican senator from Ohio, was ICA's first director. Like Dulles, Hollister believed that as long as the Soviet Union existed, American aid programs abroad were essential. Hollister's work included the organization of a public health unit initially named the Public Health Division and later called the Office of Public Health. ICA public health officers worked in various international settings for the control of specific diseases, ran environmental sanitation projects, built water systems, constructed health facilities, and trained local health personnel.[8]

American bilateral assistance also followed the Rockefeller Foundation's model of keeping a low profile and exercising control behind the scenes. The State Department praised the contributions of multilateral health agencies and let them take the credit for international programs. Because ICA was concerned about possible debates in Congress over American bilateral aid, it downplayed the financial resources given to bilateral aid by stating that such aid represented only a very small percentage of what federal and state health programs cost at home.

Eradication and the Consolidation of an Agency

The most noteworthy technocratic programs launched by the WHO during the early Cold War were disease eradication programs. This requires some explanation because the concept of eradication was anything but universally popular in the field of international health. Indeed, in the 1920s and 1930s eradication was regarded by many experts as a false hope. After vigorous but incomplete Rockefeller campaigns the goal was considered unachievable. Although anthelminthic therapy and the construction of latrines reduced the severity of hookworm infections, it failed to eliminate them entirely and thus did not

---

[7] "Public Health Termed Vital to Peace Throughout the World," *The New York Times,* August 12, 1953, p. 9.

[8] Eugene P. Campbell, "The Role of the International Cooperation Administration in International Health," *Archives of Environmental Health* 1:6 (1960), 502–511.

prevent reinfection. In the case of yellow fever, public health campaigns confronted the previously unknown sylvan yellow fever that included a cycle among primates living in forests as well as additional mosquito vectors besides the better known *Aedes aegypti*. In addition, critics believed that it was almost impossible to eliminate these diseases without expensive improvements in water systems, sewage control, and general living conditions.

A lively debate on these issues had taken place in the League of Nations Health Organization's Malaria Commission. Many experts believed that human efforts could only hope to mitigate, or control, the severity of malaria, primarily with quinine, environmental work such as the reduction of mosquito breeding places, and the integration of malaria control with the promotion of economic development. They questioned eradication because an adequate supply of quinine was not affordable by many nations and because rural health services were precarious almost everywhere. A case usually cited as an example of the success of malaria control was the work in the 1930s in the United States by the Tennessee Valley Authority, or TVA. President Franklin D. Roosevelt created the TVA with the goal of harnessing the Tennessee River's potential for hydroelectric power while improving the land around it and the standard of living of the Valley's inhabitants. An unexpected benefit was a major advance in malaria control.[9]

American, British, and some German experts believed that a good administrative structure could control the disease within tolerable limits. For them, "malaria control" meant destroying breeding places by draining marshes and clearing swamps, digging ditches and canals, using small fish with larvivorous characteristics, using petroleum oils and a copper-based powder called Paris green (aceto-arsenite of cooper) that poisoned surface-feeding mosquito larvae, and distributing quinine and other drugs. Additional control methods included the protection of humans from *Anopheles* bites by screening windows and doors and educational programs.

Some experts maintained a middle position like that of the Italian Alberto Missiroli, editor of *Rivista de Parassitologia* and later director of the malaria laboratory of Rome's Public Health Institute. Missiroli thought that elimination of malaria was possible if efforts were concentrated on mosquito control, with intensive measures such as larvae control and the screening of houses. His program, which was supported by grants from the Rockefeller Foundation, drained swamps near urban centers, provided screens for rural houses, and distributed quinine. Missiroli enjoyed respect because of his achievements, such as his antimalarial work in the Italian Pontine Marshes in the 1930s. But debates between malaria experts during the interwar period did not come to a

---

[9] Margaret Humphreys, *Malaria: Poverty, Race, and Public Health in the United States* (Baltimore: Johns Hopkins University Press, 2001).

simple resolution because experts agreed that no single method was sufficient. Not surprisingly, the first five reports produced by the WHO Expert Committee on Malaria between 1947 and 1950 subscribed to malaria control and emphasized the setting up of pilot programs, assisting in training field staff, and organizing demonstration campaigns.

A demonstration campaign that suggested malaria eradication might actually be possible had already occurred in Ceará, Brazil in the 1930s. That military-style campaign, led by Fred L. Soper, at the time with the Rockefeller Foundation, got rid of the *Anopheles gambiae* that was causing epidemic malaria. Soper secured special permission to impose his authority over provincial officials and resorted to potent larvicides that were placed in stagnant ponds and marshes. Soper successfully ended the epidemic and effectively destroyed this species of mosquito, although he did not succeed in making malaria disappear from Brazil. His principal focus was the fight against the insect, which encouraged some to believe that technical measures pushed far enough using a military regimen could ultimately eradicate the disease.

The eradication perspective received another boost in the 1940s following the control and partial elimination of epidemic malaria from areas of Egypt, Sardinia, Guyana, Argentina, Venezuela, and the British colony of Mauritius (although complete eradication of the *Anopheles* vector was not achieved). In Guyana, the Italian George Giglioli, trained in tropical medicine in London and Rome and director of the Malaria Research Unit in British Guyana beginning in 1939, organized a systematic campaign in 1944 to eradicate malaria from the densely populated coastal areas using the insecticide DDT. It had been used during World War II, mostly to protect Allied troops in different areas of the world including Africa.[10] At the time, knowledge of the insecticide was still classified by the US government as "secret war information." Giglioli and a few other health workers had learned of it confidentially and of experiments carried out by the US Department of Agriculture in Atlanta and Florida and was able to obtain half a ton of DDT.

The notion of eradicating targeted diseases grew in popularity after World War II and became a clear example of the technocratic perspective of the WHO. In the mid-1950s, Soper, now head of the Pan American Sanitary Bureau (which was simultaneously the WHO's Regional Office for the Americas), launched a campaign to make the concept a priority in international and national health programs. Soper was convinced that eradication methods could be applied to a series of diseases, such as yaws, malaria, yellow fever, and even tuberculosis. For him there were no significant technical, administrative, or economic barriers to success. He was convinced that eradication was

---

[10] James L. A. Webb, Jr., *The Long Struggle against Malaria in Tropical Africa* (New York: Cambridge University Press, 2014), p. 72.

considerably superior to traditional control measures, which implied a patch-work of methods and a long-term commitment of resources and personnel. Candau shared Soper's beliefs and later declared that most communicable diseases could be wiped out within "a foreseeable future."[11] Candau also shared Soper's conviction that malaria was an "economic disease" which slowed down agriculture, commerce, and industry because "the man who carries the malaria parasite in his blood is a man of blunted initiative. To him few things seem worth the trouble, he becomes fatalistic."[12] Thus, achieving the goal of economic growth and proactive citizenship in poor nations required lifting the burden of malaria.

The WHO completed a survey in the late 1950s of 99 countries and territories to assess the economic burden of malaria. The report identified malaria as the "most expensive disease" and argued that the cost of eliminat-ing it, however high, would be less than the economic losses produced by the disease. In India, for example, loss of wage-earning capacity due to the usual six-day attack of malaria was estimated to be USD 500 million, but if an eradication program were undertaken it would cost only USD 114 million. Thus, the WHO believed that capital invested in malaria eradication "will be regained by the community in a few years ... Development funds find their way back to industry. Improvement of health standards also implies increased demand for consumer goods." In other words, malaria eradication was business.[13]

Despite this preoccupation with malaria, in the early 1950s the WHO actually focused its first eradication campaign not on malaria but on yaws, a painful and disabling disease caused by the same treponema that was respon-sible for syphilis. The disease ate away at the skin, leaving the bones almost exposed, and in severe cases mutilating the face. The traditional response was the use of ineffective drugs made with arsenic and bismuth and, commonly, the segregation of victims in leprosaria or yaws houses, which entailed the loss of jobs, family, and social support. A first International Symposium on Yaws Control was held in Bangkok in 1953. The Symposium recognized that a single intramuscular injection of penicillin was as effective, and much cheaper, than the six required injections of arsenic and bismuth. Penicillin was one of the first broad-spectrum antibiotics used successfully in World War II and now appeared available as a new "magic bullet." One injection would usually clear

---

[11] "Disease Curb Foreseen, End of Contagious Ailments Predicted by WHO Head," *The New York Times,* May 16, 1958.

[12] "Thursday April 7 Is World Health Day 7," Press Release WHO/16, April 1, 1960, Press Releases 1960, 1–80.

[13] "Malaria, the World's Most Expensive Disease, December," in World Health Organization, Division of Public Information, *WHO Special Features* (Geneva: World Health Organization, 1953), 1–3, p. 3.

up the sores of yaws in about a week and three injections seemed to cure the disease definitively. According to the WHO symposium report, "Ehrlich's dream of a single-injection cure has come true."[14]

In the early 1950s, the number of individuals with yaws around the world was estimated at more than 20 million, most living in Haiti, Brazil, Indonesia, the Philippines, Thailand, India, Liberia, and Nigeria. The WHO campaign was designed to be implemented by mobile teams of experts traveling four in a jeep and by lay personnel who visited villages, examined the population, and gave penicillin shots to patients, their families, and neighbors. An anti-yaws campaign was launched in Haiti in 1950 after an agreement was signed between the regional representatives of the WHO, PASB, UNICEF, and the Haitian government. According to the agreement, the agencies would play a complementary role: the WHO contributed expertise; UNICEF was in charge of vehicles (jeeps and ambulances), drugs, and equipment; PASB provided technicians; and the host government provided buildings and local personnel.

The Government of Haiti, then under the rule of physician-dictator Francois "Papa Doc" Duvalier, an ally of the United States in the Cold War, established a specialized service known as *Campagne pour l'Eradication du Pian* (Campaign for the Eradication of Yaws). While subordinate to the Ministry of Public Health, the *Campagne* enjoyed a high degree of administrative and financial autonomy. Soon after work began, treatment centers were set up along with ambulatory dispensaries and a system of house-to-house visiting following a detailed epidemiological map of the country. The government paid for the health workers in charge of treatments, the conducting of surveys, and the tabulating of statistical data. Also, the government provided space, furnishings, and supplies for the program offices. The Haitian campaign was huge. Between July 1950 and March 1952 almost 900,000 people were treated, and by the end of 1954 fully 97 percent of the rural population had received penicillin injections. Samples gathered in 1958–1959 indicated that the prevalence rate of yaws in Haiti had been reduced to 0.32 percent of the population, a remarkable reduction given that at the beginning of the decade estimates of the proportion of sufferers oscillated between 30 and 60 percent.[15]

Another important yaws campaign was launched in 1950 in Indonesia, a country that had recently won its independence from Dutch colonial rule. In the early 1950s, it was estimated that out of a total Indonesian population of 70 million, 15 percent suffered from yaws, and in some rural areas the percentage was considerably higher. By 1957, more than 23 million individuals had been

---

[14] World Health Organization, *First International Symposium on Yaws Control* (Geneva: World Health Organization, 1953), p. 1.

[15] G. Samame, "Treponematosis Eradication, with Special Reference to Yaws Eradication in Haiti," *Bulletin of the World Health Organization* 15:6 (1956), 897–910.

examined and about one million people living with yaws had been successfully treated.[16] As in Haiti, a hierarchical administrative structure, house-to-house visits and detailed epidemiological mapping were developed. By the mid-1950s, the prevalence of yaws in Indonesia dropped to less than one percent.

By 1964, yaws programs existed in 46 countries, the WHO's Global Yaws Control Program had treated dozens of millions of people, and prevalence was reduced to 95 percent. Unfortunately, epidemiological surveillance was not sustained, and latent infections were overlooked.[17] As a result, the disease remains a major health problem to this day. It was discovered that humans were not the only reservoirs of the disease, as monkeys could also harbor the Treponema. The disease was still acute among rural Africans, for example in forest-dwelling Pygmy communities, on a continent that was considered the world's largest reservoir of yaws. Moreover, health workers commonly over-looked asymptomatic individuals with latent infections, and these individuals often relapsed to produce acute infectious lesions soon after control measures were withdrawn. Another issue was that health teams visited for only short periods of time, leaving little behind in terms of public health infrastructure. The infection thus reappeared in several "disease free" areas and became concentrated in the poorest sectors of some countries. Yet, yaws vanished nonetheless from the international health agenda as human and financial resources to sustain the campaign against it dwindled and disappeared (until early 2012, when with new technology the WHO decided to eradicate the disease by 2020).

Although yaws was not eradicated through a vertical campaign as was initially expected, the campaign became a model for future eradication efforts. For one thing, the yaws campaign demonstrated that two multilateral agencies – the WHO and UNICEF – could work together despite tension between them and could enlist regional assistance and the support of governments from developing countries. The work against the disease was validated by its positive impact on the economy, a justification that would be applied to malaria eradicators in subsequent years. Moreover, the administrative features of the campaign helped to shape the next WHO eradication campaign. First, it had definitive objectives and deadlines. Second, it was organized as a vertical campaign that covered whole national territories and was not deflected during its course by outbreaks or emergencies in targeted locations. Third, the emphasis was on a self-contained military-style command structure. Fourth, a characteristic focus of the campaign was the application of a simple biotechnology. The vertical

---

[16] M. Soetopo & R. Wasito, "Experience with Yaws Control in Indonesia; Preliminary Results with a Simplified Approach," *Bulletin of the World Health Organization* 8:1–3 (1953), 273–295.

[17] "Yaws: Ten Million Suffer No More," *WHO Newsletter* 8:10 (October 1955), 1.

eradication campaign did not seek integration with other health programs and did not nurture community-based programs. However imperfect the vertical eradication model now seems in retrospect, during the second half of the 1950s the WHO followed the path of the yaws campaign and launched another of even larger scope: malaria eradication.

The Boom and Bust of Malaria Eradication

Malaria eradication became the largest single undertaking of the WHO, the target of a program called the Global Program for Malaria Eradication, and a key component of the technocratic biomedical perspective. Its main underlying assumption was that medicine had at its command the knowledge and the will to eliminate this and other infectious diseases from the world. In 1954 the Pan American Sanitary Bureau preceded the WHO by launching a campaign to eradicate the disease from the Americas, basically by relying on the massive spraying of DDT. One of its differences from previous efforts of malaria control was that it relied on the use of the insecticide against adult *Anopheles* mosquitoes instead of fighting against the larvae through elimination of breeding habitats and use of larvicides. The decisive interventions were: house spraying with DDT, which as a residue on walls remained deadly to *Anopheles* mosquitoes for months, and the use of the drugs pyrimethamine and chloroquine to eliminate the Plasmodium parasite. DDT spraying worked because once parasite transmission from man to mosquito and mosquito to man was intercepted, the infection in humans would disappear within a few years as the result of the parasite's reduction to insignificant levels. The hope was that the vector would be controlled and the parasite eliminated. It was believed that treatment of human hosts solely with drugs (as had been done before with quinine) would not succeed long-term because it involved pharmaceutical availability and a health infrastructure nonexistent in developing countries.

In January 1955, the WHO's Executive Board considered a special report urging decisive action against malaria because, it was alleged, at least one-fourth of mankind was affected by the disease and there was a race against time to clean up dangerous areas before malaria-carrying mosquitoes developed resistance to insecticides. DDT resistance had already been reported in the United States, Panama, Greece, Lebanon, and Java. Another reported problem was that the success of malaria eradication in one country was jeopardized if neighboring countries did not proceed at the same pace. In a radical departure from traditional malaria control, the Executive Board urged all threatened countries to undertake total malaria eradication "before it is too late."[18] In

---

[18] World Health Organization, "Executive Board Urgency of Total Malaria Control Stressed by Board," January 28, 1955, Press Release WHO/7, Press Releases 1955.

May 1955, malaria eradication was endorsed by the Eighth World Health Assembly at a meeting held in Mexico City. The WHA decision was hailed by many malaria experts among whom were Soper, Carlos Alvarado of Argentina, Arnoldo Gabaldón of Venezuela, and Paul F. Russell of the United States, an officer of the Rockefeller Foundation who was an expert on malaria and an advisor to the WHO.[19]

Candau emphasized malaria as a major killer. It affected about 200 million people per year worldwide and killed 2 million. He also addressed concerns about the resistance of some species of *Anopheles* to DDT. Candau believed that insecticide resistance and a new "learned behavior" of some species of mosquitoes to avoid DDT-covered surfaces made imperative an immediate, coordinated campaign of malaria eradication, which, he claimed, was the only real way to proceed. Malaria work was at a "crossroads." It could either follow a path of uneven and inconsistent application of insecticides based on weak political commitments or it could pursue an all-out effort that would prevent a global malaria explosion. In Candau's mind there was "no other logical choice" but to transform malaria control programs into full-scale eradication efforts.[20] All countries should give up control efforts and concentrate instead on an energetic global eradication campaign.[21] But some European representatives at the WHA complained about the "rush to eradication." The British representative, for example, thought it would be difficult to sustain financing for such a program in its full intensity for the required number of years. Paul Russell responded to these objections by arguing that eradication was the only viable option and that it was imperative to move forward at a rapid pace.

The official US representative to WHA offered a compromise. He suggested an alternative path that would exclude parts of Africa and thereby significantly reduce the financial burden of the whole enterprise. The southern part of Africa could be excluded, he argued, because it would be "premature" to attempt eradication in an area with poor health systems and communications. Russell endorsed this plan, agreeing that African countries could wait now and, except for a few pilot programs, later follow the rest of the world, a recommendation that was embraced by the WHA.[22] Thus, the WHO's "global" malaria eradication campaign never involved a commitment to eliminate the disease in all

[19] Anne-Emanuelle Birn, "Backstage: The Relationship between the Rockefeller Foundation and the World Health Organization, Part I: 1940s–1960s," *Public Health* 128:2 (2014), 129–140.

[20] Randall M. Packard, "'No Other Logical Choice': Global Malaria Eradication and the Politics of International Health in the Post-War Era," *Parassitologia* 40:1–2 (1998), 217–229.

[21] "Marcolino Candau Intervention," Official Records of the World Health Organization, No. 63 World Health Assembly, Eighth World Health Assembly, Mexico DF Decisions and Resolutions, Plenary Meetings, Verbatim Records, Committees Minutes and Reports (Geneva: World Health Organization, 1955), pp. 65–66.

[22] "P. F. Russell Intervention," Official Records of the World Health Organization, No. 63 World Health Assembly, Eighth World Health Assembly, Mexico DF Decisions and Resolutions,

countries and on all continents at the same time. In the following years, the decision reached in Mexico by the World Health Assembly was implemented by the principal US bilateral organization, ICA, and was endorsed at the Sixth International Congress on Tropical Medicine and Malaria in Lisbon in 1958 and at the Seventh International Congress of Tropical Medicine and Malaria in Rio de Janeiro in 1963.[23]

Shortly after the Health Assembly in Mexico, the WHO opened a Malaria Eradication Special Account which was a fund to assist national eradication programs. While funding came chiefly in the form of US bilateral cooperation, UNICEF also contributed monetary resources and equipment, and the WHO provided strong leadership in the person of Emilio J. Pampana, who had been trained at the Medical School of Florence and the London School of Hygiene and Tropical Medicine and had worked at the Institute of Malariology in Rome. He served on the WHO's staff from 1947 to 1959, first as chief of the Malaria Section and later as the first director of the Division of Malaria Eradication. In the late 1950s the Division had a staff of more than 320, working in 70 countries and helping coordinate regional and national training and eradication efforts.

By the mid-1950s, DDT and other insecticides of the chlorinated hydrocarbon group such as BHC (benzene hexachloride), Aldrin, and Dieldrin, and pesticides for commercial agriculture such as Malathion, were produced and shipped to all parts of the world by US petroleum and chemical companies. In 1950, Shell Chemical – a division of the Shell Oil Company – was the exclusive seller of Aldrin and Dieldrin. Other American companies such as Monsanto and Montrose Chemical Corporation of California specialized in DDT and pesticides. These companies regularly submitted successful bids for insecticides in response to invitations by US bilateral and international health agencies. Likewise, Hudson Manufacturers of Chicago became the main supplier of spraying equipment for malaria eradication.

By the mid-1950s, Shell reported robust sales of Dieldrin and predicted that "Dieldrin would continue to experience increasing demand as a result of its successful fight against malaria."[24] By the end of 1956, ICA had purchased 22.5 million pounds of DDT or more than half of the 40 million pounds

---

Plenary Meetings, Verbatim Records, Committees Minutes and Reports (Geneva: World Health Organization, 1955), p. 205.

[23] Since 1938, tropical medical and malaria experts held joint meetings, and since 1948 these occur every five years. See *Proceedings of the Sixth International Congresses on Tropical Medicine and Malaria, Lisbon, September 5–13, 1958* (Lisbon: Instituto de Medicina Tropical, 1959), and Leonard J. Bruce-Chwatt, *Malaria at the Rio Congresses 1963: A Review of Papers on Malaria Presented at the Seventh International Congresses on Tropical Medicine and Malaria, Rio de Janeiro, September 1963* (Geneva: World Health Organization, 1963).

[24] Shell Oil Company, *Annual Report 1956* (New York: Shell Oil Company, 1956), 14.

produced for export by US manufacturers. US bilateral agencies continued buying massive quantities of insecticides in the following years. For example, in 1961 USAID purchased more than 74 million pounds of DDT, which was one-third of all the insecticide manufactured in the United States that year.[25] A letter of a USAID officer noted that "The largest proportion of AID malaria eradication funds expended during the recent years has been for DDT, accounting for more than half the dollar costs of this program to AID."[26] Thus, malaria eradication, among its other purposes, served to provide a substantial subsidy to American industries.

It is also interesting to note that only after the political decision was made to embark on eradication were the precise technical and administrative features of the program worked out. The final decision entailed that eradicators would undertake energetic but time-limited campaigns of five to eight years. Eradication would proceed in four phases: preparation, attack, control, and consolidation. Preparation lasted about a year and concentrated on exploratory surveys, recruitment and training of staff, and a pilot project. The attack phase was massive indoor DDT spraying of all rural houses in the defined malarial areas. Spraying DDT two times per year was expected to kill the female mosquitoes resting on the walls of victims' houses after their blood meals. During the third phase, any remaining cases of malaria were identified and treated with drugs.[27] The combined result of no new malaria cases and a very small number of *Anopheles* would be no new infected individuals, thus breaking the transmission cycle. A country was considered free of malaria when, for a period of three years, no inhabitant contracted the disease as a result of being bitten by an infected mosquito. The consolidation phase lasted as long as malaria existed in a neighboring country. In this phase, national health services absorbed the eradication service and acquired staff ready for other health interventions.

In February 1958, George McDonald published an article in *The Lancet* entitled "The Conquest of Malaria" that claimed that 63 countries, with a total population of 680 million at risk, had declared their policy to be the eradication of malaria. By the early 1960s, most developing countries embraced malaria eradication. National campaigns began with tripartite agreements between the WHO, UNICEF, and the host country. These agreements specified that UNICEF's responsibility was to provide vehicles, materials, and spraying equipment. The WHO's Geneva headquarters or one of its regional offices

[25] Donald Johnson & Roy Fritz, "Status Report on Malaria Eradication," *Mosquito News* 22:2 (1962), 80–81.

[26] Donald R. Johnson to Louis L. Williams, July 8, 1962. Box 1, Folder: Correspondence 1963–1967, Williams Papers, NLM, *Principal Officers of the Department of State*, p. 42.

[27] See Emilio Pampana, *A Textbook of Malaria Eradication* (London: Oxford University Press, 1963).

would provide technical cooperation and expert personnel. Finally, the governments saw to the provision of local workers, including the local campaign leaders. These agreements, moreover, specified the establishment of autonomous national entities devoted to malaria eradication. These specialized services were linked to ministries of health but with budgets outside other health programs. These National Malaria Eradication Services, as they were called, almost everywhere had significant amounts of power and prestige. These services had clear lines of command resembling military medical units or earlier Rockefeller-inspired health campaigns. The staff was generally hired on a full-time basis, departing from the tradition of part-time health work common in developing countries. The WHO also promoted a standardized vocabulary for malaria work.[28]

The transition from malaria control to malaria eradication was facilitated in some regions by meetings such as the First and Second Asian Malaria Conferences, held in 1953 and 1954 under the auspices of the Western Pacific and South-East Asia WHO regions. India actively participated in these meetings and launched its National Malaria Control Program in April 1953 when some 75 million people, or one in five of the population, suffered from the disease, and about 800,000 individuals died of it every year. The effort was supported by the National Malaria Institute in Delhi and the program proved initially successful. Within five years the incidence dropped to 2 million cases per year. Encouraged by these results, in 1958 the program was changed to a more ambitious National Malaria Eradication Program, based on DDT house spraying. By 1960, US bilateral aid had contributed more than 1 million USD and the disease's death toll dropped to fewer than 10,000 per year.[29] India was also an example of the differential impact of the campaign. The more developed Indian State of Kerala was capable of eradicating malaria in a short time because it already had good health, communication, and educational systems.[30] Good results were also achieved on islands or in regions with subtropical environmental conditions where the mosquito's survival was more challenged than in tropical regions. In 1965, Taiwan, with a population of more than 12 million people, was certified as the first Asian country to achieve malaria eradication.[31] In general, the campaigns decreased malaria mortality

---

[28] World Health Organization, Expert Committee on Malaria, *Malaria Terminology: Report of a Drafting Committee Appointed by WHO* (Geneva: World Health Organization, 1953).

[29] "More Aid Goes to India: US Grants $10,377,000 for Anti-Malaria Program," *The New York Times*, November 3, 1960, p. 15.

[30] Randall M. Packard, *The Making of a Tropical Disease: A Short History of Malaria* (Baltimore: Johns Hopkins University Press, 2007), p. 161.

[31] Discussed in From MAL to WHQ, February 9, 1967, in Malaria Eradication, Preparation of Report for the 20th World Health Assembly, M2/180/8(2) First Generation Files.

rates in developing countries but slow progress occurred in backward, isolated, and poor regions, such as the state of Chiapas in the south of Mexico.[32]

In some developing countries DDT sprayers became well-known and respected figures in their communities who helped inspire volunteers to step forward for a variety of public health roles. These volunteers included lay workers whose tasks included educating the public, reporting to health authorities any cases of malarial fever, taking blood samples, and distributing medicines (it was hoped that blood tests would alert of any asymptomatic infections). They were often schoolteachers recruited in rural communities. In Cambodia, for example, 120 *agents sanitaires* became parts of a rural health network of elementary health posts providing education, medical aid, symptomatic relief for common diseases, and the collection of statistical data on birth, mortality, and morbidity.

Enthusiastic field work was not, however, sufficient to overcome the serious political resistance that eradication began to face in the mid-1960s, not least in Geneva. Between 1958 and 1964, the Malaria Division was led by Carlos Alvarado, who was critical of Soper's aggressive tendencies (Soper's authoritative presence is suggested in Figure 4.2). The Argentinian emphasized surveillance and created a Malaria Eradication Epidemiological Assessment Unit in 1960, directed first by Y. Yekutiel and later by the distinguished British malariologist Leonard J. Bruce-Chwatt. Bruce-Chwatt had previously been a member of the WHO Expert Panel on Malaria.[33] With the support of Yukutiel and Bruce-Chwatt, Alvarado insisted that the overemphasis on spraying operations limited attention to other factors such as the investigation of the types of mosquitoes breeding and the endemicity of specific areas (the technological dimension of spraying operations is portrayed in Figure 4.3). The lack of attention to these factors was, to Alvarado, contrary to the needed flexibility and adaptability of the program. He also promoted the idea of developing rural health infrastructure to support the surveillance program. For Alvarado, surveillance was essential in the final stages of the campaign to be certain of the interruption of malaria transmission with no residual foci and no imported infections.

Geneva's approach was contrary to Soper's belief that a developing country with little sufficient resources to mount a strong surveillance program could enforce eradication and build up a rural health infrastructure at the same time. Soper also opposed Alvarado because surveillance implied the establishment

---

[32] See Marcos Cueto, *Cold War and Deadly Fevers: Malaria Eradication in Mexico, 1955–1970* (Baltimore: Johns Hopkins University Press, 2007).

[33] Leonard J. Bruce-Chwatt, "Specific Functions of the World Health Organization in the Global Malaria Eradication Program," 1962, Leonard J. Bruce-Chwatt papers, Series: Published and unpublished writings, 1950–1989, Folder, Wellcome Library, Archives and Manuscripts [hereafter WLAM].

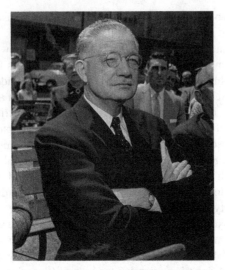

Figure 4.2 Fred L. Soper, director of the Pan American Sanitary Bureau, Regional Office of the World Health Organization between 1947 and 1959. Soper was a former officer of the Rockefeller Foundation and a champion of vertically organized malaria eradication. Photo taken at the 11th World Health Assembly, Minneapolis in 1958.
Courtesy: World Health Organization Photo Library.

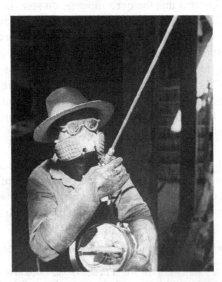

Figure 4.3 A health worker spraying Dieldrin insecticide for malaria-carrying mosquitos in the early 1960s. In most developing countries, protective gear for insecticide sprayers was not available.
Credit: Bettmann/Contributor. Courtesy: Getty Images.

[311]

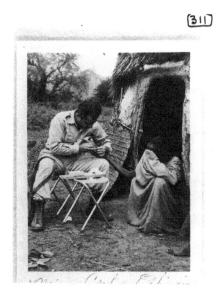

Figure 4.4 A woman, her face covered with a shawl, crouches outside a hut while a malaria control worker wearing a field uniform draws a blood sample. The blood sample taken from a finger stick on the woman's right hand was part of the malaria eradication campaign in the 1950s.
Courtesy: National Library of Medicine.

of costly good laboratory resources in several locations and the creation of a corps of personnel devoted to identifying relapses and probable malaria cases by monthly visits to families. (The difficulties of blood sampling are suggested in Figure 4.4.) For Soper, these tasks were unrealistic. He believed that the discovery of resistance by malaria in parasites and mosquito vectors demanded a rapid intensification of anti-mosquito measures and the creation of better drugs rather than, as Alvarado suggested, a thorough investigation of why resistance developed. (Eradicators' inventiveness in the face of a challenge is depicted in Figure 4.5.)

By the early 1960s two evident problems were the resistance of *Plasmodium falciparum* (the agent that causes the most serious form of malaria) to the medication chloroquine and a level of resistance to DDT that was greater than expected in some species of *Anopheles* mosquitoes. Shortly before, in country after country, mass administration of antimalarial drugs was undertaken in an unsuccessful attempt to overcome the problem. By the late 1960s, 56 species of *Anopheles* had developed resistance to DDT, and health authorities hoped to find a new magic bullet in other organophosphates or in other types of insecticides. Related challenges were the identification of changing vector

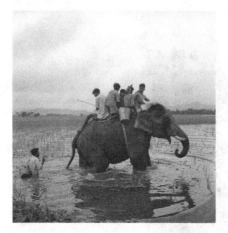

Figure 4.5 India. The mobile malaria eradication team make their way into the depths of the forests through marshes and across lakes using an elephant. Photograph c. 1950s.
Credit: WHO/P. Sharma. Courtesy: World Health Organization Photo Library.

behavior such that some mosquitoes avoided contact with insecticide-treated walls and the discovery that certain mosquito species never rested indoors in homes so that residential spraying was ineffective. An additional problem was that many rural dwellings were built of mud. These walls had a potent absorptive action that together with high temperatures diminished the effectiveness of insecticides. One temporary solution was to repeat spraying at least every three months and to increase the dosage of insecticides, which made the whole operation more expensive. In some places, such as El Salvador and India, *Anopheline* resistance was also closely related to the indiscriminate and sometimes inconsistent use of pesticides in commercial cotton cultivation as part of a "green revolution" promoted by the Rockefeller Foundation.

The difficulties with insecticides produced a swing of the pendulum from attempted preventive interventions with vectors toward chemotherapy with patients, and a growing consensus emerged that antimalarial drugs had to play a more conspicuous role in malaria eradication. But drug treatment also had problems, as no single medication was effective against all parasite species, and most drugs had relatively short-term effects and needed to be administered repeatedly in highly endemic areas. Drug treatment implied the enforcement of disciplined administration regimes such that drugs had to be taken at regular intervals of not less than once a month. Attempting to enforce these regimes augmented logistical problems in countries with a shortage of personnel and precarious public health infrastructures.

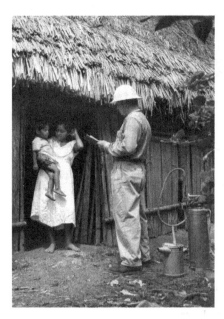

Figure 4.6 Mexico. A malaria eradication sprayer in his khaki uniform, helmet, and equipment meets a woman and his child in front of her hut in the village of Cerro Concha, a rural area of Mexico situated in a thick, tropical forest.
Credit: WHO/Eric Schwab. Courtesy: World Health Organization Photo Library.

Another challenging problem was the lifestyle of rural inhabitants. (Figure 4.6 depicts malaria eradication operations in Mexico.) This included the custom of sleeping outdoors during the summer and the movement of itinerant populations (nomads, shepherds, gypsies, and pilgrims). Nomadic populations commonly slept in tents unsuitable for residual spraying. Rural families became tired of giving their homes to spraying operations that were not working. Despite the fact that supervision of operations was technically difficult in remote areas because of poor transportation facilities, a WHO publication could not resist the temptation to blame "nomads" as a "fifth column . . . in favor of the malaria parasite" that "smuggled" the parasite into areas which had been cleared.[34]

Health personnel grew increasingly disenchanted with malaria eradication as associated problems multiplied. Bruce-Chwatt observed that local health administrators had to divide "scarce professional and auxiliary personnel

---

[34] "Guerre Mondiale au Paludisme," *Sante du Monde* no number (1958), 16–25, p. 22.

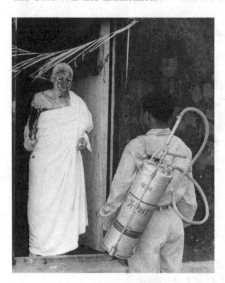

Figure 4.7 A man holding a canister of DDT explains the importance of spraying the insecticide to a shaman in Adaklu Abuadi, Ghana. Year 1965. Collection: Bettmann. Getty Images.

between general hospital care, sanitation, malnutrition, and such spectacular diseases as leprosy, trypanosomiasis, yaws, tuberculosis, smallpox, schisto-somiasis, yellow fever, cerebrospinal meningitis, relapsing fever and so on" and had no reason to believe that malaria eradication was a special key to better health and increased productivity.[35] Moreover, these administrators also had to deal with the appearance of new mosquito breeding grounds inadvertently created by road construction, deforestation, hydroelectric and irrigation projects, and with mining operations in rural areas. These activities, carried out in developing countries during the 1960s and 1970s with few public health considerations, attracted workers who became new victims of malaria. As a result, health experts became convinced that malaria work had to be associated with the development of strong rural health centers and an economic and social infrastructure for rural areas.

There were also significant technological and cultural problems. (A cross-cultural encounter associated with malaria eradication is shown in Figure 4.7.) The insecticides, especially Dieldrin, were extremely toxic and killed not just mosquitoes but also chickens, honey-producing bees, ducks, goats, and other small domestic animals. Certain species of bedbugs, fleas, and cockroaches

---

[35] Leonard J. Bruce-Chwatt, "Malaria Eradication in Africa," February 1959, Leonard J. Bruce-Chwatt papers, Series Unpublished Papers Folder: WII/LBC/F/1/14, [WLAM].

developed a resistance to DDT and became a plague in some areas, creating popular resistance to spraying. Dieldrin was also discovered to create resistance in flies, and in Nepal the insecticide was popularly known as "fertilizer of flies."[36] There were also confirmed cases of human intoxication caused by the insecticide in Venezuela, Ecuador, India, and Nigeria. To add to the complications, in some rural areas peasants strongly believed that insects came from God and that destruction of his minuscule creatures could be very dangerous. Thus, while sprayers were initially enthusiastically received, enthusiasm later wore off and spraying teams were greeted with closed doors by an increasing percentage of people.

One more serious concern still further limited the campaign's effectiveness and was perhaps its death knell: the specter of environmental contamination. The issue became particularly relevant in the United States following publication in 1962 of Rachel Carson's book, *Silent Spring*. Carson argued that DDT was endangering human life as well as poisoning wildlife and the environment. Her book quickly became the bible of an emerging ecology movement that launched a campaign to end the insecticide's use. Scientists supported Carson's claims by documenting the effects of DDT and other persistent insecticides on birds and the widespread distribution of insecticide residues throughout the world, including its accumulation in human tissue. DDT was also blamed for the decline in the peregrine falcon and bald eagle populations in North America and was attacked for contaminating drinking water and milk. A number of scientists even declared DDT a carcinogenic agent. Experts from the FAO and the WHO's Committee on Pesticide Residues, working intensely and under pressure, advised against excessive use of DDT.

The Decline of Eradication

In 1969, the US Department of Agriculture prohibited the use of DDT in some agricultural activities and in aquatic areas. In Canada, a 1969 petition to the ministers of Health and Welfare and of Agriculture resulted in a 95 percent ban on DDT announced by Prime Minister Pierre Elliott Trudeau. In 1970 Norway and Sweden forbade the use of DDT, and two years later the United Nations sponsored the first major conference on environmental concerns and created the UN Environmental Program (UNEP). The new agency had the mandate to achieve scientific consensus and encourage "sustainable development," that is, improve the standard of living of poor nations without destroying their

---

[36] "1 April–May 1957," in World Health Organization, Division of Malaria Eradication, *Monthly Letter, Division of Malaria Eradication*, WHO no number (1957), p. 3.

environment. In 1972, two years after the US Environmental Protection Agency (EPA) came into existence, DDT was the first pesticide the agency banned.[37]

In a context in which faith not only in DDT but in the power of science and "modernization" had generally begun to wane, the World Health Assembly in 1969 recognized that many countries would not achieve malaria eradication in the foreseeable future. The WHA also approved a resolution that undermined faith in free-standing eradication units and, in fact, questioned the notion of specific, vertical, disease-targeted programs. At the same time, subscriptions to the Malaria Eradication Special Account dramatically declined. Many bilateral donors, whose support had been critical at the start of the malaria campaign, now decided that they could not continue to support eradication programs. In addition, the oil crisis of the early 1970s (in 1973, the Organization of the Petroleum Exporting Countries, OPEC, launched an oil embargo, quintupling petroleum prices virtually overnight) resulted in considerable increases in the cost of DDT and other insecticides because one of its core ingredients was petroleum, which caused further reduction in insecticide use. An additional not-anticipated financial cost was the maintenance of surveillance operations.

The WHO's decision was questioned in some developing countries that tried to remain loyal to the MEP and made it clear that they also wanted to continue receiving supplies of DDT. In October 1969, the Regional Committee for South-East Asia, with representatives from India, Indonesia, Nepal, Malaysia, Ceylon, Thailand, and Burma, discussed the matter of toxicity yet made a strong plea to manufacturing companies not to stop the manufacture of DDT until an equally economical insecticide could be made available to countries where malaria was still a problem.[38] In Ceylon, for example, malaria eradication had started in 1950 and succeeded in reducing malaria to 17 cases by 1963. DDT spraying was then terminated, but as a result of this "premature" decision a large-scale epidemic of malaria started in 1967 with more than a million cases by 1968.[39] SEARO argued that while industrialized countries had good reasons for limiting the use of DDT, the insecticide still had to be used in developing countries until a more efficient and cheaper method of control was found. At the 38th World Health Assembly, there were strong statements along the same lines by several representatives of developing nations. In 1972 a consensus was shared by participants in the WHO

[37] United States, Environmental Protection Agency, DDT: A Review of Scientific and Economic Aspects of the Decision to Ban its Use as a Pesticide: Prepared for Committee on Appropriations, US House of Representatives (Washington, DC: US Environmental Protection Agency, 1975).

[38] Mentioned in James W. Wright to J. E. Scanlon [School of Public Health, University of Texas], May 18, 1970, Folder V 2/473/D/1 Toxicology of DDT, Second Generation of Files [WHO].

[39] M. Vandekar to P. Seeger, May 21, 1970, Folder V 2/473/D/I Toxicology of DDT No 2, Second Generation of Files.

Interregional Conference on Malaria Control in Countries where Time-Limited Malaria Eradication is Impracticable at Present that took place in Brazzaville: Malaria eradication as a time-limited undertaking was no longer feasible in most developing areas of the world (the conference was attended by representatives of African, Eastern Mediterranean, and Western Pacific WHO regions).

Some insecticide companies tried to influence the WHO as part of a larger effort to influence scientific societies and American universities. Max Sobelman, President of Montrose Chemical Corporation, the United States' sole DDT manufacturer, in late 1969 and 1970 wrote to Candau and other officers at the WHO. He provided testimonies of experts who were in favor of DDT and characterized the attacks on DDT as "anti-intellectualism." He asked the WHO to "restore the scientific method" in the evaluation of DDT and other pesticides.[40] In May 1970, the WHO's chief of vector biology and control, James W. Wright, accepted Sobelman's invitation to travel to the United States to confer with the British-American Thomas Jukes, professor of medical physics at the University of California, Berkeley, to discuss the problems of DDT.[41] Jukes was known for his defense of DDT as a health tool and for his argument that there was no scientific evidence of damage to the environment that would justify banning DDT.

In another 1970 letter, Sobelman requested that the WHO help restore the prestige of insecticides. He complained that the American public and politicians had been "educated" to consider DDT a deadly poison and asked the agency to "speak strongly." He considered the WHO "the only organization capable of restoring some perspective" to counteract the criticism made by environmental organizations, "assistant professors of zoology trying to make a name for themselves," and politicians and journalists "who are also jumping on the bandwagon and filling the newspapers and magazines with sensational stories about DDT."[42] Jukes wrote to Candau in June of 1970 complaining that the WHO had not done enough against "the vicious campaign to discredit and ban the use of DDT," and that more should be done by the agency because it was "almost too late."[43] A letter by James Wright reported that after conversations with Candau it was clear that the governing bodies of the agency would respect the governments' final decision "as to whether to use DDT and other insecticides." He promised to issue scientific

[40] Max Sobelman to Marcolino Candau, December 31, 1969, Folder V 2/473/D/1 Toxicology of DDT, Second Generation of Files [WHO].
[41] James W. Wright to Max Sobelman, May 18, 1970, Folder V 2/473/D/1 Toxicology of DDT folder 1 Second Generation of Files [WHO].
[42] Max Sobelman to James W. Wright, April 13, 1970, Folder V 2/473/D/1 Toxicology of DDT, Second Generation of Files [WHO].
[43] Thomas Jukes to Candau, June 26, 1970, Folder V2/473/D/I Toxicology of DDT, Second Generation of Files [WHO].

statements during the next six months "which will increasingly show the important role of DDT in public health."[44]

However, neither Montrose nor Wright could restore the prestige of DDT. This was even more difficult after 1972, when the US government prohibited the domestic usage of DDT, ending nearly three decades of massive application. Production of DDT in the United States declined, although it was still exported to developing countries for some years. During the 1970s, multilateral agencies avoided a definitive decision on DDT and on what came to be called a "circle of poison." The circle consisted in massive sales of toxic pesticides in developing nations, contamination of the agricultural products cultivated in those nations, and their consumption as food imports in developed countries.[45] But the WHO did recognize that the number of poisonings by pesticides among agricultural workers in developing countries had increased, and eventually the WHO promoted the so-called integrated pest control system that endorsed a proper, restricted, and safer use of insecticides. Yet only in 1977, after pressure by environmental groups, did USAID agree to stop exporting DDT to developing countries.

Beyond the pesticide issue, in the mid-1960s the WHO had begun to openly insist on better mechanisms for malaria's continuous assessment and surveillance and criticized the "autonomy" of malaria eradication services apart from local health services. But only a few national antimalaria programs could transform themselves and become parts of national development plans and basic health services in rural areas, largely because there were no financial resources to make this conversion. One of the exceptions was Liberia, where the Department of Basic Health Services absorbed the former malaria eradication program. Such absorption, however, typically led to the loss of focus on malaria. In 1970, when Gabaldon visited areas where malaria eradication was supposedly going on in new rural health centers, he was "unable to get any cooperation, data, or even an expression of interest [about malaria]."[46]

A factor in this outcome was the retirement of the old guard of malariologists and the absence of a new leader of eradication. PAHO's commitment to eradication was dramatically less intense after 1959 when Soper retired from the organization. Soper also lost his international authority. Shortly after his retirement, he made a two-month tour of Asia with the support of the

---

[44] James W. Wright to Thomas Jukes, Berkeley, August 12, 1970, Folder V2/473/D/I Toxicology of DDT, Second Generation of Files [WHO].

[45] See David Weir & Mark Schapiro, *Circle of Poison, Pesticides in a Hungry World* (San Francisco: Institute for Food and Development Policy, 1981).

[46] Cited in James L. A. Webb Jr., "The First Large-Scale Use of Synthetic Insecticide for Malaria Control in Tropical Africa, Lessons from Liberia," in Tamara Giles-Vernick & James L. A. Webb Jr. (eds.), *Global Health in Africa, Historical Perspectives on Disease Control* (Athens: Ohio University Press, 2013), pp. 42–69, p. 60.

Rockefeller Foundation to identify and help remove obstacles to eradication programs. But his recommendations did not receive much attention. Soper also found himself in the awkward position of disagreeing with the policies promoted by Alvarado at the WHO and Abraham Horowitz at PAHO (elected director in late 1958) yet choosing to keep his criticisms to himself because he was afraid of having his opinions used by the program's opponents.[47] Russell also withdrew from an active career, and Candau retired from the WHO in 1973. Both expressed their opposition to the change of antimalarial policies in low voices. Only Gabaldón publicly criticized the abandonment of malaria eradication and the new malaria control policies. As a consequence of the loss of these leaders, the number of experts in malariology dramatically decreased as the field lost the prestige that it previously had. The British Leonard S. Bruce-Chwatt, a WHO malaria officer and supporter of the old priorities, deplored the negative perception of malariologists as "sorcerers' apprentices" unable to control the forces they unleashed.[48] It is revealing that the WHO asked Rene Dubos to give the first "Jacques Parisot Lecture" in 1969. Dubos was then developing his idea that health workers would never "master nature" by eliminating infectious diseases and that their best hope was, instead, to maintain control. This was in striking contrast to Soper who had hoped that spraying and good administration would perform miracles.[49]

By the end of the 1960s, malaria eradication seemed hopeless; the sense of urgency of the technocratic perspective disappeared and international funding rapidly fell off. UNICEF decided that proposals for support of health projects should be an integral part of overall national health development plans. USAID ended its annual contribution to PAHO's Special Malaria Fund in 1970, a decision that led to cutbacks in several national programs. A *Lancet* editorial, as well as articles in a variety of academic and public health journals, questioned the rationale of the program and suggested that the effort was over.[50] In March 1973 the WHO Division of Malaria Eradication merged with a unit on parasitic diseases to create a new WHO unit for malaria and other parasitic diseases but with no reference to eradication. In 1974, a new director-general asked the WHO Executive Board: "Was malaria eradication a foolish

---

[47] See Socrates Litsios, "The Health, Poverty and Development Merry-Go-Round, the Tribulations of WHO," in S. William Gunn (ed.), *Understanding the Global Dimensions of Health* (New York: Springer, 2005), pp. 15–34, p. 25.

[48] Leonard J. Bruce-Chwatt, "Malaria Eradication at the Crossroads," *Bulletin of the New York Academy of Medicine* 45:10 (1969), 999–1012, p. 1009.

[49] His presentation appeared in Rene Dubos, "Human Ecology," *Chronicle of the World Health Organization* 23:11 (1969), 499–504.

[50] "Editorial, Epitaph for Global Malaria Eradication?" *The Lancet* 2:7923 (July 5, 1975), 15–16.

enterprise? Where, when and how did the program go wrong?"[51] A WHO officer described the atmosphere inside the WHO in the years leading up to this moment as a time when many "were struggling to face the implications of the failure of malaria eradication ... [and] were out looking for ... scapegoats to blame."[52]

Another reason for the decline of malaria eradication was linked to Cold War politics. In some countries, massive American aid had not prevented the influence of communism and malaria grew. In India, for example, malaria grew from 100,000 cases in 1965 to more than a million in 1971, and at the same time the influence of the Indian Communist party and of the Soviet Union also grew, demonstrating that the campaign had not been an effective tool to eliminate communism as its American designers expected.[53] President Johnson lost interest in malaria eradication as he became more deeply immersed in fighting communism via the war in Vietnam. During Johnson's administration (1963–1968) the US government progressively shoved aside bilateral health and aid to multilateral programs and returned to unilateralism and cheaper health interventions such as smallpox eradication and family planning (discussed in the following chapters).

On the Soviet side, the aggressive foreign policies that included USSR-sponsored international health programs reduced their scale after Nikita Khrushchev was removed as Soviet leader and replaced by Leonid Brezhnev in 1964. Brezhnev was concerned with the domestic economic challenges of his country, increasing its military expenditures, specific interventions such as that of the invasion of Czechoslovakia in 1968, and control of any political dissidence on the Soviet bloc. These priorities meant a retreat from global health initiatives such as the malaria eradication program.

Long Term Perspectives

Despite its failings and abandonment, it is important to note that the malaria program achieved its goal in all developed countries where the disease was still endemic, mainly Mediterranean countries. It also succeeded in interrupting malaria transmission in some developing countries. Although not all malaria areas of the world were covered by eradication programs, in 1960 more than two-thirds of the population in these areas (1,336 million out of 2,872 million) were covered. Estimates of the positive effects varied. According to a British

---

[51] Cited in "Leonard J. Bruce-Chwatt, "Need for New Weapons," *World Health Forum* 1 (1980), 23–24, 24.

[52] Kenneth Newell, "Selective Primary Health Care: The Counter Revolution," *Social Science and Medicine* 26:9 (1988), 903–906, p. 903.

[53] World Health Organization, Regional Office for South-East Asia, *Health Care in South-East Asia* (New Delhi, WHO Regional Publications South-East Asia Series No 14, 1989), p. 88.

expert, in 1955 there were 250 million cases of malaria with 2.5 million deaths, whereas in 1959 there were only 140 million cases with 980,000 deaths. This was an impressive reduction.[54] An optimistic assessment by the same British malariologist in 1965 estimated that – not including China, North Korea, and North Vietnam for which figures were not available for political reasons – about 74 percent of the population living in the originally malarious areas of 1955 were free from the disease or in the process of becoming fully protected by malaria eradication programs.[55]

It is also important to note that malaria eradication campaigns stimulated greater awareness of health issues faced by rural populations. Most of the health interventions at the turn of the twentieth century in many colonial and postcolonial nations had concentrated on ports and cities, but malaria eradication efforts had directed greater attention to the countryside where the majority of the population of these countries lived. It is true that certain local organizations had already done valuable work in remote rural areas of developing countries, but it was only with yaws and later malaria eradication programs that significant professional and financial resources became available for many disadvantaged populations. Malaria eradication efforts also produced benefits in terms of training senior and junior health workers, physicians, entomologists, sanitary engineers, and sprayers not only from their own country and region but from other WHO regions. During MEP's first years, there was a marked decline of malaria cases and deaths, and success was achieved in some regions and islands where indigenous malaria cases ceased to exist by the mid-1960s. Despite these successes, however, eradication efforts did not become an entry point for comprehensive public health reform as some of the program's leaders had expected.

By the late 1970s, health leaders around the world were convinced there was no "magic bullet" for malaria. It had become clear that technologically driven "vertical" campaigns were not sustainable and could only deliver temporary success at best. Instead, malaria needed to be attacked on many fronts, and antimalaria efforts had to adapt to diverse ecologies and cultural contexts and should be linked to the creation of permanent rural health services and significant improvements in the rural poor's living conditions. The most far-seeing experts in the late 1950s and early 1960s argued that malaria was associated with low socioeconomic levels and "could only be fully abolished

---

[54] Leonard J. Bruce-Chwatt, "The Role of the World Health Organization in the Evolution of Malaria Eradication," 1961, p. 18, Leonard J. Bruce-Chwatt papers, Series: Published and unpublished writings, 1950–1989, Folder WTI/LBC/F/1/58, [WLAM].

[55] Leonard J. Bruce-Chwatt, "Malaria Eradication in Today's Africa," p. 1, 1967, Leonard Jan Bruce-Chwatt papers, Series: Published and unpublished writings, 1950–1989, Folder WTI/LBC/F/1/39, [WLAM].

by a long-term policy of improvements in education, economic development and living conditions."[56]

The malaria campaign was a learning experience for the WHO's staff in Geneva, which by the mid-1960s began to emphasize the development of basic health services as a requisite for any mass campaign. They also began to emphasize the need for a close connection between disease-control programs and general public health systems. A growing conviction emerged that any health program needed integration with general health services and a strong system of supervision and evaluation of operations. But only in the 1990s, when Roll Back Malaria was launched, did the WHO and other agencies attempt a new coordinated attack on malaria.

Yet even though malaria eradication had failed in the 1960s and 1970s, the concept of eradication through vertical programs was not completely discredited. A few individuals and institutions made special efforts to retain the essence of these programs and achieved some significant progress with modified vertical techniques. Their efforts will partly explain the success attained with other infectious diseases that plagued the world. This was especially the case in the smallpox eradication program examined in the next chapter.

---

[56] Leonard J. Bruce-Chwatt, "Malaria and Public Health," p. 4, 1962, Leonard J. Bruce-Chwatt papers, Series: Published and unpublished writings, 1950–1989, Folder WI/LBC/F/1/25, [WLAM].

5   Overcoming the Warming of the Cold War: Smallpox Eradication

Smallpox eradication, achieved in 1980, was a landmark historical event for several reasons. First, it was the first human intervention to eradicate a major infectious disease. Second, it suggested that "technical cooperation" between the United States and the Soviet Union was possible during the Cold War despite the tension between the two superpowers. Third, the WHO was able to transcend Cold War bipolarity by acting as a supranational organization and a leader in global affairs. Fourth, the WHO worked successfully with governments and health officers of developing countries. Fifth, smallpox eradication proved to be a useful learning experience for science and public health, as the campaign demonstrated that success could be achieved not by applying a fixed technology forcefully but by testing, changing, and improving tools, administrative methods, and epidemiological strategies as time went on (a depiction of the success of the campaign can be seen in Figure 5.1). The smallpox campaign was not a last gasp of the obliterating-disease-through-eradication era. Rather, despite some similarities with earlier eradication campaigns, smallpox eradication introduced several innovations in public health and medical politics. The difference between malaria and smallpox eradication was in kind not of degree. The purpose of this chapter is to describe and analyze this remarkable experience that was inspired in some of the best features of both perspectives of the agency.

Background to the Smallpox Eradication Program

For centuries, smallpox was feared because of the death, suffering, and disfigurement it caused. It was endemic in China and India since ancient times, and from these seats it spread globally. It was the disease that devastated the Americas during the sixteenth century Iberian conquest, being largely responsible for the native demographic collapse. By the nineteenth century, the disease was known to have two forms: variola major, with a high fatality rate, and the milder but more prevalent variola minor, with a low fatality rate (however, for the eradication program of the 1960s and 1970s, the distinction was not relevant nor entailed the use of two different techniques). A common

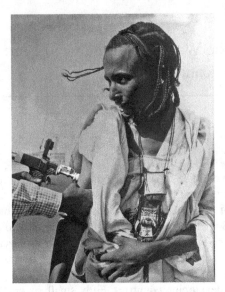

Figure 5.1 Photograph taken during Smallpox Eradication and Measles Control Program in Niger, West Africa, February, 1969. The health worker carries a vaccine injector gun.
Credit: J. D. Millar, 1969/Smith Collection. Source: Getty Images.

technique against the two forms of smallpox since ancient times was "variolation," which consisted in taking the dried-up scabs of smallpox patients recovering from the disease and introducing them in some form into healthy individuals or making healthy individuals inhale powder made from smallpox patients' scab crusts. These procedures, when successful, created a mild smallpox infection and lifelong immunity, but variolated individuals were still contagious. A more effective medical intervention was introduced in late eighteenth-century Britain by Edward Jenner, who noticed that fluid from the pustules produced in a closely related but humanly harmless disease, cowpox, somehow produced immunity to smallpox. Jenner's injection of cowpox materials – his "vaccination" method – proved more effective than "variolation." A number of European governments embraced the new technique.[1]

During the nineteenth and early twentieth centuries, western countries enacted compulsory vaccination laws and created laboratories to prepare smallpox vaccine from bovine lymph. With this legislation and methodology, the disease was gradually eliminated from industrial nations. But smallpox

---

[1] Donald R. Hopkins, *Princes and Peasants: Smallpox in History* (Chicago: University of Chicago Press, 1983).

flared up following World War I in Italy, Portugal, Germany, and the Soviet Union. Smallpox disappeared again from Europe by the late 1930s, with the exception of Spain and Portugal. On the other side of the continent, Stalin's regime vaccinated millions, and in the mid-1930s the USSR celebrated smallpox's elimination as an achievement of socialism. During and shortly after World War II, northern Africa suffered significant smallpox epidemics that reached the south of Italy. A devastated Japan was also affected by smallpox in the wake of World War II. In 1949, the PASB Executive Committee approved a Plan for the Eradication of Smallpox in the Americas. Within a short time, Mexico, Guatemala, Chile, and Argentina eliminated the disease within their borders, and most other Latin American nations significantly reduced its incidence. The success was due to firm political decisions and the use of lyophilization, designed in Paris in the 1910s, which could preserve the vaccine with little refrigeration facilities. In 1953, WHO Director-General Brock Chisholm proposed a campaign for the elimination of smallpox worldwide, but the 1955 World Health Assembly turned the proposal down as "unfeasible."

Détente

Perceptions of the feasibility of smallpox eradication changed dramatically in the 1960s. This decade was characterized by the contradictory coexistence of seemingly idealistic beliefs grounded in the power of science and technology and the sometimes cynical commitment to the pragmatic policy of "Détente." Supporting scientific optimism were successes in the race to reach outer space and, in the case of medicine, achievements such as the first heart transplant and the control of previously rampant bacterial and viral diseases thanks to new drugs and vaccines. In often quoted 1969 testimony before Congress, US Surgeon General William Stewart asserted that, thanks to antibiotics and vaccines, it was time to "close the book on infectious disease." Idealism, humanitarianism, and dreams of progress were all parts of the UN's "Development Decade," launched by President John F. Kennedy at the UN General Assembly in 1961. Moreover, the Peace Corps, an international development program inaugurated by Kennedy in 1961, and the Fulbright educational and cultural exchange program approved in the same year empowered young American professionals to help poor countries.

These hopes coexisted with a novel phase of the Cold War, Détente, or the relaxation of tension between the United States and the Soviet Union. Under its more benign definition, Détente was a political initiative to limit the spread of nuclear weapons before proliferation led to a final deadly global war. Its origins can be traced to the mid-1960s, when US President Lyndon Johnson sought strategic disarmament and the UN sponsored a Non-Proliferation of

Nuclear Weapons Treaty. Détente between the United States and the USSR became more prominent with the start of President Richard Nixon's first term. Détente was embraced by the USSR when, after the overthrow of Khrushchev as the Russian Communist party's leader in 1964, Brezhnev, general secretary of the Communist Party of the Soviet Union, started supporting a foreign policy of "peaceful coexistence."[2] In reality, Détente with regard to nuclear weapons coexisted with the covert continuation of military build-up by both the United States and the Soviet Union and with the open pursuit of proxy wars such as in Vietnam. Beginning in the mid-1960s, the United States and the Soviet Union had regular weapons-control conversations and signed agreements while at the same time continuing to invest in strengthening their military arsenals well into the seventies. The contradictions of Détente became more visible in President Jimmy Carter's administration (1977–1981). Though initially willing to put a lid on the increase of military spending, after a few years Carter's administration became hostile toward the Soviet Union after the USSR's War in Afghanistan, begun in 1979. But it was only in the early 1980s with the election of President Reagan, seconded by Western European leaders such as Margaret Thatcher, that Détente collapsed.

Although Détente did not ultimately prevent either nuclear proliferation or the unilateral actions of the superpowers, one of its by-products was the belief – which the superpowers tried to live up to – that collaboration between heavily armed states of radically different ideologies was possible, especially in technical areas. International health was one such area, and collaboration here turned out to be critical for launching smallpox eradication. As in other international initiatives promoted by the Soviet regime or the US State Department, government officials worked intensely in launching and budgeting the smallpox program but later left it on its own, partly because "technical cooperation," unlike military aid, was frequently difficult to manipulate for political ends. Thus, to a large extent smallpox eradication was fortuitously left in the hands of medical experts who emphasized the technical and humanitarian dimensions of the program.

The WHO used this window of opportunity to make progress with a campaign directed at smallpox. The WHO's Soviet-inspired campaign was actually launched at two different times.[3] First, the Soviets won approval from the World Health Assembly in 1958, but this vote of approval did not mean much as sufficient funds were not initially available. Funds were tight because in that pre-Détente phase of the Cold War the United States did not desire to

---

[2] Raymond L. Garthoff, *Détente and Confrontation: American-Soviet Relations from Nixon to Reagan* (Washington, DC: The Brookings Institution, 1994).

[3] The official history is F. Fenner, D. A. Henderson, I. Arita, Z. Jezek, & I. D. Ladnyi, *Smallpox and Its Eradication* (Geneva: WHO, 1988), pp. 366–371.

support a USSR initiative and was already investing considerable resources in the US-inspired malaria eradication program. The second approval at the World Health Assemblies of 1966 and 1967 was more definitive because it followed important changes in both US and Soviet foreign policy. The super-powers were now experimenting with Détente and sought WHO approval for a collaboration consisting of the USSR contributing the lion's share of smallpox vaccine and the United States making sizeable donations to the WHO's budget and providing expert staff.

It took some time for this collaboration to coalesce. In 1958, Viktor M. Zhdanov, deputy minister of Health of the Soviet Union, had argued in the 11th World Health Assembly that it was feasible to eradicate smallpox worldwide. At that time smallpox afflicted about 15 million people annually, of whom 2 million died. Zhdanov believed that smallpox eradication could be achieved in five years if compulsory vaccination was carried out in endemic countries. Three factors explain the USSR's intense interest. First, this was the first Health Assembly that the Soviets attended since their reincorporation in the WHO in 1956, and a number of representatives made a special effort to demonstrate their openness to Soviet proposals that the Soviets did not want to pass up. Second, the Soviets wanted to challenge US influence in the WHO and make their own mark on international health. Third, the Soviets were concerned about smallpox importation from two of their endemic southern neighbors, India and Pakistan. The USSR promised 25 million doses of freeze-dried vaccine which had the advantage of being heat-stable for several weeks, thus allowing health personnel to work in remote, rural areas far from refriger-ation facilities.

Another solid basis for the Soviet proposal were biomedical realities that potentially made smallpox vaccination effective and cheap. First, the human body was the sole transmitting agent and reservoir of smallpox virus, unlike the case in malaria where an insect acted as the vector for transmission of the parasite that could also infect other animal species. Second, smallpox victims were easily identified because those who were infected displayed a distinctive rash, usually in the face, and their homes had a unique fetid odor (from puss-filled pustules). These facts facilitated the identification of cases. Finally, the disease spread slowly not explosively, a disseminating pattern that could be readily traced or anticipated.

During the early 1960s, the WHO conducted studies to learn more about the disease and help standardize the vaccine in developing countries where previ-ously a diversity of vaccines existed. The WHO provided not only technical advice and laboratory equipment, but also organized regional meetings in Asia and Africa, provided training courses, and stressed the importance of proper planning and staffing before national programs were launched. The first meeting of a WHO expert committee on smallpox took place in 1964, where experts agreed that worldwide eradication was possible as long as some fundamental problems were solved first, especially bad reporting.

The WHO committee was aware that in addition to the freeze-dried smallpox vaccine, a second tool for mass vaccination was now available – the intradermal jet injector. The jet injector had been developed for the US Army during World War II and was improved by the early 1960s after testing against diphtheria on an American Indian reservation and against diphtheria and tetanus in Jamaica, Tonga, Brazil, and in US prison populations (in an era of few concerns regarding human medical experimentation).[4] A difference between the jet injector and traditional immunization methods was that it used high pressure to get the dose instantly under the skin, rather than relying on a needle to inject the vaccine through the skin. Thus, the quickness and efficacy of vaccination increased and costs diminished considerably. The first injector models had depended on electricity and their maintenance was difficult, but later the foot-powered "ped-o-jet" became the jet injector of choice because it did not require electricity and its maintenance was easier. An American company, the Scientific Equipment Manufacturing Corporation of New Jersey, mastered ped-o-jet production and an American pharmaceutical company, Wyeth, produced a pure and potent vaccine required for the ped-o-jet. The basic assumption was that trained teams of health workers could now vaccinate up to one thousand persons in an hour, with a goal of reaching 80 percent of national populations (the percentage that was believed to be sufficient for stopping smallpox transmission).

The hopes raised by new medical technologies allowed the notion of smallpox eradication to make some progress at the WHO, even though the agency still had malaria eradication as its priority. Progress was possible thanks to experts such as Czechoslovakian epidemiologist Karel Raška, director of Prague's Institute of Epidemiology and Microbiology, who arrived at the WHO in 1962 and a year later was appointed director of the Division of Communicable Diseases. Raška visited smallpox countries in Africa and Asia and returned to Geneva believing in the feasibility of smallpox eradication. He trusted in the power of medical science and technology and was also a pioneer in careful epidemiological surveillance, a key strategy that helped smallpox eradication achieve its goal even though he had to leave the WHO early in the smallpox campaign because of his open disapproval of the Soviet suppression of the Prague revolt in 1968.[5]

[4] Horace G. Ogden, *CDC and the Smallpox Crusade* (Washington, DC: US Department of Health and Human Services, 1987), p. 16.

[5] Walter W. Holland, "Karel Raška – the Development of Modern Epidemiology, the Role of the International Epidemiology Association," *Central European Journal of Public Health* 2010, www.szu.cz/svi/cejph/archiv/2010-1-11-full.pdf, last accessed August 1, 2016, and Norman

Yet despite the growing enthusiasm for smallpox eradication in the first half of the 1960s, the WHO's smallpox program in reality had few resources and staff. It was found that only a small percentage of the donated vaccine was sufficiently potent to be useable. The WHO's expectation that countries would themselves take responsibility for the implementation of their smallpox campaigns was never fully realized. The US representatives to the World Health Assembly remained mostly silent about smallpox eradication, which they still considered a Soviet initiative. Their attitude was also explained by the fact that the US-backed malaria eradication program was still lumbering forward in the early 1960s on a much larger scale. This meant that the WHO had to keep an interest in smallpox eradication alive, despite the fact that industrial countries opposed increases in the agency's budget that might have been used for the smallpox program, and despite UNICEF's lack of enthusiasm for smallpox vaccination. The Soviet Union complained that the WHO did little to convince UNICEF or other agencies and was not moving rapidly enough to obtain the financial resources required for the program. In confirmation of the Soviet perception was the fact that from 1960 to 1966 smallpox eradication expenditures amounted to 0.6 percent of the WHO's total expenditures.[6]

The Second Launching of Eradication

In a dramatic turn of events in the mid-1960s, at almost the exact time that malaria eradication was encountering colossal difficulties in the field, the American government became interested in smallpox eradication. The WHO's smallpox program was, as a result, invigorated with significant donations and resources. The United States' shift in priority was most immediately inspired by foreign policy considerations, but already in the early 1960s some US medical experts had begun to envision the possibility of global smallpox eradication because of the end of endemic transmission in developed nations, in most of Latin America, and in a few Asian and African countries. Some of the countries that eliminated smallpox managed this through intensive vaccination campaigns even though they lacked adequate medical infrastructures. An early indication of support for the notion of global smallpox eradication was the response by many members of the American Public Health Association to a question posed by James Watt, director of the Office of International Health of the US Public Health Service.[7] To APHA members, the technical challenges

---

D. Noah, "Key Figure in World Smallpox Eradication Receives Jenner Medal," *Journal of the Royal Society of Medicine* 78:4 (1985), 344.

[6] Gian Luca Burci & Claude-Henri Vignes, *World Health Organization* (The Hague: Kluwer Law International, 2004), p. 175.

[7] Cited in Erez Manela, "A Pox on Your Narrative: Writing Disease Control into Cold War History," *Diplomatic History* 34:2 (2010), 299–323, p. 308.

were less daunting for smallpox than for malaria, and epidemiological trends indicated an ongoing decline of smallpox worldwide. In 1964, the acting director of the CDC wrote a memo to the US surgeon general outlining a program for smallpox eradication in the Americas by 1970 that would concentrate on Brazil, the remaining endemic country in the region.

European governments' concern with global smallpox eradication was related in part to endemic smallpox in former colonies in Africa and Asia, which had continuing contacts with European capitals. The massive international migration and jet travel of the 1960s increased the risk of inadvertently importing cases of smallpox. For example, in 1963, 116 cases and 11 deaths followed from the importation of one case from Pakistan to Poland.[8] Although the United States had not had a smallpox case since the late 1940s, it had experienced a few "smallpox scares" in the following years and spent more than 140 million dollars per year during the early 1960s on routine vaccination. Some American pediatricians, such as Henry Kempe, were openly against immunization, arguing that the number of child deaths due to the complications of vaccination was much higher than deaths from the disease. Global smallpox eradication was perceived by the United States, the USSR, and many European countries as an investment to save money still being spent on domestic immunizations and to protect their citizens from possible outbreaks coming from abroad.

Worldwide smallpox eradication was also justified in the United States by foreign-policy considerations. The US government did not want the USSR to claim unchallenged recognition for its leadership role in the WHO eradication effort and was interested in the possible political payoff of the program in terms of gaining the loyalty of developing countries. The US government thought of its aid to health programs as a way to modernize societies, minimize communist infiltration, and bolster capitalist economic growth in poor nations. In addition, the initial smallpox eradication design, with a clear goal and deadline, fit the mold of international cooperation preferred by those in charge of American bilateral assistance. Another draw for US experts was that smallpox eradication was a matching program, with the United States providing expert personnel and a percentage of the budget (about 25 percent), while the multilateral agency and developing nations paid for the local expenses, estimated at about 75 percent of the total budget. The WHO was willing to allow that US funds be spent on American medicines, equipment, and materials, as required by a resolution of the US Congress.

The World Health Assembly in May 1965 approved a resolution stating that smallpox eradication was one of the main goals of the agency, thus reviving

---

[8] WHO Expert Committee on Smallpox, *Review of the Smallpox Situation in the World Presented by the Secretariat*, September 1963, Smallpox/WP/12 24 Geneva, WHO Library, p. 3.

the 1958 resolution. At the same time, President Lyndon Johnson's administration issued a press release pledging its support for smallpox eradication. WHO officers promptly moved to confirm the US decision. In August 1965, Raška and the WHO's Assistant Director-General Milton Siegel, an American who had worked at the WHO for more than 20 years, traveled together to Washington, DC, to talk to administration officials and to request more funds for the smallpox program. In November of that year Candau was in Atlanta and in a conversation with a CDC officer praised the work the CDC was organizing in Africa as "a working model of the fully organized smallpox eradication campaign which we [in the WHO] aim to launch on a much wider basis."[9]

Other accounts, including one by the American architect of the program, suggest that Candau and other WHO officers did not believe in smallpox eradication. Most likely, they were reluctant to commit the WHO to a new global eradication campaign that might, like the malaria program, lead to another embarrassing failure. But multilateral agencies are not monolithic institutions. They harbor different perspectives and their leaders might need to be ambiguous for political reasons. The persistence, persuasiveness, and seniority of Raška were crucial for the re-creation of a consensus within the WHO to pursue smallpox eradication. Evidence suggests that Candau was positive, although not wildly enthusiastic.

African medical leaders were part of the process of promoting global immunization. In 1960, four African health ministers, including Paul Lambin from Upper Volta (today Burkina Faso), who had trained as a medical doctor in Paris, visited the US National Institutes of Health thanks to a grant provided by the American government. They met with microbiologist Harry Meyer, who was in charge of a section on viral-vaccine research and who was working on a measles vaccine which was partially tested but not yet licensed in the United States. Measles was a killer in Africa, with a mortality rate of about 25 percent. Industrial interests were also involved since the pharmaceutical company Merck Sharp & Dohme wanted to confirm the validity of a measles vaccine that would be effective and have few side effects.

In response to Lambin's request, a NIH mission was sent to Upper Volta in 1961, which by 1963 had vaccinated 700,000 children with the Merck vaccine in a field trial. Neighboring African countries learned about the successful field trial and requested that the project be extended. Astute and assertive African health ministers played the superpowers against one another and in this case asked the United States to provide more assistance and funds. Thus, programs were quickly planned for six more countries – Dahomey, Guinea, Ivory Coast,

---

[9] Ogden, CDC and the Smallpox Crusade, p. 32.

Mali, Mauritania, and Niger – because the US State Department was now convinced that measles vaccination was an excellent way to cement friendly relationships with African recipients.

In 1966, President Johnson proposed to Congress a USD 1 billion International Health Act whose goal was to "wipe out" smallpox and malaria and to control yellow fever over the next decade. Johnson was toying with the idea of promoting a "Global Great Society" where want and infectious disease would not exist (an effort that encountered resistance in the US Congress, as described by Reinhardt).[10] There was also hope that a healthy "Global Great Society" would enhance the number of global consumers of American goods and of regimes loyal to the United States.

The State Department instructed American representatives to the 19th World Health Assembly in 1966 to support the smallpox eradication initiative and the creation, for the first time, of an item on smallpox eradication in the WHO's regular budget. An astute Candau presented a significantly increased budget proposal for 1967 to the WHA and included in it about two and a half million USD for the smallpox eradication program. Representatives from the United States complained that the budget increase was larger than usual and did not correctly estimate the effects of inflation. Candau responded that to carry out smallpox eradication effectively, his proposed budget was essential. He got support from developing countries in the Health Assembly, which took at face value the statement by President Johnson. Candau's budget was approved by a small margin of votes, and the United States acceded after the decision was reached.

In 1967, the WHA formally approved the formation of the Smallpox Eradication Program, SEP, whose mission was to lead an "intensified" global program. In that same year the Soviet Union donated 75 million doses of vaccine for the first three years of a projected ten-year campaign organized by the SEP. The term "intensive" was literal because in some cases SEP health workers would work for three months on a seven-day work week schedule of fifteen hours a day. In that year the disease was endemic in 31 countries with a total population of more than 1 billion, and in that year alone between 10 and 15 million people were stricken with smallpox. Yet by 1967 there were two smallpox eradication programs underway, one based on US bilateral assistance in Africa, and the other one led by the WHO. It is important to turn to the African program first in order to understand the full development of the SEP.

---

[10] See Bob Reinhardt, *The End of a Global Pox, America and the Eradication of Smallpox in the Cold War Era* (Chapel Hill: University of North Carolina Press, 2015).

The Centers of Disease Control in Africa

Because of the central importance of the CDC in the WHO's smallpox eradication work, some background information is needed on the agency.[11] Its origins can be traced to World War II and the establishment in 1942 of the office of Malaria Control in War Areas (MCWA) as an arm of the US Public Health Service. Based in Atlanta, Georgia, in 1946 MCWA was renamed the Communicable Disease Center (CDC) and was transformed into a federal agency that would support state and local health units in investigating and controlling communicable disease outbreaks. Beginning in the 1950s, the CDC began to accumulate even broader functions, such as the control of venereal diseases that might come across the Mexican border, and in 1962 President Kennedy signed the Vaccination Assistance Act which gave the CDC national responsibility for mass immunization campaigns. Three years later the US Public Health Service transferred national quarantine responsibilities to the CDC.

The CDC's interest in smallpox can be traced to Alexander Langmuir, the creator of the agency's Epidemic Intelligence Service (EIS), established in 1951. This unit, born during the Cold War in an atmosphere of anxiety about biological warfare, trained health professionals for rapid dispatch to the sites of epidemic outbreaks in the United States. But Langmuir's imagination carried him beyond the borders of the country. He was one of the few American epidemiologists in the 1950s with direct experience of smallpox, which he acquired while working in a bilateral vaccination program in East Pakistan in 1958.[12] He also mentored talented young epidemiologists, among whom were J. Donald Millar, who investigated smallpox around the world; William H. Foege, an epidemiological officer in Colorado and later a medical missionary of the Lutheran Church in Africa who subsequently returned to the CDC; and Donald A. Henderson, future head of the WHO Smallpox program. Critical to these efforts was David Sencer, head of the CDC from 1966 to 1977, who was convinced that the best way to protect the United States was to get rid of epidemics abroad.

In September 1965, representatives of the CDC and the African regional office of the WHO met to discuss the CDC's immunization efforts in Africa. The meeting was instrumental in convincing USAID, the principal funder of

---

[11] The following paragraphs are based on Elizabeth Etheridge, *Sentinel for Health: A History of the Centers for Disease Control* (Berkeley: University of California Press, 1992); Mark Pendergrast, *Inside the Outbreaks: The Elite Medical Detectives of the Epidemic Intelligence Service* (Boston: Houghton Mifflin Harcourt, 2010).

[12] Paul Greenough, "'A Wild and Wondrous Ride': CDC Field Epidemiologists in the East Pakistan Smallpox and Cholera Epidemics of 1958," *Ciência & Saúde Coletiva* 16:2 (2011), 491–500.

the measles program, to enlarge the initial effort to 18, later 19 nations, all located in West and Central Africa. The area occupied by these countries was inhabited by 100 million people and had clear geographic boundaries: on the west the Atlantic Ocean, on the north the Sahara Desert, on the east Sudan, and on the south the Congo basin. The CDC and the WHO also convinced USAID to combine measles immunization with smallpox eradication for five years. A simple biological fact cemented that connection: Measles and smallpox were both believed at the time to be highly contagious and clearly recognizable by distinctive rashes. According to a CDC officer, a large budget was submitted to USAID with the expectation that the US government would never fund such an ambitious program. But the WHO and CDC were pleasantly surprised and by 1966 began to prepare for a measles-smallpox eradication program in West and Central Africa. For US policy makers, health work in the region seemed to provide an extraordinary opportunity to demonstrate the power of American technological expertise, to forge a link between health programs, moderniza-tion and anticommunism, and to develop an influence in newly independent developing countries.

Shortly after the beginning of the program, the measles arm was dropped. The reasons were unanticipated side effects (such as vomiting) of the vaccine being used and that it soon became clear it would be impossible to wipe out the disease in just a few years as expected. Another reason was that the measles program suffered from foolish logistical mistakes, such as trying to use refrigeration units not designed for African climates of above 100 degrees or using American-made trucks in francophone countries where there were few US-trained mechanics or spare parts. More importantly, the Merck vaccine was simply not good enough, for by the late 1960s the vaccine was no longer in use, and in 1971 the US government authorized a new Merck measles, mumps, and rubella vaccine, known as MMR.

After 1968, the CDC had an often-tense relationship with USAID and the US Department of State. There were tensions between CDC staff and USAID concerning to whom the CDC reported. Also, the CDC's priority was to expand the budget of the program, whereas USAID wanted to constrain it. In addition, the CDC concentrated on the disease, and local politics only mattered if it interfered with medical interventions, whereas USAID officers preferred to concentrate on countries loyal to the United States. As an example, the United States had no diplomatic relationship with the People's Republic of Congo. The CDC did not care, but the State Department did. In another example, Guinea and Mali had left-wing regimes, which did not prevent CDC epidemiologists from forging working agreements with local health workers who happened to be members of the Communist party. In another telling example, a CDC field worker was asked by locals to vaccinate individ-uals who he later found out were members of a guerrilla movement that fought against the government of a neighboring country. While vaccinating, he remembered that an American diplomat had asked him to "inform him about any military movements." He decided not to do so because "our surveillance was very different from his surveillance."[13]

Other difficulties derived from subtle political differences between countries. For example, in the decentralized former British colonies it was crucial to gain the consent·of local tribal chiefs because they still enjoyed a great deal of authority. But in former French colonies the chiefs had been subordinated to the centralizing regime of French imperialism with its civil servants in the villages. In order to make progress, these civil servants had to be dealt with. The Americans also had to adjust to two different French bilateral agencies: the *Organization de Coordination et de Cooperation pour la Lute contre Grandes Endemies* (OCCGE), with headquarters in Upper Volta, and the *Organization de Coordination pour la Lute contre les endemies en Afrique Centrale* (OCEAC), based in Cameroon. In addition, AFRO's new director, Alfred C. Quenum from Benin, was suspicious of US intentions. It was also difficult for Americans to visit Brazzaville, the headquarters of AFRO, because of poor relations between the United States and the Congo. Henderson and George I. Lythcott, a CDC African American pediatrician, met with Quenum in 1966 and elicited formal cooperation but little enthusiasm.[14]

Beginning in 1967, hundreds of US physicians, statisticians, technicians and other personnel from the CDC and USAID (plus a few from the WHO and other agencies) began to work in West and Central Africa. By 1970, 19 African countries had eradicated smallpox with the help of the CDC, and the experience became the model for the global smallpox eradication program developed by the WHO. An indication of the operation's dimension is that between 1967 and 1972, more than 153 million smallpox vaccinations were administered.[15] In many rural villages, people endured long lines for vaccinations, and each individual vaccinated received a certificate. Initially, the strategy was "mass vaccination" of at least 80 percent of national populations. According to the "herd-immunity" theory, this was required for the virus to die off.

A key event occurred in 1966 in eastern Nigeria, where Foege was working as a medical missionary. His experience there created fatal dissonances for the herd immunity theory and the linked strategy of mass vaccination. Foege

---

[13] Joel G. Breman, "A Miracle Happened There: The West and Central African Smallpox Eradication Programme and Its Impact," in Sanjoy Bhattacharya & Sharon Messenger (eds.), *The Global Eradication of Smallpox* (New Delhi: Orient BlackSwan, 2010), pp. 36–60, p. 54.
[14] Ogden, *CDC and the Smallpox Crusade*, p. 28.
[15] William Herbert Foege, John Donald Millar & Donald Ainslie Henderson, "Smallpox Eradication in West and Central Africa," *Bulletin of the World Health Organization* 52 (1972), 209–222.

found that he did not have sufficient resources for mass vaccination.[16] Of necessity, he decided to use his limited supply in the villages where outbreaks had occurred and in immediately neighboring villages, hoping that this intervention would contain the disease. In about four weeks there were no reports of smallpox in Nigeria's eastern region, in contrast to other regions of the country. Shortly thereafter and guided largely by intuition, Foege convinced the Nigerian minister of health to abandon mass vaccination. His alternative plan was to focus on the prompt identification in homes, markets, and schools of individuals exhibiting rashes and to vaccinate compulsorily people in and around these locations. Foege's hunch was that smallpox could be made to disappear with a fraction of the vaccinations required for a mass campaign.

Because of the secessionist Nigeria-Biafra civil war between the eastern and western regions of Nigeria, Foege had to leave Nigeria for about a year. He returned to CDC headquarters in Atlanta, where he criticized the flaws in the mass vaccination strategy and promoted the advantages of his new methods. He convinced CDC officer Donald R. Hopkins, who was about to travel to Sierra Leone – the country with the highest smallpox rate in West Africa – to use the new strategy from the start. Foege also convinced Donald Millar, who was in charge of the whole West Central African program, of the advantages of the new strategy.

A growing consensus developed in the CDC that herd immunity did not work in Africa for two reasons. First, Africans lived in isolated communities, and migrants, nomads, and traders moved from one region to another, which made them difficult to vaccinate. Even if the 80 percent target were reached, the possibility existed for smallpox to break out in regions previously vaccinated because of itinerant populations. Foege's strategy made it easier to assign officers to follow these itinerant groups. Some years later, Isao Arita, a Japanese epidemiologist, developed the notion of "density of unvaccinated susceptibles" and argued that because a few susceptibles could generate an outbreak there should be surveillance and containment in endemic regions.[17] Enforcing mass vaccination for an entire country or region discouraged good reporting because if this target were not achieved it was usually considered a "failure" of the vaccination teams, which led many field workers to send in unreliable records.

When Foege returned to eastern Nigeria, the region was still free of smallpox. His innovative strategy – a creative response to an insufficient supply of

---

[16] Interview with Dr. William H. Foege by Victoria Harden, July 13, 2006, Centers for Disease Control and Prevention [last accessed July 15, 2016]; Foege, Millar, & Henderson, "Smallpox Eradication in West and Central Africa," 209–222.

[17] Isao Arita, John Wickett & Frank Fenner, "Impact of Population Density on Immunization Programs," *Journal of Hygiene* 96 (1986), 450–466.

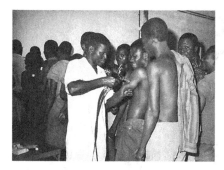

Figure 5.2 Smallpox Eradication worker vaccinating a group of local
residents in Benin, Africa in 1968.
Credit: Centers for Disease Control/Smith Collection (CDC). Source: Getty Images.

vaccine – was initially called "ring vaccination" or the "eradication escalation
strategy." The term "surveillance and containment" came to replace these.
Foege presented his strategy in African regional meetings, such as in Abidjan,
Nigeria, in 1968, and discussed it with CDC and African health officers, many
of whom still preferred mass vaccination. But the new strategy was accepted
and accelerated the program's achievements. By 1970, when West and Central
Africa were rendered smallpox-free using fewer financial resources and vaccines than originally planned, Foege's strategy had become incontestable.

After their experience in Africa, all of the CDC officers promoted surveillance and containment, and their African program became a model for the
WHO to follow (Figure 5.2 depicts some of the work in Africa). In 1972,
American officials declared that their bilateral assistance was over and their
work in West and Central Africa finished. They next turned their attention to
the WHO, where the CDC had already made considerable inroads and where,
in fact, a CDC officer had been the head of SEP since 1966. His name was
Donald A. Henderson.

Henderson's Leadership

In 1964, while in the United States, Candau insisted to US Surgeon General
Luther Terry that an American be assigned to direct the WHO's smallpox
program. It is not clear if Candau did it to ensure US support or to blame the
United States in the case of a possible failure. In any case, it was an intelligent
move. After additional conversations in Geneva and Washington, it was
agreed that the CDC's Henderson was the man for the job. D. A., who had
prepared the plan for the CDC's intervention in Africa and was ready to direct
the African program, was asked – ordered, really – to assume responsibility in

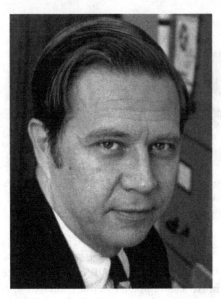

Figure 5.3 Donald A. Henderson, an American physician and epidemiologist, who was an officer of the US Centers for Disease Control and Prevention. In 1966 he became head of the World Health Organization's global smallpox eradication program. He would direct the program until 1977.
Courtesy: World Health Organization Photo Library.

Geneva, which he did in October of 1964. Henderson (see Figure 5.3) went to work at the WHO while formally "on loan" from the CDC, his salary being paid by the US government and not by the WHO. During those years, the CDC also provided more than a hundred experts for the program.

At first disappointed that a Russian was not selected, the USSR acceded to the choice of Henderson. A Soviet health officer told him that his government considered him a good scientist and a person with whom they could work.[18] Most likely, Raška supported Henderson in Geneva and in communist circles; the Czech had known Henderson since a 1957 international meeting of epidemiologists in the Netherlands and had maintained correspondence with him afterwards.

Henderson headed the World Health Organization's SEP from 1966 to 1977 and proved to be an effective and tireless administrator. He would travel to where he was needed, was capable of winning over skeptics inside and outside the WHO, and demonstrated that he could be at the same time a no-nonsense

---

[18] Donald A. Henderson, "Smallpox Eradication: A Cold War Victory," *World Health Forum* 19:2 (1988), 113–119, p. 118.

manager and a masterful diplomat, working intimately and effectively with his Soviet counterparts to secure vaccines, funds, and personnel and to smooth out problems. He orchestrated diplomatic pressures from the US and USSR embassies to obtain confidential information worldwide and to secure cooperation from governments reluctant to cooperate with the WHO. Henderson kept close ties with the CDC, exchanging information and closely monitoring its work against smallpox in Africa. Largely thanks to Henderson, "surveillance of communicable diseases" was the main issue discussed in the 1968 World Health Assembly in Geneva.

That meeting marked a transition at the WHO from "mass vaccination" to a "surveillance and containment" strategy. The emphasis in mass vaccination projects had been on how many people received the vaccine. Little attention was paid to the identification of cases that reappeared in the wake of campaigns. The new strategy involved identifying individuals with smallpox and vaccinating all members of their immediate family, their close contacts, and everyone within a radius of a few miles from the initial case. The strategy required careful supervision. This meant collecting small human scabs and sending them as soon as possible to the laboratory for diagnosis and careful house-to-house and village-to-village searches.

Surveillance and containment signaled also the relative autonomy of international health from the politics of the Cold War. Malaria eradication was launched when the United States was in active competition with the Soviet Union. From the US perspective, MEP could win "hearts and minds" in the battle against Communism by delivering benefits but without enlisting the participation of local populations in planning or implementation. In contrast, smallpox eradication through surveillance and containment empowered medical experts who believed that their technical knowledge and the interaction with locals were crucial factors for success. This more cooperative strategy was able to gain space in the international arena because of the politics of Détente, when the superpowers declared their willingness to limit their own nuclear arsenals and coexist peacefully while collaborating on humanitarian programs.

We still know little about the transition from mass vaccination to surveillance and containment within the WHO, but it's clear that there was at least extensive discussion and some resistance. But SEP personnel who had done mass vaccination in the past came to subscribe to the new strategy for three reasons. First, it made sense to concentrate attack and resources in specific locations and seasons when smallpox was at its lowest point. Second, most SEP members were young, adaptable, and highly motivated. Many were willing to sleep in any place and eager to develop a spirit of camaraderie. Even Henderson, born in 1928, was in his 30s when he went to Geneva. No less important was the hunger for learning and the eagerness to innovate on the

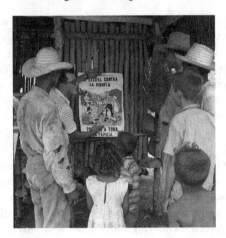

Figure 5.4 Poster "Vaccine against Smallpox: Protect all your Family" displayed by a health worker in a rural area of Barranquilla, Colombia in the 1960s.
Credit: WHO/Paul Almasy. Courtesy: World Health Organization Photo Library.

part of local health workers. For example, in the absence of a telephone system, teenagers became messengers and informants. In addition, local health workers learned how to say a few words in different languages and dialects, such as: "Has anyone seen a child like this?" (showing a "recognition card" depicting a smallpox case). Health workers were willing to learn from endemic populations that had lived with smallpox for centuries (another example of work with local communities can be seen in Figure 5.4). For example, in parts of India it was traditional to mark homes infected with smallpox, a system later adopted by the SEP despite its stigmatizing implications.[19] As the campaign built momentum, many sensed that the WHO was about to accomplish a historical goal and wanted to be part of that achievement. Finally, because several of the SEP staff were former CDC staff who arrived at the WHO with confidence in, and sometimes devotion to, Henderson, the transition to surveillance and containment was relatively easy. By the mid-1970s, the WHO made popular two new phrases in the anti-smallpox vocabulary: "intensive search and containment" and "target zero."[20]

A telling anecdote took place in India where Foege was stationed beginning in 1973. He confronted skeptics, including the Indian minister of health, who

---

[19] Robert Holbrook Reinhardt, "Remaking Bodily Environments: The Global Eradication of Smallpox," PhD Dissertation, University of California, Davis, 2012, p. 205.
[20] "WHO Reports Dread Diseases Are Soaring in the Region of India," *The New York Times*, September 18, 1973.

believed that surveillance and containment would not work because of the nation's very large population (about 600 million people in the early 1970s), its cultural and linguistic division into 21 states, the strong autonomy of local authorities, and the high incidence of smallpox. The minister wanted mass smallpox vaccination, but Foege explained firmly: "When a house is on fire, you pour water on that house, not in the neighborhood."[21] His resolution convinced some Indian health workers and helped keep SEP on its new path. Only then did Indian health leaders and other members of SEARO embrace surveillance and containment as the proper strategy for smallpox eradication.

Henderson should be given credit for the discipline to sustain the course of SEP when the program was approaching its goal. After a successful few years with a small number of smallpox cases, national health authorities were eager to move on to other health problems. Henderson distributed among SEP workers a quote from *The First Circle* (1968), written by Russian dissident author Aleksander Solzhentitsyn: "In that moment of fatigue and self-satisfaction it is especially tempting to leave the work without having attained the apex of quality ... the rule of the Final Inch consists in this: do not shirk this crucial work. Not to postpone it ..."[22] According to Henderson, in the final years of the program his staff was frequently urged to recall "the final inch rule" as a reminder to resist complacency.

The principal test for the "final inch" occurred in the 1970s in India and Ethiopia (other remaining endemic countries were Nepal, Indonesia, Brazil, and Somalia). The situation in India, with by far the largest number of cases, was breathtaking. An Indian national smallpox eradication program had begun in 1962 based on mass vaccination. By this time, the CDC and the WHO used a new vaccination technique that replaced the jet injector: the bifurcated needle. It was a small piece of steel shaped like a miniature pitchfork and designed to hold the right amount of freeze-dried smallpox vaccine between its two prongs. It was simpler to employ than the jet injector, easier to clean, cheap, and ideal for a massive global campaign. The Indian National Smallpox Eradication Program, NSEP, vaccinated more than 20 million people in 1961, then obtained more funds from the government, the USSR, and the USAID. Nevertheless, evaluations completed some years later revealed that there had been loose work in remote rural areas, a lack of potency of the vaccine used, outbreaks not identified in their early stages, inadequate storage of vaccine, concealed cases, unmotivated health workers, and, worst of all, a hiatus

---

[21] Donald A. Henderson, *Smallpox: The Death of a Disease – The Inside Story of Eradicating a Worldwide Killer* (Amherst, MA: Prometheus Books, 2009); William Foege, *House on Fire: The Fight to Eradicate Smallpox* (Berkeley: University of California Press, 2011).

[22] Cited in Henderson, "Smallpox Eradication," p. 118.

between 1966 and 1969. In spite of all this, NSEP still eliminated smallpox from the southern region of India.

Indian health authorities decided around 1970 to "nationalize" the smallpox program by removing responsibility from the states and passing it to a central program. In the early 1970s, some states had interrupted transmission, but others had not. A careful search revealed that the problem was of considerable magnitude, with almost 6,000 cases distributed among about 1500 villages in Uttar Pradesh and another 3,800 cases in Bihar. The WHO helped reorganize the Indian program in 1973 with the aid of experts of different nationalities but with a core of Indian health experts. These included epidemiologist Mahendra Dutta; R. R. Arora, deputy director of the National Institute of Communicable Diseases of India; M. L. D. Sharma, director of the Institute of Communicable Disease at SEARO; and Indian Health Minister Karan Singh. Another positive factor was the arrival of new donors, such as Swedish and Danish bilateral agencies, Rotary International, and the Tata industrial consortium of India. To this support were added donations from Austria, Canada, Denmark, and Japan. US donations continued but did not increase, partly because of the conservative political climate in the American Congress in the late 1970s.

The work of the reorganized smallpox eradication program in India was also daunting from a regional political perspective. A war in East Pakistan created Bangladesh in December 1971. After the war, thousands of refugees and soldiers who had previously moved to India suddenly returned home, some carrying the smallpox virus with them. In 1971, Bangladesh did not register a single case of smallpox, but a year later 11,000 cases were reported.[23] A presidential decree declared smallpox a national emergency, and Swedish bilateral funds supported surveillance teams working with SEP officers to apply surveillance and containment methods. By August 1974, smallpox was restricted to two northern districts and eradication appeared near. Unfortunately, a flood produced migration that disseminated the disease again. In January of 1975, a radical decision was made to demolish the slums of Dacca and of three other cities. About 1 million former slum dwellers were forced to move back to their native villages. Other directives of the government were also quite strict: Outbreaks had to be detected within a period of 15 days, and 21 days was the maximum allowed to complete containment measures. The implementation of these strict measures was facilitated by a new radio network and by a network of 14,000 family welfare workers who

---

[23] The World Health Organization, *A Decade of Health Development in South Asia 1968–1977* (New Delhi: WHO, Regional Office for South-East Asia, 1980), p. 197.

made monthly house-to-house searches. Compulsion apparently worked, as Bangladesh's last case of variola major was identified in October 1975.[24]

One of the political obstacles to reorganizing smallpox eradication services in India was the country's proud tradition of autonomy. The head of the government from 1966 to 1977 was Indira Gandhi, daughter of the former prime minister Jawaharlal Nehru. She had a difficult relationship with President Nixon, was suspicious of his motives for developing friendly ties with China, and was happy to have the USSR as India's largest arms supplier and commercial partner. The antagonism between India and the United States was sometimes so intense that the US government considered closing its Indian embassy. Foege knew about this possibility and convinced the American Ambassador Daniel Patrick Moynihan, who served in India from 1973 to 1975, to maintain the US embassy. The Ambassador also played a critical role in easing the work of the eradicators in India.

Indira Gandhi was persuaded by Indian and foreign physicians to support smallpox eradication in order to bolster her political position. In May 1974, India had its first underground nuclear detonation, creating fear in members of the US government that suspected it had been done with Soviet aid (for others, the detonation had been assisted by the United States). Journalists commented on the irony that a poor country that spent millions of US dollars on nuclear tests was still threatened by a preventable disease such as smallpox. In 1975, Gandhi announced a 20-point development program to increase agricultural and industrial production and fight poverty, but smallpox eradication did not appear in the program. The French physician Nicole Grasset, a WHO officer posted to SEARO, met with Gandhi directly to request that smallpox eradication be added as the 21st priority because it was a serious menace to the country and the world. Gandhi was convinced and included smallpox eradication as the 21st priority.

During 1974 and 1975, 250 million smallpox vaccine doses were produced and distributed in India. By late 1974, 93 WHO epidemiologists were working in India and Bangladesh in 115 special teams headed by Indian physicians. In 1970 India had about 75 percent of the more than 218,000 total smallpox cases worldwide. In February of 1975 it recorded only 216 cases.[25] Surveillance and containment had produced a rapid decline and the country had its last case of smallpox in May of 1975, that of Saina Bibi, a poor young teenager from Assam.

[24] A. K. Joarder, D. Tarantola, & J. Tulloch, *The Eradication of Smallpox from Bangladesh* (New Delhi: WHO, South-East Regional Office, 1980).

[25] "WHO Foresees Conquest of Smallpox this Year," April 4, 1975, Press Release WHO/16, *WHO Press Releases 1973–1976*, WHO Library.

By late 1974 it was clear to Gandhi and to Ambassador Moynihan – not yet to Henderson – that smallpox was very close to its end in India. Henderson stuck to international rules and asked for an "epidemiological silence" of two years after the last identified case before confirming eradication. Gandhi did not want to wait and sent a contradictory message to Geneva requesting the celebration of smallpox eradication yet demanding more WHO assistance.[26] As the celebration of India's independence approached (August 15), Gandhi decided to change the official date's name: It would be commemorated as "Independence *from smallpox* day." On Independence Day, a ceremony in New Delhi was attended by director-general Mahler, Henderson, and local health authorities. Most staff at WHO headquarters in Geneva and in the regional offices truly believed that eradication was going to happen very soon – even in 1975, despite a dramatic epidemic outbreak in Pakistan the year before.[27]

Mahler's support of smallpox eradication was not limited to his participation in ceremonies. In November 1974, he invited diplomatic representatives of 18 countries, including some from the industrialized nations, to a meeting in Geneva where he asked for a sum of between USD 2.2 million and 3.3 million to support eradication work on Bangladesh, India, and Ethiopia in 1975. He argued that the amount represented a small fraction of what the United States currently spent on routine immunization – 150 million. He also reported that the cost of the campaign thus far had been about 50 million, of which 22 million came from the WHO's regular budget supplemented by 31 countries making donations, while endemic countries such as India made up the difference.

The Horn of Africa had fewer cases than India in the 1970s but was a concern and a test for the "final inch" doctrine because of the open borders between countries, the dispersion of population, and rudimentary health infra-structures. The situation in Ethiopia was complicated by its large number of cases, its vicinity to Somalia with its high incidence of smallpox, occasional armed conflicts with Somalia, and the misery that plagued many of its 70 million people. Moreover, up until the early 1970s Ethiopian health resources had been concentrated on malaria eradication, and malaria personnel boycotted the smallpox eradication campaign because they perceived it as competition. Eventually, Emperor Haile Selassie was persuaded to pursue eradication, and Japanese and Austrian bilateral agencies were willing to provide funds

---

[26] "Annex 1 Message of Indira Gandhi dated July 1, 1975," in R. N. Basu, Z. Jezek, & N. A. Ward, *The Eradication of Smallpox from India* (New Delhi: World Health Organization South-East Asia Regional office, 1979).

[27] "WHO Foresees Conquest of Smallpox This Year," April 4, 1975, Press Release WHO/16 *WHO Press Releases 1973–1976*, WHO Library.

beginning in 1971. By the end of that year the program reported more than 26,000 cases. Vaccination made rapid progress, but in 1974 a communist revolution deposed the emperor and US Peace Corps volunteers and American diplomats left the country. Most UN offices were closed, and two vaccinators were killed. Fortunately, the SEP continued and after a few months the Ethiopian communist government, pressured by the Soviet Union, established order and kept the WHO smallpox program as a priority.

In Somalia, the political situation was difficult, too. In 1975, the country experienced a severe drought and massive internal migration. The following year, the one-party regime proclaimed its adherence to Marxism and Islamism and emphasized self-sufficiency. The new government decided to concentrate its limited public funds on education and literacy, reducing assistance to public health to a minimum. Somehow, the health work continued. A SEP team relied on a workforce of schoolteachers, police, a Somali Women's organization, and members of a Red Cross organization to manage a surveillance and containment program with 3,000 Somalian health workers searching for rashes and fever cases. There was even a "smallpox rumor register."[28] Incredibly, this work was accomplished during the 1977–1978 war between Somalia and Ethiopia. The world's last case of smallpox was reported in Somalia in October 1977, the case of a 23-year-old hospital cook, Ali Maow Maalin. It was ironic and revealing of the contradictions of the campaign that not only had Maalin worked at a hospital, but he had also been employed as a vaccinator without being himself successfully vaccinated.

Also, in 1977, Henderson left SEP to take up the deanship of the Johns Hopkins School of Hygiene and Public Health, although he remained as an advisor to the WHO. The SEP stayed on track under the command of the experienced Japanese physician and virologist Isao Arita, who had been deputy head of SEP under Henderson. In 1978 the SEP hired James Magee as an information officer to prepare press releases and organize radio and television programs that would mark the anticipated formal achievement of eradication.

Somalia and the SEP had to wait two more years to confirm that smallpox had in fact been eradicated. The two-year waiting period was established because it was found that in some countries where smallpox supposedly no longer existed, the disease reappeared after approximately six months. Between 1975 and 1979, various international commissions visited several countries but mainly Asian and African countries to examine documents, field reports, and epidemiological information.[29] In 1978, the WHO created

---

[28] Isao Arita, *Worldwide Smallpox Eradication Program, Last Known Foci and Global Certification*, SMWE/78.21 Global Commission WP/78.1, November 1978, WHO Library, p. 2.

[29] The Global Eradication of Smallpox: *Final Report of the Global Commission for the Certification of Smallpox* (Geneva: WHO, 1980).

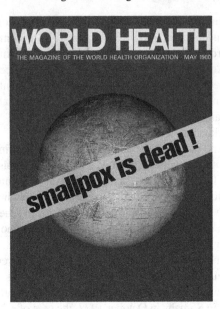

Figure 5.5 Front cover of the May 1980 issue of *World Health*, a WHO journal. The global eradication of smallpox was certified by an independent panel of scientists drawn from 19 nations in December 1979.
Courtesy: World Health Organization Photo Library.

the Global Commission for the Certification of Smallpox Eradication, and the Commission concentrated its work on Somalia.

In May 1980, the 33rd World Health Assembly "solemnly" declared that the global eradication of smallpox had been accomplished. No cases had been discovered for more than two years (as seen in Figure 5.5, the achievement was celebrated on the cover of an important illustrated publication of the WHO). The Australian virologist Frank Fenner, chairman of the Global Commission for the Certification of Smallpox Eradication, presented the official certificate of eradication to the World Health Assembly. His Commission transmitted its final reports and recommendations and was dissolved.

A cost estimate of the WHO's smallpox program for the period 1967 to 1980 totaled 98 million US dollars, of which a third was provided by the WHO and other UN agencies and two-thirds by individual countries (mainly the United States, the Soviet Union, and Sweden). A *New York Times* article claimed that USD 2 billion yearly savings could be expected from the eradication of smallpox. It was estimated that had smallpox not been eradicated, the

20-year period between 1978 and 1998 would have witnessed approximately 350 million new cases and 40 million deaths.[30]

Regional Dissonance, Resistance, and Participation

The response was different in each WHO region, with some quite reluctant regional offices. PAHO headquarters was then under the command of the Chilean Abraham Horwitz, who believed in the advantages of balanced transformations in public health systems over "vertical" programs. He formally agreed to work with SEP and distributed the limited financial and human resources for smallpox among all countries of the region. But he dismissed Geneva's request to concentrate on the more than 4,000 Brazilian cases that existed in 1967 and that potentially could expand, given that Brazil shares borders with almost every other South American country. SEP subtly sidestepped PAHO and worked out an agreement directly with the Brazilian Ministry of Health to launch a *Campanha de Erradicacão da Variola* (CEV). CEV undertook to vaccinate millions of people, delivering about 30 million vaccinations in 1970.[31] Thanks to these efforts, the last case of smallpox in the Americas was recorded in April 1971 in a Rio de Janeiro slum.

The archipelago of Indonesia, part of the WHO's Regional Office for South-East Asia (SEARO) and one of the world's most populous countries with about 135 million inhabitants, was another trouble spot. During the pre–World War II colonial period, it had virtually eliminated smallpox with mass vaccination. But the misery produced by Japanese occupation and the Dutch attempt to re-colonize led to the reintroduction of smallpox. A new national program based on mass vaccination began in 1967 and with little outside support managed to control smallpox in the major urban centers. Only in the late sixties did local health workers learn about surveillance and containment and begin to implement that strategy successfully. In 1972, an outbreak of more than 100 cases occurred in a remote location. Thanks to the surveillance and containment strategy, the outbreak was ended and no new cases occurred after 1972.[32]

The WHO's Western Pacific Region was never an active participant in the program because smallpox was minimal in the region. Most WPRO countries

---

[30] Donald A. Henderson, "Smallpox Eradication: A Cold War Victory," *World Health Forum* 19:2 (1988),113–119, p. 118; "$2 Billion Yearly Saving Expected from the Eradication of Smallpox," *The New York Times,* November 7, 1978.

[31] Gilberto Hochman, "Priority, Invisibility and Eradication: The History of Smallpox and the Brazilian Public Health Agenda," *Medical History* 53 (2009), 229–252.

[32] Vivek Neelakantan, "Eradicating Smallpox in Indonesia: The Archipelagic Challenge," *Health & History* 212:1 (2010), 61–87.

had enforced compulsory vaccination since the 1950s. In the late 1970s, it was confirmed that some countries in the region suspected of harboring smallpox were actually free of the disease: Cambodia, Vietnam, and China. In these countries late certification was due to political reasons. The People's Republic of China first joined the WHO's Western Pacific Region in 1972, a year after being admitted to the UN in place of Taiwan. Cambodia and Vietnam were involved in the Vietnam War until 1975. Cambodia had its last smallpox case in 1959, and after the end of the war the WHO initiated a program in Vietnam to terminate smallpox there.

The region where the complex relationships between SEP and local health authorities have been most extensively studied is SEARO, thanks to the work of Bhattacharya. It was in the highly endemic South Asian subcontinent, for example, where SEP officials had the complex task of negotiating with SEARO but also with officers from the Eastern Mediterranean Regional Office, EMRO, which included Pakistan. Bhattacharya argues that "adequate" technologies were not enough in this politically highly charged region, that adaptation was common, and that dissonance was not rare. His work demonstrates that Geneva officers did not have always full control of what happened in the field and suggests that the WHO's eradication program should be understood as a series of diverse local eradication campaigns.[33] Intensive and diverse negotiations in different regions of India also became obligatory because of the differing importance of political parties opposed to governments that chose whether or not to collaborate with eradication, and because an unexpected by-product of better surveillance was the surfacing of more small-pox cases, which some thought were evidence of a dramatic epidemic surge. But medical experts believed that the "surge" had to be seen against the low number of cases registered in the past due to underreporting. In the context of a 1974 outbreak of smallpox, the Indian Communist Party accused the United States of spreading the disease, and the SEP had to reach agreements with local communist cells to work in some regions. Negotiations were essential for the work in India to proceed.

A questionable method that demanded special negotiations was the more intensive use of cash rewards in the final stages of the program. Initially, small financial incentives to encourage people to report active cases were part of the WHO's intervention. The rewards became larger as the campaign developed. It was more commonly used in South-East Asia than in other regions but evidence suggests that it existed everywhere and was used by SEP officers willing to reach the target zero by any means necessary. They offered cash bounties to people who reported the first case of smallpox in a village, but they

---

[33] Sanjoy Bhattacharya, *Expunging Variola: The Control and Eradication of Smallpox in India, 1947–1977* (New Delhi: Orient Longman, 2006).

also resorted to coercive vaccinations carried out in military-style raids. These "carrot and stick" methods were promoted at SEP's highest levels because it was believed that local health workers were not always disseminating the information among the public because some were afraid the promised rewards would not materialize. But instructions came down the command chain that rewards were to be publicized via posters on walls, placards on public health vehicles, banners in fairs and festivals, and via radio, cinema, and press announcements. SEP leaders were convinced that it was a necessary step to transform a "passive" system of surveillance into an aggressive surveillance intervention, and aggressive surveillance sometimes was coupled with coercion. According to Greenough, the system of rewards and compulsory vaccination left a troubled legacy in some locations, compromising popular support for future immunization efforts.[34] For Reinhardt, although members of the SEP preferred persuasion and to "be nice," they did resort to coercion. In Somalia, for example, they set up isolation camps to hold the nomads for some days – although they did pay those nomads who worked in the construction of the camps and provided all who were isolated with free clothing at the end of their stay.[35]

The SEP sometimes confronted silent barriers and open skepticism on the part of local health organizations that believed that smallpox eradication was a misplaced priority. Some local health authorities would have preferred that the WHO emphasize basic health care or that the SEP would limit itself to providing the vaccine to health centers and hospitals, leaving to locals the task of vaccination. SEP's leaders believed that this would be a waste of resources because local health workers were frequently overwhelmed by competing health concerns. There was also jealousy among health programs because the smallpox program existed outside of routine services and enjoyed privileges in terms of resources and autonomy.

Africa was the scene of another kind of resistance to smallpox eradication, one inspired by popular cults and religious beliefs. Lay medical men called *fetisheiurs* believed that the disease was the expression of a deity, called *Saphona* in some African countries, that demanded worship. According to this belief, smallpox was impossible to defeat by human means alone because it was only this deity that could cause and cure smallpox.[36] *Fetisheiurs* relied on herbs and incantations as treatments and sometimes even used variolation, but the main "cure" consisted in reestablishing a balance between the patient, his family,

[34] Paul Greenough, "Intimidation, Coercion, and Resistance in the Final Stages of the South Asian Smallpox Eradication Campaign, 1973–1975," *Social Science and Medicine* 41:5 (1995), 633–645.

[35] Reinhardt, *The End of a Global Pox*, p. 145.

[36] Bernard D. Challenor, "Cultural Resistance to Smallpox Vaccination in West Africa," *Journal of Tropical Medicine and Hygiene* 73:3 (1971), 57–59.

his community, and nature. Other Africans distrusted any medical intervention, especially if it meant using a syringe, and believed that smallpox was lethal only to bad people who had used magic against others.[37] SEP officers confronted these beliefs head on and accused *fetisheiurs* of having vested interests since they inherited the possessions of people who died of smallpox.

India too had popular religious traditions that affected smallpox vaccination efforts.[38] Many Indians believed that smallpox's source was a capricious goddess, commonly called Sitala, who could prevent, mitigate, or in wrath, produce smallpox. People celebrated an annual festival for this deity and kept shrines and places of worship. As a result, in certain areas of India some simply refused vaccination. In other areas, communities were reluctant to allow their women or children to be examined by outsiders and resisted the isolation enforced on sick individuals. Isolation was resisted because in many rural areas relatives and friends were the safety net of the sick and there was a tradition to care for sick patients. An Indian health worker was convinced that religious resistance was the main obstacle to effective surveillance.[39]

In Ethiopia, smallpox vaccinators who tried to enter rural communities that had never before received Western medical doctors were driven away with sticks and stones. In one instance, a religious leader denounced the vaccinators as heretics who wanted to change local religious beliefs – and threw a hand grenade (kept from the Italian invasion during World War II) at a SEP helicopter. Fortunately, the health workers jumped and saved their lives.[40] In Bangladesh SEP members realized that they needed to supplement their helicopter visits with chocolate for children, which would facilitate the acquiescence of the population.[41] Religion was also used to advantage by SEP workers. For example, among Muslims religious events such as Ramadan and preparations for pilgrimage to Mecca were used as occasions to deploy vaccinators in strategic locations. Much of the progress in Ethiopia was possible thanks to a Brazilian, Ciro de Quadros, who was chief epidemiologist for the WHO's smallpox program in this country from 1970 to 1977 (and later applied the lessons he learned to eradicate polio in the Americas).

Thanks to SEP's achievements, the United States ended domestic smallpox vaccination in 1972, assuming that, although the disease still existed overseas,

---

[37] Richard Pankhurst, "The History and Traditional Treatment of Smallpox in Ethiopia," *Medical History* 9:4 (1965), 343–355.

[38] See Babagrahi Misra, "Sitala: The Smallpox Goddess of India," *Asian Folklore Studies* 28:2 (1969), 133–142.

[39] Interview with Zafar Husain, Smallpox Campaigner, India, *PBS* Series, www.pbs.org/wgbh/peoplescentury/episodes/livinglonger/husaintranscript.html, last accessed December 1, 2017.

[40] Ciro de Quadros, "The Last Challenge, the Horn of Africa," in Bhattacharya & Messenger (eds.), *The Global Eradication of Smallpox*, pp. 84–105, p. 93.

[41] Reinhardt, *The End of a Global Pox*, p. 143.

the likelihood of smallpox coming to the United States was small. At the same time, the UK, Chile, and Portugal, among others, made routine smallpox vaccination no longer obligatory. In 1981, the WHO removed smallpox from the international list of quarantinable diseases. By 1984 all countries had ceased smallpox vaccination of the general public and withdrew the requirement of a smallpox vaccination certificate for international travelers. In a related development, a discussion began about what to do with the variola virus still kept in laboratories.

Following a request made by the WHO, more than 75 laboratories began to destroy their samples or send them to the two most secure labs, collaborating WHO centers that kept them in liquid-nitrogen freezers. The locations of those two laboratories embodied the Cold War: the US Centers for Disease Control and Prevention laboratory in Atlanta and the laboratory of the State Research Institute for Viral Preparations in Moscow. Some experts considered the mere existence of the virus a menace and urged the destruction of all samples. The World Health Assembly and scientific task forces commissioned by the WHO recommended that the smallpox virus stocks be destroyed. Unfortunately, the distrust between the Soviet and American governments was still strong and became an obstacle to implementing this recommendation. The Americans and the Soviets both claimed that the virus was necessary for the design of antiviral drugs and diagnostic tools.

The 1990s and early twenty-first century witnessed a growing concern over the virus' weaponization. In 1992, Kanatjan Alibekov, Russia's biological warfare program's chief scientist, defected to the United States and revealed that, during and after the Cold War, the USSR had secretly used the smallpox virus to design a biological weapon. This was a matter of great concern in the West because of fears that this and other biological weapons existed in laboratories, perhaps in China, North-Korea, India, Iran, or even maintained by terrorist groups. People were now generally unprotected against smallpox because physicians and nurses were no longer familiar with the disease, routine immunization had stopped, and young people were still vulnerable. Since the mid-1990s, the Pentagon pushed to retain the smallpox virus for the development of biological defenses.

A unusual turn of events came a month after the terrorist attacks on the World Trade Center and the Pentagon in September 2001. A series of anthrax-laced letters in the United States created a wave of fear and an upsurge of profound concern about "bioterrorism." Shortly thereafter, the US military reinstituted smallpox vaccination for its personnel, and President Bush asked Henderson to head a new office of public health preparedness. Henderson, however, did not approve the initial plans – never actually implemented – to vaccinate the entire US population because in his mind the possible side effects of vaccination outweighed the harm that could possibly result from bioterrorist attack. He also had serious reservations about the medical value of research that could be conducted with the smallpox virus. Some physicians, scientists, and politicians, mainly from the United States, now proposed at world health forums that preserving and studying the smallpox virus was crucial because the danger existed of reintroducing the disease. The 2002 World Health Assembly yielded to American concerns and conceded that smallpox research programs be allowed at authorized laboratories for an indefinite period. At the same time, many former members of SEP remained proponents of destroying the known stocks of the virus and insisted that no containment system was free of risk for accidental or deliberate release. The issue is still pending to this day.

Final Remarks

A contentious debate has developed in public health over the merits of global smallpox eradication. Critics argue that it was wrong to use scarce funds to concentrate efforts on one disease in countries where people suffered many illnesses. The same critics claim that the eradication program diverted the best staff and resources and led health systems to ignore other needs. Cynics believed that people were spared smallpox deaths only to fall to other deadly diseases. But supporters of smallpox eradication were convinced that SEP added resources to existing health services, that their work emphasized adaptation to local conditions, and that enhancing pride in the achievement was good for everyone involved in public health because it generated momentum for broader programs.

A statue commemorating the 30th anniversary of the eradication of smallpox was unveiled in front of the agency's headquarters in 2010, confirming a landmark moment in the memory of the WHO. Yet smallpox eradication's success was anything but clear and straightforward. It began with a World Health Assembly resolution in 1958 that was not supported with an adequate budget. The initiative gained momentum in the mid-1960s with US support, a concurrent US bilateral program in Africa, and the rapid and successful transition from mass vaccination to the surveillance and containment strategy. SEP flourished in the 1970s, not least because of Henderson's leadership and strong US-Soviet collaboration. There were moments when success appeared uncertain and contradictory declarations dominated. For example, jubilant WHO officials announced in November of 1975 that the Asian continent was free of smallpox and just a few days later had to take back the statement when new outbreaks appeared.[42]

---

[42] Barry Kramer, "UN Agency Says Asia Is Smallpox-Free with Total Eradication Just Weeks Away," *The Wall Street Journal*, November 14, 1975; "WHO Takes Back Statement That Asia Is Free of Smallpox," *The Wall Street Journal*, November 24, 1975.

Unanticipated political and cultural victories marked the path of smallpox eradication success. The program began as a bilateral initiative linked to a conventional model of development, but SEP's staff gained relative autonomy and overcame the tradition of multilateral agencies being subservient to political powers as they increasingly exercised legitimate international authority. SEP was thus one of the few examples in the WHO's history where the agency transcended its conventional role as the coordinator of a collection of national initiatives and conducted a successful program at least partially in what Akira Iriye calls "global space."[43] In addition and at the same time, thanks to the smallpox program political and medical leaders in developing countries came to understand the power of their nations as political actors. They enhanced their people's health status but also learned how to behave to negotiate successfully with multilateral agencies and to play the United States and USSR off one another. Finally, it is necessary to emphasize that the smallpox program's success derived significantly from human agency. Lambim, Foege, Henderson, Candau, de Quadros, Mahendra Dutta, and the WHO's Director-General Half-dan Malher, among others, were compelling charismatic leaders who convinced political and medical leaders, tribal chiefs, and local vaccinators to persist in pursuing the goal of worldwide eradication. Their examples suggest that outstanding international public leaders can make a real difference.

---

[43] Akira Iriye, *Global Community: The Role of International Organizations in the Making of the Contemporary World* (Berkeley: University of California Press, 2002).

6 The Transition from "Family Planning" to "Sexual and Reproductive Rights"

During the 1960s, as the global malaria eradication program waned and smallpox eradication began to take shape, international and national health agencies focused on a new priority: the impact of population growth on health and development. This meant reorganizing international health and involved calling into question some of the basic assumptions of public health. In most countries, it was also seen as an example of the technocratic perspective that hoped to solve social problems by means of a magic bullet that drew on medical technology.

Public health has traditionally been pronatalist and has supported population growth for both its economic benefits and as a means of protecting the well-being of mothers and children. In around 1960, there was a revival of Malthusianism (Thomas Malthus published his *Essay on Population* in the eighteenth century). Unprecedented rates of population growth were perceived by sociologists, demographers, and economists as hindering economic development because they drew scarce resources to "nonproductive" segments of society (such as the elderly and children), contributing to underemployment and more uneven distributions of income. Foreign-aid programs for poor countries were thought to be nullified by the rapid pace of population growth. Population control was portrayed as a necessary condition for development. A by-product of the revival of Malthus' ideas was that disease-control activities in developing countries were perceived as counterproductive because they decreased the death rate and led to a rise in the number of poor people and an increase in their life spans.

Between 1950 and 1980, first private philanthropic organizations, then bilateral and multilateral organizations disseminated effective and low-cost contraceptive devices for birth control across the globe. These devices were usually tested in developing countries, under the title of "family planning" programs. During the 1980s, these programs suffered critiques and pronatalist policies were revived, in line with the conservative ethos of the decade. By the mid-1990s, new concern with population issues emerged and the terms "family planning" and "birth control" were replaced by new concepts advocated by the UN, including "sexual and reproductive health," "women's rights," and "sexual and reproductive rights," pointing to a paradigm shift. The purpose of this chapter is, first, to analyze the transition from the family-planning programs of the 1960s, which received belated and only tepid support from the WHO, to the sexual and reproductive health perspectives of the 1980s and 1990s, which were embraced by the health agency.

Preparing a Consensus

Concerns about implementing population programs in the early twentieth century can be traced to a number of sources, including the work of feminist Margaret Sanger, the influence of eugenics (a controversial "socio-medical" perspective held by right-wing and leftist doctors, intellectuals, and politicians), and to a few developing countries, such as India, that established birth-control clinics in the 1930s. Another advocate of birth control during the interwar period was the Planned Parenthood Federation, a private organization that expanded after 1952 when it created an international branch called the International Planned Parenthood Federation, IPPF. Much of this work did not became public policy until the late 1950s for several reasons: the baby boom in the United States gave credence to the idea that a family with several children was good per se; the expectation that women had to fulfill traditional domestic roles such as motherhood; and on account of a generalized belief in many countries that birth control and sex education were too sensitive as social and religious issues in opposition to Christian beliefs.

During the 1950s, private organizations and scholars from developed nations pushed back against the prevailing view that was pronatalist. Together, they created a core body of knowledge and expertise and provided the basis for policies implemented by US federal agencies in the 1960s.[1] Among these agencies was the Population Council, that had been established in 1952 by John D. Rockefeller III as an autonomous nonprofit organization that was independent of the Rockefeller Foundation whose trustees did not wish to focus on population control and whose members had held different opinions on the issue. The Council placed an emphasis on research. It also distributed a small number of contraceptives. This agency was convinced that the solution to backwardness in developing countries was a reduction in their rate of fertility, ideally via voluntary family planning. The Council was helped by the Ford Foundation (FF), which had been created in 1936 but only became an international philanthropic organization around 1947 (a change reinforced by the decision to transfer its headquarters from Michigan to New York City in 1953). The FF was convinced of the need for a worldwide reduction in fertility.

---

[1] See Marshall Green, "The Evolution of US International Population Policy, 1965–92: A Chronological Account," *Population and Development Review* 19:2 (1993), 303–321.

Thanks to grants from the Population Council and the Ford Foundation, researchers developed new contraceptives, such as the intrauterine contraceptive device (known as the IUD) and launched new public family-planning programs. Between 1952 and 1968, the FF gave about USD 100 million to population programs all around the world, donations that were coordinated by a Population Office established in 1963. Three years later, in 1966, the program became a subdivision of an international division of the Foundation (and remained so until 1981, when it once again became an independent program after the Foundation was restructured). India, the second most populous country in the world after China, received significant aid from the FF. The Foundation provided USD 9 million to India in the year 1958 alone.[2] This aid was welcomed by the Indian government of Pandit Nehru (1947–1964), who believed that economic development without birth control would be futile because any increase in productivity would be absorbed by the growing number of people. Nehru was going against the ideas of Mahatma Gandhi, the leader of Indian independence, who was opposed to contraception. Initially the family-planning program consisted of a series of specialized clinics opened in the country by the government and voluntary organizations that provided conventional contraceptive services and devices for women such as diaphragms. In the 1960s, a more energetic campaign promoted the notion of an ideal family with few children and provided more contraceptive methods, relying on auxiliary nurse-midwives for women and family planning health assistants for men. Later, the Indian family program became an integral part of maternal and child health care services. Along with India, only a few other developing countries launched population programs, including Pakistan (1960) and South Korea (1961). In 1962, the Chinese government began to promote sterilization and intrauterine devices, using its own resources to curb a fertility rate that was the highest in the developing world and was particularly acute among rural populations, which accounted for about 80 percent of the country's inhabitants.[3] In sum, the Population Council, the FF, and to a lesser degree the IPPF, helped to create a consensus among policy makers in industrialized countries and provided the funds to develop the first international family-planning programs.

A number of scholars, activists, and popular authors of the late 1950s and 1960s reinforced the Neo-Malthusian-inspired idea that the race between the production of natural resources and population growth was going to end in a

---

[2] A discussion of the work of the Ford by its leaders in the field is Oscar Harkavy, Lyle Saunders, & Anna L. Southam, "An Overview of the Ford Foundation's Strategy for Population Work," *Demography* 5:2 (1968), 541–552.

[3] See Tyrene White, *China's Longest Campaign: Birth Planning in the People's Republic, 1949–2005* (Ithaca: Cornell University Press, 2006).

global disaster. A popular study was the 1968 best-selling book *The Popula-tion Bomb,* authored by Stanford University's Professor Paul R. Ehrlich.[4] The World Bank's president, Eugene Black, endorsed another book, by the econo-mist Joseph M. Jones, titled *Does Overpopulation Mean Poverty?* Black's preface urged for the restraint of population growth in order to maintain hopes of economic progress in Asia and the Middle East.[5]

The concern about overpopulation was linked to a criticism of the work done by the WHO and other health organizations. Despite the fact that the global malaria eradication program had fallen short of its objectives, many experts blamed "miracle drugs and insecticides" for the decline in infectious diseases within a context of high birth rates and poor living conditions. For these critics, malaria eradication had incited a "population explosion" in developing countries with concomitant pressure on subsistence resources. A newspaper article attributed the decline in the death rate to: "an increase in trained medical and paramedical personnel, DDT spraying, vaccination for tuberculosis, the services of trained midwives" and held US bilateral aid and the World Health Organization responsible.[6]

In the late 1950s, the US government commissioned a report on population growth, an indication that interest in this theme had passed from private to federal agencies. The report ended by affirming that assistance to economic growth in poor nations might be eroded by the rapid pace of population growth. Its author was General William Draper, an investment banker who had formerly served as undersecretary of the US Army and played a leading role in population control discussions. Initially, in 1959, President Eisenhower did not endorse the report and declared that birth control was not the responsi-bility of the federal government, but after a few years the US government, and Eisenhower himself, began to support family-planning programs. The motiv-ation for US foreign policy makers was a fear that communism could gain a foothold among desperate people in poor overcrowded nations where demands for social services could not be met. During the early 1960s, the US govern-ment began to promote family programs at home and in developing countries. An early decision in this direction was made by the Food and Drug Adminis-tration, FDA, which in 1960 approved the marketing of the oral contraceptive pill, Enovid, that in a few years would become a multimillion dollar business (subsequently, in 1968, a modernized intrauterine device was approved). Both were portrayed as effective, harmless, and low-cost technological fixes to the

---

[4] Paul E. Elrich, *The Population Bomb* (New York: Ballantine Books, 1968).

[5] Joseph M. Jones, *Does Overpopulation Mean Poverty? The Facts about Population Growth and Economic Development* (Washington, DC: Center for International Economic Growth, 1962), p. 35.

[6] S. Chandrasekhar, "A Billion Indians by 2000 A.D.?" *The New York Times*, April 4, 1965, p. 32.

population problem. It is worth pointing out that the global population in 1960 was approximately 3 billion and the number of women in developing countries who were not using any form of contraception was around 350 million. These figures were striking at the time, and there was a fear that they would grow rapidly.[7] New drugs and interventions complemented sterilization (forced or voluntary) and became a panacea for overpopulation problems all over the world.

In 1963, Dean Rusk, President Kennedy's secretary of state and the former head of the Rockefeller Foundation, issued a memorandum to USAID missions abroad stating that they should assist requests for family-planning services. This was even before bilateral European agencies, notably the Swedish International Development Agency, SIDA, supported family planning. A symbolic decision occurred a year later: Eisenhower became honorary co-chair (with former President Truman) of the Planned Parenthood Federation. Both former presidents called for expanding family-planning programs, at home and abroad. These activities were based on the premise that women from poor nations wanted contraception methods. A corollary development was USAID's creation of an Office of Population in 1965. By the end of 1966, officers from USAID, the Peace Corps, the US Information Agency, and the State Department (including ambassadors) were instructed to pay careful consideration to help any country to limit "excessive rates" of population growth.[8] These events marked a departure from the traditional, cautious, American foreign policy toward birth control. During its first eight years, USAID's Population Office granted about USD 500 million for contraception methods and family-planning programs all over the world.[9] This figure was more than half of the international assistance provided from all sources for these types of programs during the period from 1965 to 1973.

Between 1965 and 1968, the US congressman and physician Ernest Gruening organized a series of "Population Crisis" hearings at the US Senate, with support from the Government's Operations Committee on Foreign Aid Expenditures. These hearings attracted public attention and press coverage and created a favorable climate of opinion about birth control.[10] USAID spent vast sums convincing developing country governments that family-planning programs were key to their economic growth. The trend was reinforced with

---

[7] Alexander Kessler, "Family Planning and the Role of WHO," *World Health* 47:3 (1994), 4–6.

[8] United States Agency for International Development, *Population Program Assistance, Annual report 1975* (Washington, DC: USAID, 1976), p. 12.

[9] B. Mass, "A Historical Sketch in the American Population Control Movement," *International Journal of Health Services* 4:4 (1974), 651–676, p. 663.

[10] United States, Congress, Senate, Committee on Government Operations, Subcommittee on Foreign Aid Expenditures, *Population Crisis: Hearings, Eighty-Ninth Congress, First Session* (Washington, DC: US Government Printing Office, 1966).

President Johnson's 1965 State of the Union address where he referred to the menace of global population growth.[11] In the same year, he addressed a UN meeting celebrating its 20th anniversary with a statement that made clear that family planning was a cost-effective priority: "Less than five dollars invested in population control is worth a hundred dollars invested in economic growth."[12] Johnson's administration's use of family planning as a cheaper foreign-policy "silver bullet" program was important because his government was tied up in the Vietnam War, social protests at home, and other urgent domestic problems such as the provision of civil rights to ethnic minorities in the United States. Johnson also found a domestic dimension to his support of family planning. His "war on poverty" implied the "assistance" of poor families to reduce the number of children they had.

Toward the end of his administration, President Johnson directed USAID to move decisively into population programs all over the world. In his 1967 State of the Union message, he again dealt with population programs, which he considered to be key to the "pursuit of peace" (a Cold War euphemism). Johnson also created the post of deputy assistant secretary for population and family planning in the Department of Health, Education, and Welfare (HEW). In 1968, he enacted a Foreign Assistance Act that gave the Congress a specific mandate to carry out family-planning programs in developing countries and earmarked USD 35 million for worldwide family-planning programs.[13]

Under presidents Richard Nixon, Gerald Ford, and Jimmy Carter, curbing population growth in developing nations became a common bipartisan issue. USAID's Population Office received substantial resources and personnel. In 1969, President Nixon delivered to Congress the first specific presidential message on population growth, calling it a crucial issue and urging the UN to respond to the challenge.[14] Following Nixon's lead, in 1970 the US Congress approved a Population Research Act that created an Office of Family Planning and ensured federal legislation for enlarging subsidized population control programs. As a result, the American FDA, and its advisory Committee on Obstetrics and Gynecology, adopted a more lenient attitude toward the use of new oral contraceptives and intrauterine devices (by the late 1960s, contraceptive methods included IUD insertion, tubal ligation, vasectomy, oral pills,

---

[11] Mentioned in United States Agency for International Development, *Population Program Assistance Report 1975* (Washington, DC: USAID, 1976), p. 11.

[12] Johnson's statement of January 12, 1966, in United States Agency for International Development, *Population Program Assistance, United States Aid to Developing Countries* (Washington, DC: US Government Printing Office, 1974), vol. 2, p. 20.

[13] United States, Department of State, *The Foreign Assistance Program, Annual Report to the Congress, Fiscal Year 1968* (Washington, DC: US Government Printing Office, 1968), p. 11.

[14] United States Agency for International Development, Committee on Government Operations, Subcommittee on Foreign Aid Expenditures, *Population Crisis: Hearings, Eighty-Ninth Congress, First Session* (Washington, DC: US Government Printing Office, 1966), vol. 1, p. 7.

condoms, and spermicides). Around the same time, the Supreme Court made a landmark decision in the Roe versus Wade case (1973) that recognized a woman's right to choose abortion to terminate her pregnancy. As a result, most American medical doctors were no longer reluctant to perform the procedure, resulting in the opening of abortion clinics across the United States.

Although, by the end of 1969, more than seventy USAID officers worked with family-planning activities and contraceptives were eligible for financial assistance in overseas programs, initially much of the work of the bilateral agency was carried out by international NGOs, such as the Pathfinder Fund, a Massachusetts-based group. USAID supported Pathfinder in opening regional and country offices in Africa, Asia, and Latin America. By 1973, the USAID budget for population activities was almost USD 2 billion, or 6.3 percent of its total foreign aid. Ray T. Ravenholt, a controversial epidemiologist who strongly believed in contraceptives and was accused of portraying pregnancy of poor women as a disease to be eradicated, headed USAID's Population Office during its most active years (1976–1979).

In this new political atmosphere, governments from developing countries embraced population-control and birth-control policies to reduce fertility, with a more rapid uptake in Latin America and Asia, compared with Africa. Nonetheless, abortion – which was removed from the criminal code in the United States, Canada, and Western Europe – continued to be a controversial theme. Most developing countries only authorized it when it was necessary to preserve the life of the pregnant woman, rarely when pregnancy was the result of rape, and usually required the spouse's permission. In Muslim countries, repressive legislation on abortion persisted. During the 1970s and 1980s, many poor nations began to revise their population legislation and policies and launched family-planning programs to limit population growth, with the possibility of resorting to abortion. According to a 1974 USAID report: "Ten years ago comparatively few nations and organizations were tackling the problem. Today there are many."[15]

The governments of developing nations targeted poor women and marginalized ethnic minorities for contraception and sterilization that frequently was forced upon people. The decision to target women was based on male resistance, technological advances, and gender and even race discrimination. Male physicians, who were usually white and part of the middle class or the elite, targeted poor women for sterilization or IUD insertion while withholding access to short-term oral contraceptive measures (under the assumption that the poor were not disciplined enough to stick to the pill). With the exception of

---

[15] United States Agency for International Development, *Population Program Assistance, United States Aid to Developing Countries* (Washington, DC: US Government Printing Office, 1974), p. 1.

India, which encouraged surgical sterilization of men (vasectomy), most governments were reluctant to accept this contraceptive intervention, one of the reasons being that men feared impotency resulting from what was then an irreversible procedure. India was an exceptional case, reaching more than 1 million vasectomies in 1970, and thereby exceeding the total number of sterilized males in the rest of the world. However, the Indian program had a social and race component because it focused on lower-caste untouchables and poor Muslims.

Technology and market demands also helped. First, during the 1970s, modern lubricated condoms for men were developed, restrictions to condom sales were lifted in many countries, and advertisements made them popular. Secondly, laparoscopic sterilization became popular in the 1970s. This novel and cheap surgical technique consisted of an operation in the woman's abdomen by means of small incisions that made the tubal ligation procedure easier and more popular among physicians since it could be made under local anesthesia and on an outpatient basis. By the mid-1970s, a significant number of middle- and upper-class women in the industrialized world and in middle-income countries used the pill, and most poor women in developing countries resorted to sterilization and IUD as means of contraception. For many private and multilateral agencies, this was the result of years of preaching for world-wide awareness of the population problem.

During the late 1960s and early 1970s, a number of American scientists strongly believed that compulsory sterilization was the only sound method of birth control in poor countries. A newspaper article explained the advantage of sterilization: "it solves the problem, once and for all."[16] One study reported that during the 1970s there was a global fivefold increase in the number of sterilizations and that in 1977 alone, 75 million couples had chosen sterilization.[17]

In 1971, the Population Council organized a small meeting on population growth and economic development at the Rockefeller Foundation Center in Bellagio, Italy. The speakers were leaders of the population movement: Bernard Berelson, president of the Population Council and former officer of the Ford Foundation; the economist David Bell, former officer at USAID and the Ford Foundation; Oscar Harkavy, who had been with Ford's population programs since 1953; Joel Bernstein, a senior officer at USAID; and Allan Barnes from the Rockefeller Foundation. They discussed a report that predicted that population growth would be the second biggest global problem

---

[16] Chandrasekhar, "A Billion Indians by 2000 A.D.?" p. 34.

[17] P. Bordahl, "Tubal Sterilization: A Historical Review," *Journal of Reproductive Medicine* 30:1 (1985), 18–24, and Joanne Omang, "Sterilization Is Top Method of Birth Control in America," *The Washington Post*, May 22, 1977, p. 3.

after a possible "nuclear catastrophe."[18] Although a WHO officer attended this meeting, the health agency was a late entrant to the population field and followed the lead of private and bilateral organizations.

The UN, the WHO, and Population Debates

With the exception of the World Bank, which supported family-planning programs in the early 1960s, most organizations within the UN system, such as the WHO, were slow, reluctant even, to respond to the challenges posed by population growth. As mentioned elsewhere in this book, Brock Chisholm was unable to establish a population program at the WHO basically because of Catholic opposition. Communist nations shared with Catholic governments their opposition to working with population issues, if for different reasons. In the first instance, Marxists had traditionally dismissed Malthusian ideas. The Soviet Union considered concerns with high rates of population growth to be a bourgeois excuse for the inadequacies of capitalism and family-planning programs to be a capitalist diversion to stop potential revolutionaries from being born in the developing World. During the postwar period, the Soviet Union and communist Eastern European nations adopted pronatalist population policies and restricted access to contraception because their populations had declined dramatically during World War II. The Soviets had legalized abortion in the 1920s but Stalin then made abortion illegal in the late 1930s, a prohibition that persisted for decades.

In the same way, in developing nations, nationalist, anti-imperialist, and populist regimes and independence movements embraced pronatalist arguments in the belief that their countries ought to be more populous because their main problems were related to social exploitation and not to an excess number of inhabitants. African nationalists in Zimbabwe, for example, were hostile to family planning upon its introduction in the late 1950s, arguing that it was part of a plot to control the black population. These opinions paralyzed the WHO from taking any definitive stand on population issues.

During the 1960s, UN agencies – and the WHO in particular – avoided active participation in the "overpopulation debates," considering such debates to be a scientific issue that was only of interest to demographers.[19] For some

---

[18] The Population Council, "Status Report," p. 6, March 30, 1971, Meetings of the Interim Committee of the Bellagio Population Group, Folder P/13/80/7, Second Generation of Files [WHO].

[19] See Gary R. Kyzr-Sheeley, "The Evolution of Population Policies in the World Health Organization, the World Bank and the United Nations Fund for Population Activities," unpublished PhD Dissertation, Indiana University (1980), and Stanley P. Johnson, *World Population and the United Nations: Challenge and Response* (Cambridge: Cambridge University Press, 1987).

time, the UN argued that they could not take a stand because there was insufficient information on population size, rate of growth, and distribution in developing countries. They subscribed to modest demographic goals such as carrying out at least one reliable national population census every ten years, an objective difficult to achieve in some regions because many African nations had never taken any population census at all. Another reason why UN specialized agencies resisted supporting family-planning programs was that they implicitly suggested that the disease-control and nutritional programs that had been an integral part of the WHO's work could still be a priority.

The health and nutritional programs launched by the WHO and the UN Food and Agriculture Organization, FAO, were based on the assumption that they would protect and increase the populations of middle-income and developing countries. In response to the argument of the growing gap between population size and natural resources, these agencies asserted that new technologies would solve the problem. Until the mid-1960s, the WHO's director-general, Marcolino Candau, was convinced that a separate family-planning program in the agency would lead to a reduction in funding for the control of malaria and other infectious diseases. In a 1954 dinner with officers of the Rockefeller Foundation, he avoided questions on birth control and insisted that he had to act according to instructions received from the General Assembly, for the moment had to "stay away" from birth control, and saw this as a program more suited to private agencies.[20] A US proposal for making the agency the leader in family-planning programs was rebuffed at the World Health Assembly of 1966, which approved a watered-down resolution offering advice upon request by member nations. Candau also had some doubts about the new contraceptive techniques that became popular in the 1960s. A newspaper article from 1967 quoted Candau as saying that "oral contraceptives," such as the pill and IUD, were not "ideal," and their use demanded careful study in developing regions.[21]

It took some negotiating to convince the WHO. According to a memorandum of 1968, John D. Rockefeller had lunch with Marcolino Candau and other population experts in New York City, where the "very sensitive and cautious" director-general understood the problem but explained that he doubted very much whether the WHO could help in family-planning programs and suggested that the work should be carried out by private agencies. In the memorandum, Candau is described as prepared "to take WHO as far as abortion, but not sterilization," since the Brazilian believed that an attempt to move faster might result in a setback for the "whole family program." He also believed that

[20] A brief report of the dinner is in "Marcolino G. Candau, New York, October 14, 1954," RFA, RG 2–1954, Series 100, Box 8, Folder 57, RAC.
[21] "WHO Head Asks Study of Contraceptive Means," *The New York Times*, May 4, 1967, p. 9.

abortions could be carried out for personal or medical reasons where it was legal and that it was necessary to make abortions safe, especially in countries where abortion was legal in a limited number of circumstances. In the long term, Candau's priority was to educate doctors, "who had never before thought of [family planning]," and draw a connection with maternal and child health.[22] His remorse was based on the likely resistance of members of the world health assemblies.

During the mid-1960s, the WHO was under pressure from member countries and bilateral agencies and from the UN. In 1969, the head of the USAID population office described the relationship between his organization and the UN in a cordial but patronizing tone, saying that his organization was ahead of the UN, which would "follow trails blazed" by USAID.[23] The WHO yielded to pressure but maintained its emphasis on a comprehensive approach, kept a clear link with Family Health (emphasizing the health risks of adolescent pregnancy and little spacing between births as well as pre- and postnatal care), and did not promote sterilization programs. (Figure 6.1 depicts a health center setting.) The pressure came from some member countries such as Sweden, India, and the United States, and later, Japan, West Germany, Norway, and Canada. The WHO's friendlier attitude toward family planning was encouraged by a change in the Soviet Union's traditional position on the issue. In the late 1960s, the USSR sought methods for curbing birth as a means of addressing the high rate of illegal and unsafe abortions that had unofficially become a means of birth control. By the late 1960s, the Soviet Union and other communist countries had begun to view family planning – which they preferred to call "demographic development" – in a more positive light. Demographic development meant combining family planning with development policies in the belief that the economic development of a country would bring a drop in its birth rate, in line with what had happened in most industrialized countries. In 1965, the UN General Assembly took a major step in support of family planning when it passed a resolution calling all agencies to assist in developing family-planning training facilities, information, and services when requested by governments. The resolution was carefully phrased to specify that no operational activities would be imposed.[24] In 1966, UNICEF followed suit with a similarly cautious decision in the wake of an Executive Board meeting that was devoted to the discussion of family planning. Henry R. Labouisse, UNICEF's executive director, had no intention of persuading any country

[22] "Memo 25 October 1968," Collection Population Council, Series Administration Files, Box 34, Folder WHO correspondence, RAC.

[23] Cited in Mass, "A Historical Sketch," p. 667.

[24] "WHO Authorized to Give Members Birth-Control Data," *The New York Times*, May 22, 1965, p. 33.

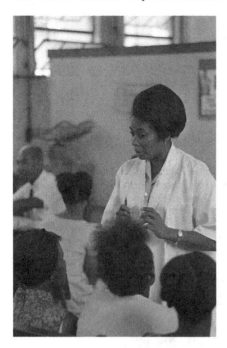

Figure 6.1 Women are shown various contraceptive methods at the Victoria
Jubilee Maternity Hospital in Kingston, Jamaica, in 1970. This was part of the
family-planning campaign of the Pan American Health Organization, the
Regional Office for the Americas of the World Health Organization.
Credit WHO/Edward Rice. Courtesy: World Health Organization Photo Library.

to adopt population control policies, nor of providing technical advice or
supplying contraceptives.[25]

From the late 1960s onward, World Health Assembly resolutions have
recognized the importance of family planning, but as part of the delivery of
maternal and child services (that were usually dismissed in traditional vertical family-planning programs). A 1968 World Health Assembly Resolution
recognized family planning as a component of "basic health services," or
balanced health infrastructures. The health agency was concerned about the
vertical implementation of family-planning programs and about coercive
methods that might be imposed on parents. The following year, the World

---

[25] Henry R. Labouisse, "Family Planning, Introductory Statement to the Executive Board," May
25, 1966, Collection Henry R. Labouisse Papers MC199, Mudd Manuscript Library, Series
2 United Nations, Subseries 2C: United Nations Children's Fund (UNICEF), Box 20, Folder 2,
Princeton University Library, Department of Rare Books and Special Collections
[hereafter PUL].

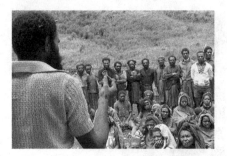

Figure 6.2 A heath worker in Papua Guinea demonstrates a contraceptive device before an attentive audience of both sexes in 1976.
Credit WHO/Jose Abcede. Courtesy: World Health Organization Photo Library.

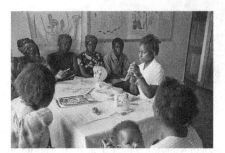

Figure 6.3 A class on the use of contraceptives in a specialized clinic in Kampala, Uganda, in 1968.
Credit WHO/Eric Schwab. Courtesy: World Health Organization Photo Library.

Health Assembly underlined that family size should remain a matter of parental choice but recognized the need to provide information on different methods and was careful to recognize that it was not the responsibility of the organization to endorse any specific population policy. The issues that the WHO considered to be of special interest were maternal and infant health care and infertility programs (meaning antenatal care), and natal and post-natal care, as well as child immunization. For WHO officers, family planning was seen as a means to reduce both maternal mortality caused by the growing number of illegal abortions and infant mortality. (Examples of the educational dimension of the campaign on family planning appear in Figures 6.2 and 6.3.) They emphasized the need for a medical framework of family-planning services because only when parents were certain that their children would survive the diseases that used to plague them in their early years, would they be willing to embrace the ideal of a small family. According to the WHO, these findings reinforced the idea that holistic medical services

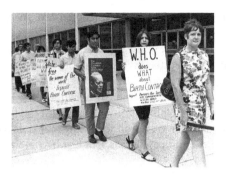

Figure 6.4 Pro–birth control demonstrators protest outside the 22nd World
Health Organization Assembly taking place at the War Memorial Auditorium
in Boston on July 23, 1969. They protest against the WHO's timid role in
family-planning and birth-control programs.
Photo by Jack O'Connell/The Boston Globe via Getty Images.

were better prepared to reach women and provide care, advice, and postpartum family-planning services. In 1969, the WHO supported 20 countries
in the introduction of family-planning activities. (However, as Figure 6.4
indicates, American pro–birth control activists believed the WHO was not
doing enough in family planning.) A decisive move by the WHO into
population themes came a year later with the creation of the Special Program
of Research, Development and Training in Human Reproduction (also
known as Special Program of Research in Human Reproduction, HRP). Its
first director was the American physician Alexander Kessler, who had trained
in New York and Harvard universities and had worked at the WHO's
Division of Family Health since 1966. The program was "special" because
it was to be funded from outside the regular WHO budget (like most of the
malaria eradication operations). One of the program's innovations was its
focus on research and training. It signaled a moment at which the WHO was
willing to tie the voluntary contributions and financial resources of other
agencies to specific objectives. HRP trained thousands of experts and coordinated and evaluated international research in human reproduction.[26] Initially, the Program concentrated on support for fertility research, studies on
effective, safe, and acceptable contraceptives, the improvement of maternal
and infant care, and the control of sexually transmitted diseases. It also
helped to establish a global network of research centers. One of the first
was the WHO Collaborating Centre in Research and Research Training in

---

[26] A. Kessler, G. W. Perkin, & C. Standley, "The WHO Expanded Research Programme in
Human Reproduction," *Contraception* 5:5 (1972), 423–428.

Human Reproduction in Stockholm. The Program organized an epidemiological study, codirected by the noted epidemiologist Abdel R. Omran, to examine the relationships between family formation, family health, and socioeconomic conditions that favored the involvement of women in family-planning programs. Another theme examined by the Program was the declining birthrate, a matter of growing concern in industrial nations. By 1971, the WHO had begun to actively seek funds for family planning for the first time. This turn of events revealed another motivation for the agency's decision to embrace population control: the significant funds that had become available for these programs.

Although the WHO made considerable progress, its position was seen as too cautious by other organizations. Some bilateral officers and population experts did not want population programs to be in the hands of physicians. Critics believed that health officers might downgrade demographic targets or dilute family planning in clinical services. As a result, the WHO was not fully trusted to conduct family planning, and in 1969, private donors and bilateral agencies created the United Nations Population Fund, UNFPA.[27] This new multilateral agency was given the mandate to coordinate government efforts on family planning and to operate through country offices. In 1971, the UN General Assembly designated the new agency as responsible for playing a leading role in promoting population programs across the world. Its budget was made up of voluntary contributions and the organization received sizeable funding from USAID. University professor, diplomat, and government official Rafael Salas from the Philippines was the organization's first executive director, holding the post from 1969 to 1987. He stressed the dangers of an urban population boom, at a time when many experts forecast that by the year 2000, most of the world's population would live in overcrowded cities.

After some initial tension and negotiations, the UNFPA found its niche in the web of international agencies. In the early 1970s, a World Bank-UNFPA project began to support Indonesia in limiting its population growth. The project was aligned with the ideas advocated by the WHO and included the construction of maternal and child-care services and family-planning clinics, activities that would normally be considered to be under the remit of the WHO. After some negotiations, the WHO convinced the UNFPA and the World Bank that its participation was important in all projects with a health component, so that subsequently any overlap between the UNFPA and the WHO was

---

[27] Created as the United Nations Fund for Population Activities and renamed in 1987 as the United Nations Population Fund, but the acronym UNFPA remained unchanged, see Rafael M. Salas, *International Population Assistance: The First Decade: A Look at the Concepts and Policies Which Have Guided the UNFPA in Its First Ten Years* (New York: Pergamon Press, 1979).

deliberately avoided. However, the role of the UNFPA was hegemonic because it provided much of the funds earmarked for the WHO's population programs. In November 1973, the WHO signed an agreement with the World Bank, negotiated by Mahler and Robert S. McNamara, former secretary of defense in the Kennedy and Johnson administrations and, since 1968, president of the World Bank, to develop population programs. As a result, health experts were added to the Bank's population missions, and regional offices and country representatives worked together with these missions. Three years later, the WHO signed a Memorandum of Understanding with the IPPF that established the basis for close consultation and collaboration. However, it was the UNFPA that maintained supremacy over population programs during the first half of the 1970s.

The year 1974 was designated "World Population Year" by the UN General Assembly as a way of driving forward population policies and catalyzing the work of various agencies and organizations. In the same year, the UN sponsored a World Population Conference in Bucharest, Romania. The conference, which was inaugurated by UN Secretary-General Kurt Waldheim, occurred at a time when experts predicted a world population of 6.5 billion by the year 2000, an unprecedented figure.[28] The Bucharest Conference was different from previous demographic conferences organized by the UN because it focused on how to encourage developing countries' governments to embrace more fully family-planning programs. Delegates from industrial nations were in favor of these programs, but they had to confront resistance from representatives of most developing nations that criticized the imposition of isolated population-control programs to the exclusion of overall socioeconomic aid for development. In a famous statement, the minister of health of India affirmed at this meeting that "development" was the best contraceptive. The final document produced by the conference, which had the telling title of "Action Plan," was a compromise between the two approaches and established a link between "development" and "family-planning programs."[29]

In 1975, the WHO's Special Program of Research in Human Reproduction launched a task force for the development of long-acting contraceptives that were not produced by the established pharmaceutical industries. The WHO helped to demonstrate the safety and reliability of Depo-Provera (depo-medroxyprogesterone acetate), an injectable contraceptive that offered women

---

[28] Susan Greenhalgh, "The Social Construction of Population Science: An Intellectual, Institutional, and Political History of Twentieth-Century Demography," *Comparative Studies in Society and History* 38:1 (1996), 26–66.

[29] Carl Wahren, secretary-general, International Planned Parenthood Federation: "Bucharest 1974, Mexico City 1984: World Population Growth, a Ten-Year Perspective," in Carl Wahren-Secretary-General, International Planned Parenthood Federation Papers, Box 3, Folder SA/PGP/B/1/13, [WLAM].

the option of a long-acting method that lasted a month (although until 1992 it was banned in the United States by the FDA because of its side effects). During the late 1970s and early 1980s, a time in which religion played a less prominent role in population debates, the WHO's Program supported research on contraceptive drugs, on different methods to regulate fertility, and even on the controversial issue of induced abortion. In principle, the WHO had no definitive position on abortion, but after an initial rejection in the 1960s, by the 1970s it came to accept and endorse the procedure in those countries in which it was legal. Although the WHO never fully endorsed sterilization, during the 1970s it became less critical of the procedure. A report produced in the 1970s pointed to a possible association between vasectomy and prostate cancer, thereby generating some fears among physicians.[30] By 1975, the WHO was providing technical assistance to more than 60 countries in different areas of family planning. This development occurred in parallel to a dramatic increase in expenditure on population issues by the WHO (coming chiefly from the UNFPA and the World Bank). Between 1973 and 1994, the WHO spent more than USD 300 million on maternal and child health care and family-planning projects.[31] The WHO's proactive approach to the issue led to an increase in the production of contraceptives and their large scale use in developing countries, contributing to decreases in fertility rates in the late 1970s and early 1980s. The World Health Assemblies of the early 1980s considered family planning to be a key component of health systems and advocated for the development of family planning alongside maternal and child health services and for the recruitment of nurses, midwives, and health auxiliaries to educate the public and to make family planning more socially acceptable in developing countries. The WHO organized a meeting in 1985 in Brazzaville to discuss how to implement family-planning programs in sub-Saharan Africa. Two years later, a conference organized by the WHO's African Regional Office (AFRO) on Safe Motherhood was held in Nairobi at which a call was issued to reduce maternal mortality in developing countries by 50 percent in the subsequent decade, a goal that would be maintained until the turn of the twenty-first century. Another important program was launched in 1987, the WHO's Safe Motherhood Initiative, to reduce maternal morbidity and mortality by 50 percent by the year 2000. (However, these targets were not reached and maternal health continues to be a concern of global health.)

Nevertheless, the political climate that sustained national and international population programs was set to change once more.

---

[30] Hajo I. J. Wildschut & Wilma Monincx, "Vasectomy and the Risk of Prostate Cancer," *The Bulletin of the World Health Organization* 72:5 (1994), 777–778.

[31] Kessler, "Family Planning and the Role of WHO," p. 6.

Conservativism and the 1980s

Population debates changed course in the 1980s. Sterilization, which had been one of the methods advocated by family-planning supporters, came to face vigorous criticism from human rights organizations and American neoliberal and religious conservative groups. These critics argued that bilateral and multilateral organizations, such as the World Bank and USAID, had placed too much emphasis on population control, even setting quotas for sterilizations in poor nations as a condition for aid, and had prompted developing country governments to produce compulsory legislation with little regard for informed consent. The countries that received the most criticism were China and India, although only India had received international aid. The critics pointed out that the Indian government had provided financial incentives to men who underwent sterilization and made sterilization a condition for basic goods such as electricity, while health officials resorted to unethical tactics such as bribery and threats to promote sterilization; in some cases, even jail sentences were given to couples where both partners remained unsterilized after the birth of their third child. In 1971, abortions were legalized in India, a country in which an estimated 12.6 million sterilizations were carried out between 1974 and 1981. The program met with such fierce opposition domestically and abroad that Prime Minister Indira Ghandi was compelled to scale it back drastically and eventually withdraw it completely.[32] Fear and criticism explain the significant decline in the number of vasectomies worldwide, including in India.

China, which was home to around a quarter of the world's population (about 800 million people) in the mid-1970s, was also criticized for its stringent birth-control policy. From the early 1960s onward, the Chinese regime had encouraged late marriage, condemned premarital sex, distributed contraceptives, and made abortion legal. In 1979, China established a one-child-per-couple policy for families living in urban areas with the goal of preventing the total population from reaching 1.2 billion by 2000. The Chinese constitution stated that both husband and wife were responsible for practicing family planning by using different contraceptive measures. At the same time, radio, films, and newspapers continuously promoted the Chinese population control program across rural villages, urban residential areas, factories, mines, and military units. Although the Chinese government stated that its family-planning program was voluntary and flexible and there were no economic penalties, it was impossible to deny the existence of an organized system that put pressure on

---

[32] See Sanjam Ahluwalia & Daksha Parmar, "From Gandhi to Gandhi: Contraceptive Technologies and Sexual Politics in Post-Colonial India, 1947–1977," in Rickie Solinger & Mie Nakachi (eds.), *Reproductive States: Global Perspectives on the Invention and Implementation of Population Policy* (New York: Oxford University Press, 2016), pp. 124–155.

couples. Families with one child, for example, received special allowances from the state, including preferential treatment for educational and medical services, employment opportunities, and housing. Furthermore, in cases where couples had a second child, they usually had to refund any support they had received for the first child. Another serious human rights violation was that women who had unauthorized pregnancies often had to undergo abortions.[33]

During the mid-1980s, US foreign policy makers pointed to the excesses and wrongdoings of the coercive family-planning policies in order to promote new pronatalist population programs. Programs implemented in developing countries were also accused of being medically negligent – even those supported with funds of the United States or Western Europe – because frequently life-endangering operations were performed in unsafe conditions and because they used experimental or unapproved supplies and equipment banned in industrialized nations. Another criticism was that these programs were racist, with a hidden agenda of cutting the reproduction of nonwhite populations, and were abusive because in rural areas and shantytowns of poor nations women were sterilized without consent, usually in the aftermath of childbirth.

The administrations of Ronald Reagan and George H. W. Bush, which had the support of conservative Christian groups, ended the previous bipartisan agreement on population control and changed the international population agenda. These groups, and President Reagan himself, considered contraceptives to be a sin and portrayed them as being abortifacient. Reagan subscribed to the work of the neoliberal economist, Julian Simon, who was professor of business administration at the University of Maryland and questioned the negative correlation between economic development and population growth that had been the backbone of population control programs. Simon's 1981 book, *The Ultimate Resource*, argued that the scientific evidence proved that earlier fears of a population explosion were unfounded and that population growth was good for the economy because it created more producers and consumers and encouraged technological innovations and a diversification of markets.[34] Under the influence of Simon, the Reagan administration withdrew the federal government from previous domestic birth-control programs.

In 1984, at the UN's International World Population Conference that took place in Mexico City, Reagan took his concerns to the international stage. Senator James L. Buckley, a staunch opponent of abortion, was the head of the US delegation to the Mexico Conference, and Simon was his advisor. The American representatives announced that US bilateral aid could not be used in any abortion-related activity. Paradoxically, this occurred when most families all over the world and many governments in developing nations were

[33] See White, *China's Longest Campaign*.
[34] Julian L. Simon, *The Ultimate Resource* (Princeton: Princeton University Press, 1981).

accepting of family-planning methods, including abortion. Representatives from these countries argued that family planning was still necessary because the world's population was growing, and couples in the developing world, many of whom were from poor rural areas, did not want more children but had no access to contraception programs.

Nevertheless, the Reagan administration remained committed to the radical reversal of American family-planning programs. It reduced funding for family planning in general and imposed a gag rule on abortion referrals. This rule prohibited physicians in clinics or NGOs that received funds from the United States from practicing, informing, or discussing abortion as an option. The gag rule meant that recipients of American funds could not engage in any activity related to abortion, even if these activities were done with their own funds or if abortion was legal in the country where they operated.[35] Any refusal to comply led to the termination of American bilateral aid. The decision had a significant impact internationally because the United States was the main donor in the field, contributing more than half of all international funds used in family planning. In 1985, shortly after the Mexico Conference, the Reagan administration ended US contributions to the UNFPA and withdrew its support for IPPF, accusing these organizations of using American funds for abortion programs. This represented a 180-degree turnaround in USAID's population programs.

President George H. W. Bush (1989–1993) continued the trend that had begun under Reagan. He defiantly demanded assurances from the WHO that no part of the agency's work on human reproduction supported research on RU-486, a French commercial drug discovered in the early 1980s and later known as Mifepristone, that could induce early abortion (Bush had banned importation of the drug in 1989 because it was considered an abortifacient).[36] A corollary development was the decision by American companies to abandon research and production of contraceptives and restrict their sales because of fears of antagonizing the federal government, legal liabilities, and ideologically based boycotts.

If Reagan's policies were difficult to accept in developing countries, the same was not the case in all industrialized countries, not only because some had conservative governments like the United States, but also because they were experiencing a marked decline in the fertility rate. In 1984, the minister of the interior of the Federal Republic of Germany caused a sensation when he predicted that the number of German citizens would decrease from

[35] B. Crane & J. Dusenberry, "Power and Politics in International Funding for Reproductive Health: The US Global Gag Rule," *Reproductive Health Matters* 12:24 (2004), 128–137.

[36] Lawrence K. Altman, "US Quizzes WHO on Abortion Pill," *The New York Times*, April 7, 1991, p. 8.

56.9 million to 38.28 million by 2030. At the same time, other European countries began to report a spectacular fall in fertility and mortality rates, increased aging of the population, and the prospect of a reduction in populations. In France, for example, the fertility rate was 1.8 children per woman, i.e., less than the 2.1 children required for each generation to replace its numbers. Thus, for many of these governments deterring family planning, contraception and abortion became a matter of national interest.[37]

Despite growing conservatism on population issues in some industrial countries, NGOs, feminists, human rights movements, and multilateral agencies, including the WHO, began to pursue a new and more progressive direction on population themes. They recognized the grave mistakes of India's and China's coercive population policies but believed that these did not justify dismissing family-planning programs altogether and received a boost when the political context changed again with the election of Bill Clinton in 1993. During his two terms in office, Clinton's administration moved away from the gag rule and developed a friendlier attitude toward the UN and its population programs. At the same time, families around the world continued to use contraceptive devices. A UN report estimated that 381 million people used contraception in developing countries from 1985 through 1990, a significant increase from the 31 million during the period 1960–1965.[38]

The WHO and the Emergence of Sexual and Reproductive Health

In 1993, American support to the UNFPA and the IPPF was restored, and, in the subsequent years, additional funding was provided for international population programs. A critical change was that significant funds were provided to NGOs and grassroots organizations, rather than to governments of developing countries, as a way of circumventing red tape and local bureaucracies. By the mid-1990s, a broader approach to population issues was promoted at two landmark meetings in which the WHO participated: the International Conference on Population and Development, held in September 1994 in Cairo (known as ICPD-Cairo), and the Fourth World Conference on Women, held in Beijing the following year. Both meetings took place when "overpopulation" was no longer perceived as an imminent threat on account of a significant reduction in fertility rates and average family sizes in developing countries.

---

[37] Carl Wahren, secretary-general, International Planned Parenthood Federation: "Bucharest 1974, Mexico City 1984: World Population Growth, a Ten-Year Perspective," 1983, Box 3, Folder SA/PGP/B/1/13 (WLAM).

[38] "U.N. Agency on Sex: Pitfalls and Promise," *The New York Times*, October 15, 2007, p. 3.

However, abortion was still a concern because unsafe abortions represented one of the main causes of maternal mortality in developing countries. At these meetings, the notion that women were passive recipients of population programs was criticized, and participants urged for the empowerment of women's organizations. Another novelty of these meetings was the frequent use of a series of terms previously promoted by feminists. Some terms were new, such as "reproductive rights," which evoked the notion of citizenship, equity between men and women, and human rights. "Reproductive rights" also meant a condemnation of compulsory sterilization and that women had the right to exercise voluntary choice in marriage, to determine the number and spacing of children, and to have access to information and the means for making a choice about abortion. Another new term was "sexual health," which implied the search for fulfilling and healthy lifestyles. Some terms acquire a more complex meaning, such as "gender," which replaced "sex" and was used to emphasize that gender orientation could be different to an individual's sex. It was also a term that suggested diversity, tolerance, and respect. An all-encompassing term that replaced "family planning" and "population control" was "sexual and reproductive health" (to be replaced in the early twenty-first century by "sexual rights" in order to encompass gays and other sexual minorities).

The WHO and other agencies embraced and supported the new vocabulary and mindset prompted by the meetings in Cairo and Beijing.[39] A 1995 World Health Assembly resolution declared "reproductive health" a priority area, urging member countries to organize or strengthen their reproductive health programs, paying particular attention to equity and human rights. A year later, the health agency organized two new units: Family and Reproductive Health (FRH), and Gender, Women, and Health (GWH). The first unit was required to link the management of childhood diseases with overall child development (known as Integrated Management of Childhood Illnesses, IMCI) in order to improve the prevention and treatment of reproductive tract infections, including cervical cancer and sexually transmitted diseases. In addition, it was responsible for identifying key interventions to decrease maternal morbidity and mortality. The second unit had a broad mandate, requiring all programs to disaggregate data by sex (something that had not always been done in the past) and to integrate a "gender perspective" into new guidelines, manuals, training programs, and policies.[40] The decision was instrumental in demonstrating that some health issues such as tobacco consumption, domestic violence, and

---

[39] Rebecca J. Cook & Mahmoud F. Fathalla, "Advancing Reproductive Rights beyond Cairo and Beijing," *International Family Planning Perspectives* 22:3 (1996), 115–121.

[40] A discussion of the policies and programs of the health agency appears in World Health Organization, Department of Women's Health, Review of WHO's work related to the implementation of the Program of Action of the International Conference on Population and Development (ICPD) (Geneva: World Health Organization, 1999).

HIV/AIDS had a different impact on women, compared to men. Thanks to the second unit, during the mid-1990s the WHO made some progress in implementing a UN resolution that sought to establish parity in gender distribution among officers by increasing the number of women, especially in the leading positions of the agency. However, these developments would face a challenge from the international political context at the turn of the twenty-first century.

In another turn of political events, there was a return to religious conservatism on the part of the US government. The Republican George W. Bush, first elected in 2000 and reelected in 2004, reinstituted the "Mexico City Policy," or gag rule, on his first day as president, denying assistance to governments and organizations that provided abortion information or services, except in cases of rape where the woman's life was at risk. President Bush also cut millions from the budgets of the UNFPA and IPPF, accusing them of supporting abortions abroad.[41] In addition, he increased funding for domestic and international "abstinence-only" sexual education programs that promoted abstinence as the only acceptable sexual behavior for young people. It is interesting to note that President Bush found unexpected allies not only in the Vatican but also in Islamic governments, which opposed abortion, artificial conception, and feminism. The backlash led to opposition from experts and other organizations. In the 2004 Health Assembly, the WHO confirmed its adherence to the Cairo and Beijing meetings and approved a progressive health strategy on population issues, a definitive change from its more cautious position of the 1960s.[42] The Strategy established five priority areas: improving antenatal, delivery, and postpartum care; providing high-quality services for family planning; eliminating unsafe abortions; combating sexually transmitted infections; and promoting sexual health. A publication that reinforced the strategy was the 2005 World Health Report entitled "Make Every Mother and Child Count," which proposed a new global partnership for maternal, newborn, and child health, and established as a target universal coverage of maternal, newborn, and child health interventions.[43] Nonetheless, the struggle between the two ideas and policies on population health would continue. In 2009, President Barak Obama reversed the "global gag rule" on family-planning organizations and restored support to the UNFPA. In January 2017, the Trump administration reinstated the Mexico City Policy, which requires foreign NGOs to abstain from informing or advocating for abortion services as a condition

[41] Barbara Crossettte, "Implacable Force for Family Planning," *New York Times*, July 30, 2002, p. F7.

[42] World Health Organization, Department of Reproductive Health and Research, Reproductive Health Strategy, to Accelerate Progress toward the Attainment of International Development Goals and Targets (Geneva: World Health Organization, 2004).

[43] World Health Organization, *The World Health Report, 2005 – Make Every Mother and Child Count* (Geneva: World Health Organization, 2005).

of receiving US global health assistance. The administration also ended US funding for the UNFPA.

Final Remarks

During the second half of the twentieth century, the relationship between population growth, health, and economic development was one of the main debates of international health. Initially, the WHO did not play a leading role in these debates. In spite of its mild criticism of self-sufficient, top-down vertical population programs, the WHO followed the lead of private and bilateral American agencies. Toward the turn of the twenty-first century, the WHO, with the help of the UN, became an important player in its own right and helped to reframe and intertwine population themes with broader notions of women's rights and gender. In order to understand better the coexistence in the agency with a non-vertical program, it is necessary to return to the late 1970s and examine the emergence of a revolutionary socio-medical perspective in international health: Primary Health Care.

7   The Vicissitudes of Primary Health Care

In the late 1970s and 1980s, the WHO saw the emergence, influence, and decline of a novel and powerful concept: Primary Health Care, PHC. Although PHC encountered obstacles and opposition, its goals became compelling aspirations for health workers around the world, stimulating collaboration between physicians and lay health workers and increasing people's self-reliance in health. PHC served initially as a glowing ideal and as a source of energy and was in its original version one of the clearest expressions of the social medicine perspective that surfaced from time to time in the agency's history.

PHC developed from a critique of the short-sighted export of technologically intensive health care from developed to developing countries. This critique led to new proposals for health and development, such as those in American physician John Bryant's book *Health and the Developing World* that questioned the transplantation of hospital-based health care systems in developing countries and the lack of emphasis on prevention. From a similar mindset, Carl Taylor, chairman of the Department of International Health at Johns Hopkins University, published a book that offered Indian rural medicine as a general model for poor countries.[1] Another influential work was by Kenneth W. Newell, a WHO staff member from New Zealand who had worked in Indonesia, became familiar with the experiences of medical auxiliaries in developing countries, and argued that a strict health sectorial approach was ineffective.[2] He published articles and books that stated that in rural areas better food and improved income, without any major changes in health service, could result in a decrease in infant death rates.

In a more developed setting, the 1974 Canadian Lalonde Report (named for the minister of health who commissioned it, Marc Lalonde) deemphasized the importance of high-tech medical institutions and proposed four determinants

---

[1] John H. Bryant, *Health and the Developing World* (Ithaca: Cornell University Press, 1969); Carl E. Taylor (ed.), *Doctors for the Villages: Study of Rural Internships in Seven Indian Medical Colleges* (New York: Asia Publishing House, 1976).
[2] Kenneth W. Newell (ed.), *Health by the People* (Geneva: World Health Organization, 1975).

of health: biology, health services, environment, and lifestyle.[3] According to the report, a balance between these four factors – and not only a concentration on health services – explained the good health of a population. Other studies were also influential in challenging the assumption that health improvement resulted exclusively from doctors or medical technologies. The British physician and demographer Thomas McKeown argued that overall health was less related to biomedical advances than to improved standards of living and nutrition. More aggressively, Austrian philosopher Ivan Illich's *Medical Nemesis* contended that medicine was not only often irrelevant but frequently detrimental because doctors were too commonly guilty of iatrogenesis, namely, patients suffering from new illnesses caused inadvertently by medical treatment. This book became a bestseller and was translated into several languages.[4]

Another inspiration for primary health care came from the experience of missionaries. The Christian Medical Commission, a specialized organization of the World Council of Churches, was created in the late 1960s by medical missionaries working in developing countries.[5] This new organization emphasized the training of village workers at the grassroots level and urged that they be equipped with essential drugs and simple methods. In 1970, the CMC created the journal *Contact*, which regularly used the term "primary health care." It is worth noting that Bryant and Taylor were members of the Christian Medical Commission and that in 1974 collaboration was formalized between the Commission and the WHO. In addition, in Newell's book *Health by the People,* published in 1975, several of the examples cited were Christian Medical Commission programs that are presented as models to follow in developing countries.

A further inspiration for primary health care was the new global visibility of China's "barefoot doctors." This visibility coincided with China's entrance into the United Nations (UN) system and the WHO. The barefoot doctors, whose numbers increased dramatically between the early 1960s and the Cultural Revolution (1964–1976), were village health workers who lived in the community they served, stressed rural rather than urban health care and preventive rather than curative services, and combined Western and traditional medicines. In other countries of the world, innovative primary care initiatives also existed. For example, in rural South Africa in the 1940s and 1950s, the physicians Sidney and Emily Kark implemented a comprehensive approach to

[3] Canada, Department of National Health and Welfare, *A New Perspective on the Health of Canadians/Nouvelle Perspective de la Sante des Canadiens* (Ottawa: n.p., 1974).
[4] Thomas McKeown, *The Modern Rise of Population* (New York: Academic Press, 1976); Ivan Illich, *Medical Nemesis: The Expropriation of Health* (New York: Pantheon Books, 1976).
[5] Socrates Litsios, "The Christian Medical Commission and the Development of the World Health Organization's Primary Health Care Approach," *American Journal of Public Health* 94 (2004), 1884–1893.

population health and primary care, taking into account the socioeconomic and cultural determinants of health, identifying health needs, and working with the communities.[6] In addition, Cubans made primary care a priority after their 1959 revolution.

Primary health care was also favored by a new political context characterized by the emergence of decolonized African nations and the spread of national, anti-imperialist, and leftist movements in less-developed nations. These movements demanded an equitable distribution of resources, real political and economic independence from foreign powers, radical agrarian reforms, and increased opportunities for employment, housing, and education for society's poorest sectors. These political realities led to new proposals for development made by some industrialized countries. In 1974 the UN General Assembly adopted a resolution on the "Establishment of a New International Economic Order" to uplift less-developed countries. Modernization was no longer seen as the replication of the model of development followed by the United States. This was a trend promoted by a number of conferences and reports. For example, Prime Minister Lester B Pearson of Canada and Chancellor Willy Brandt of West Germany chaired commissions on international development emphasizing long-term socioeconomic changes instead of specific technical interventions and called for a large-scale transfer of technical and financial resources to developing countries.

The Organization was moving in a similar direction since the early 1970s. New leaders and institutions embodied the new academic and political influences. Prominent among the new leaders was Halfdan T. Mahler of Denmark, who was elected the WHO's director-general in 1973.[7] Mahler was later reelected for two additional five-year terms, remaining as the WHO's director-general until 1988. He had received his MD from the University of Copenhagen in 1948 and had a postgraduate degree in public health. His first international activities were in tuberculosis and community work in less-developed countries. Between 1950 and 1951, he directed a Red Cross anti-tuberculosis campaign in Ecuador and later spent several years (1951–1960) in India as the WHO officer in the National Tuberculosis Program. In 1962, he became chief medical officer of the Tuberculosis Unit at WHO headquarters.

[6] Sidney & Emily Kark, *Promoting Community Health: From Pholela to Jerusalem* (Johannesburg: Witwatersrand University Press, 2001).
[7] Information on this page is from Marcos Cueto, "The Origins of Primary Health Care and Selective Primary Health Care," *American Journal of Public Health* (2004), 1864–1874; Peter Bourne, Memorandum for the President, November 17, 1977, Jimmy Carter Presidential Library Collection: Office of Staff Secretary, Series: Presidential Files, Folder 11/18/77, Container 51, www.jimmycarterlibrary.gov/digital_library/sso/148878/51/SSO_148878_051_08.pdf, last accessed January 3, 2018; and Theodore M. Brown, Elizabeth Fee, & Victoria Stepanova, "Halfdan Mahler: Architect and Defender of the World Health Organization 'Health for All by 2000' Declaration of 1978," *American Journal of Public Health* 196 (2016), 38–39.

In anticipation of an idea of Primary Health Care, in 1966 Mahler proposed that tuberculosis programs should be integrated within general public health services so that each would strengthen the other. In 1969, he was appointed as director of the systems analysis project of the WHO, a program that aimed to improve national capabilities in health planning. Beyond his technical expertise, Mahler was a charismatic figure and a compelling speaker who believed that "social justice" was a holy term and was described by one advisor to President Jimmy Carter as "a saint."[8] His father, a Baptist minister, and his mother, who came from a German family of physicians, helped shape his personality. The impression he produced in some people is well illustrated by a religious activist who met Mahler in the 1970s: "I felt like a church mouse in front of an archbishop."[9] Mahler (see Figure 7.1) believed – like Chisholm – that the main advice of the WHO to his staff and health officers of developing countries was "Adapt, don't adopt."

Mahler had excellent relations with older WHO officers. The Brazilian Candau, for example, appointed him as an assistant director-general in 1970, responsible for the Division of Research in Epidemiology and Communications Science. Thanks to this close relationship with the WHO's old guard, Mahler could ease a transition in the agency as he gradually took command and some of these changes occurred before Mahler assumed the post of DG. From the late 1960s, there was an increase in the WHO of "basic health services" projects for the provision of public services (education, adequate water and sewage systems, sanitation, and electricity) which were understood to be essential to improve the health of the poor. These projects were institutional predecessors of the primary health care programs that would later appear. Until this time, the level of health of a given country was associated with the number of hospitals, health professionals, laboratories, and medical schools. Since developing countries did not have sufficient resources to increase their health resources, they began to demand help to initiate infrastructural development programs, especially in rural areas, where the majority of the population lived. Mahler also pursued excellent relations with world leaders (his conversation with President Jimmy Carter was the first meeting between a US President and the head of the WHO in 13 years). In addition, the WHO began to recognize the contributions made by traditional medicine over thousands of years in a variety of therapies and practices in developing countries.

The creation in 1972 of a division for "Strengthening Health Services" was an early expression of change in the WHO. Newell, a strong academic and

---

[8] Jimmy Carter Presidential Library Collection: Office of Staff Secretary, Series: Presidential Files; Folder 11/18/77, Container 51.
[9] G. Paterson, "The CMC Story, 1968–1998," *Contact* 161–162 (1998), 3–18, p. 13.

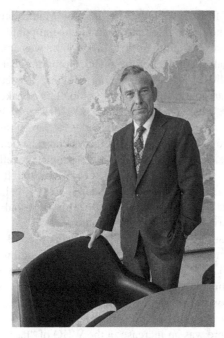

Figure 7.1 Halfdan T. Mahler, architect of Primary Health Care, was elected director-general of the World Health Organization in 1973. Mahler was the third director-general and served in this position from 1973 to 1988.
Credit: WHO/Erling Mandelmann. Courtesy: World Health Organization Photo Library.

public health voice for primary health care, was appointed director of this division. In 1973 the Executive Board of the WHO issued the report "Organizational Study on Methods of Promoting the Development of Basic Health Services."[10] This report was the basis for a new collaboration between the WHO and UNICEF. Mahler established a close rapport with Henry Labouisse, UNICEF's executive director between 1965 and 1979, who had his own rich experience with community-based initiatives in health and education and promoted comprehensive, multisectoral, and low-cost basic services at the district and provincial levels. In 1976, UNICEF approved the basic services strategy as a means of meeting the essential needs of children and mothers in rural communities and urban slums and in the same year the strategy was endorsed by the General Assembly of the United Nations. Other agencies such

---

[10] "The Work of WHO in 1972: Annual Report of the Director General to the World Health Assembly," in *WHO Official Records* 205, 1973, Geneva, WHO Library.

as USAID also shifted emphasis to what was called a "basic human needs" approach, which included food and nutrition, population planning, health, education, and human resources development.

The agreement between the WHO and UNICEF produced a 1975 joint report, *Alternative Approaches to Meeting Basic Health Needs in Developing Countries.*[11] The term "alternative" was meant to underline the shortcomings of traditional vertical programs concentrating on specific diseases. In addition, the assumption that the expansion of "Western" medical systems would meet the needs of common people was highly criticized. According to the document, the principal causes of morbidity in developing countries were malnutrition and respiratory and diarrheal diseases, which were the results of poverty, squalor, and lack of education. The report also examined successful experiences in Bangladesh, China, Cuba, India, Niger, Nigeria, Tanzania, Venezuela, and Yugoslavia to identify the key factors in their success. This report shaped the WHO's ideas on primary health care. The 28th World Health Assembly in 1975 reinforced the trend, declaring the construction of national programs in primary health care a priority matter. *Alternative Approaches* became the basis for a worldwide discussion. The 1976 World Health Assembly approved "Health for All by the Year 2000" as a moral imperative and a commitment to achieve universality and equity rather than a specific deadline when miraculously all disease and disability would vanish. For Mahler, this target required a radical change, a social revolution in public health.[12]

The landmark event for primary health care was the International Conference on Primary Health Care that took place at Alma-Ata from September 6 to 12, 1978. Alma-Ata was the capital of the Soviet Republic of Kazakhstan, located in the Soviet Union's Asiatic region (the idea of such a meeting had been proposed by the World Health Assembly of 1975). Tension among communist countries had helped in the selection of the site. The Chinese delegation to the WHO introduced the idea of an international conference on primary health care. Initially, the USSR opposed the proposal and defended a more medically oriented approach. However, after noticing that the primary health care movement was growing, the Soviet delegation, headed by the talented deputy health minister Dimitri Venediktov, declared that his country was eager to hold the meeting and offered USD 2 million to help fund it. The Soviet Union had one condition: The conference must take place on Soviet

---

[11] V. Djukanovic & E. P. Mach (eds.), *Alternative Approaches to Meeting Basic Health Needs of Populations in Developing Countries: A Joint UNICEF/WHO Study* (Geneva: World Health Organization, 1975).

[12] Hafdan Mahler, "A Social Revolution in Public Health," *Chronicle of the World Health Organization* 30:12 (1976), 475–480.

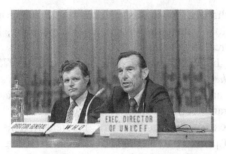

Figure 7.2 Senator Edward M. Kennedy of the United States of America with Halfdan T. Mahler at the International Conference on Primary Health Care at Alma-Ata (USSR) organized by the WHO and UNICEF, September 1978. Courtesy: World Health Organization Photo Library.

soil. For a while, the WHO searched for an alternative site in Iran, Egypt, and Costa Rica, but no country could match the economic offer of the Soviet Union. Finally, the WHO accepted the Soviet offer but asked for a different location than Moscow, suggesting a provincial city. After some negotiation, Alma-Ata was selected because of the remarkable health advances that had been achieved there by its dynamic health authorities.

About 3,000 delegates attended the conference. They came from 134 governments and 67 international organizations from all over the world. Details were orchestrated by the Peruvian David Tejada-de-Rivero, the WHO's assistant director-general since 1974, who was responsible for the logistics of the event. Most of the delegates came from the public sector, primarily from ministries of health but not from planning, finance, or education ministries as expected by the organizers. (One important exception was the American politician, Senator Edward M. Kennedy, seen in Figure 7.2.) The meeting was also attended by representatives from the UN and international agencies such as the International Labor Organization (ILO), the Food and Agriculture Organization, and the Agency for International Development. Nongovernmental organizations, religious organizations (including the Christian Medical Commission), the Red Cross, Medicus Mundi, and political movements such as the Palestine Liberation Organization and the South West Africa People's Organization were also present. But because China had strained relations with the USSR, China was absent. At the opening ceremony, Mahler challenged the delegates with eight compelling questions that called for immediate action. Two of the most audacious were as follows:

Are you ready to introduce, if necessary, radical changes in the existing health delivery system so that it properly supports primary health care as the overriding health priority?

Are you ready to fight the political and technical battles required to overcome any social and economic obstacles and professional resistance to the universal introduction of primary health care?[13]

When the conference took place, primary health care had already been "sold" to many participants. From 1976 to 1978, the WHO and UNICEF organized a series of regional meetings to discuss "alternative approaches." The conference's document, the Declaration of Alma-Ata, whose draft was previously known by many participants, was approved by acclamation. "Declaration" suggested high importance, like other momentous declarations of independence and human rights. The intention was to create a universal and bold statement for health equity. Three key ideas permeated the Declaration: appropriate technology, opposition to medical elitism, and health as a tool for socioeconomic development. Regarding the first issue, there was criticism of the negative role of "disease-oriented technology."[14] The term referred to technology, such as body scanners or heart-lung machines, that was too sophisticated, expensive, or irrelevant to the common needs of the poor. The term implicitly criticized the proliferation of urban hospitals in developing countries that used this technology to promote a consumer culture, benefiting only a wealthy minority and drawing a substantial share of human and financial resources. "Appropriate" medical technology was presented as an alternative to fulfill the needs of the people. This kind of technology would be scientifically sound and financially feasible. In addition, the construction of health facilities in rural areas and shantytowns was emphasized rather than urban-hospital construction. In addition, the competition between separate disease-control programs was portrayed as detrimental to the goal of integrated approaches to address the multidimensional common health needs of poor people.

The Declaration's second key idea, its criticism of elitism, meant a disapproval of the overspecialization of health personnel in developing countries and of top-down health campaigns. Instead, training of lay health personnel and self-reliant community participation were stressed. In addition, the need for working with traditional healers such as shamans and midwives was emphasized. Finally, the Declaration linked health to a number of intersectoral activities and to development. Health work was perceived not as an isolated intervention but as part of a process of improving living conditions. Primary

---

[13] "Intervention of Director General of WHO, H. Mahler," September 6, 1978, p. 4, Folder ICPHC/ALA/78.1–11 Folder "Alma-Ata 1978, International Conference on Primary Health Care, September 6–12, 1978, Statements by Participants in the Plenary Meetings," Second Generation of Files.

[14] See Hafdan Mahler, "Health – A Demystification of Medical Technology," *The Lancet* 2:7940 (November 1, 1975), 829–833.

health care was designed as the new center of the public health system. This required an intersectoral approach, with public and private institutions working together on health issues (e.g., on health education, adequate nutrition, housing, safe water, and basic sanitation). Organizationally, this meant that the WHO could play a leading role in the organization of meetings and activities with other UN agencies such as FAO, UNESCO and the UN Office for Development and International Economic Cooperation. Furthermore, the link between health and development had political implications and encouraged links with NGOs working on health and development. Mahler was convinced that health should be an instrument for development and not merely a by-product of economic progress. This change in emphasis would make health workers "the *avant garde* of an international conscience for social development." According to Mahler, PHC was a means to project worldwide new visions of well-being, human development, and human dignity.[15]

The 32nd World Health Assembly that took place in Geneva in 1979 endorsed the Alma-Ata conference's Declaration. The assembly approved a resolution stating that primary health care was "the key to attaining an acceptable level of health for all." In 1981, the health agency proclaimed its "Global Strategy for Health for All," using the same term "global" that had been used in its malaria program of the 1950s. In the following years, conferences, seminars, and workshops targeted at different audiences in various cities of the globe articulated the aims and features of Primary Health Care. Mahler tried to advance the cause by becoming a sort of global spokesman for PHC, publishing articles and giving speeches on such topics such as "Health and Justice" (1978), "The Political Struggle for Health" (1978), "The Meaning of Health for All by the Year 2000" (1981), and "Eighteen Years to Go to Health for All" (1982).[16] Nonetheless, despite initial enthusiasm, it proved difficult to implement primary health care after Alma-Ata.

A New Context

The principal challenges to implementation came from changed political circumstances in the eighties, and much of that change was symbolized by Ronald Reagan's election as President of the United States in November 1980. Reagan's election was part of a global revival of conservatism and an assertion of neoliberal economic policies. This revival was ushered in by Margaret Thatcher's electoral victory in the United Kingdom in 1979 (and her reelection

---

[15] Hafdan Mahler, "WHO's Mission Revisited: Address in Presenting His Report for 1974 to the 28th World Health Assembly," May 15, 1975, n.p., 10, Box 1, Geneva, Hafdan Mahler papers [WHOA].
[16] Mahler articles in Mahler papers [WHOA].

in 1983 and 1987). She and Reagan led national and global crusades to limit government programs and expenditures, cut taxes, promote widespread privatization, and – contradictorily – increase spending on national defense. Neoliberalism was also the dominant political ideology in other industrial nations such as the Federal Republic of Germany that in 1982 elected the Christian-Democrat Helmut Kohl as chancellor, and in Canada where in 1984 the Conservative Brian Mulroney became prime minister.

With regard to foreign policy, Reagan aggressively confronted the Soviet Union by providing support to anticommunist forces in Central America, the Middle East, Asia, and Africa and by denouncing the USSR as an "evil empire." He also brushed aside schemes for indigenous social change in developing nations and distinguished implausibly between "authoritarian" and "totalitarian" regimes. The former could be allies as long as they endorsed market capitalism and had friendly relations with the United States. The latter were pernicious if they were communist or close to the Soviet Union. Reagan's policies for developing countries assumed that what was good for America was good for poor nations, namely acceptance of largely unregulated markets as indispensable to prosperity, general reduction of the dimensions of the state, privatization of state enterprises, and the removal of restrictions on foreign investors. It was expected that economic growth would trickle down to the poor and solve their problems, including their health problems. Neoliberalism, promoted by the World Bank and USAID, meant a sharp decline in the funding of public health services, an increasing trend toward privatization, and the preeminence of profit-driven health provider and insurance organizations.

Reinforcing Reagan's policies were disillusionment with communism caused by the perceived lack of democratic rights in communist regimes as well as economic crisis and technological stagnation in the Soviet Union. Central planning by the State – typical of the Soviet system – was increasingly perceived as overly bureaucratic and incapable of providing decent housing, sufficient food, and quality goods. Not even General Secretary of the governing Communist Party of the Soviet Union Mikhail Gorbachev could solve the economic and political problems of the Soviet system during the years 1985 to 1990, when he unsuccessfully tried to reform the system from within. In addition, the confrontation between the USSR and the Polish trade union Solidarity during the 1980s, the coming down of the Berlin Wall in 1989, and the defeat of the Soviet Union in Afghanistan against multi-national insurgent groups were severe blows to Soviet communism around the world. In the same period, several other Soviet-style regimes collapsed. In 1991, the Soviet Union and the Warsaw Pact ceased to exist, inaugurating a unipolar international system centering on an apparently triumphant United States.

US foreign policy makers now believed that they could ignore or radically transform international institutions. These ideas were generalizations of the Reagan administration's criticism of the UN and its specialized agencies. This criticism was similar to that directed by neoliberalism against national state or governmental institutions that had been used to legitimize structural adjustment programs that shrank health budgets. The UN was considered a bloated bureaucracy with no accountability and unable to provide clear reports to donor nations on how their money was being used. This criticism was fueled by the loss of US dominance in UN forums. American proposals were outvoted in the General Assembly by the increasing number of developing countries that used the one-country, one-vote system to assert their authority and autonomy. Reagan's appointment of political scientist Jeane Kirkpatrick, an outspoken critic of "anti-American" and "anti-free enterprise" currents, as UN ambassador in 1981 began the overt assault on "politicized" multilateral agencies. The Reagan administration withdrew from UNESCO in 1985, accusing the multilateral agency of politicizing educational and cultural themes and doing very little to restrain its budgetary expansion, and created the strong suspicion that the United States would withdraw from several other international agencies. During the Reagan presidency, the United States reduced and delayed its payments to the UN. Beginning in the mid-1980s, American delegates to the World Health Assembly and other bodies of the WHO likewise complained of "improper" political debates in what was supposed to be an apolitical "technical" agency. Alleged examples of the latter were an attempt to hold a World Health Assembly in Cuba, a call for "cessation" of the arms and nuclear "race," and a call for assistance to Middle Eastern and African national liberation movements.[17] Using these WHA debates as a pretext, the Reagan administration allowed a widening gap to develop in its relationship with the WHO and other UN organizations created after World War II.

Selective Primary Health Care

Thus, when Primary Health Care was about to be implemented, a different political climate prevailed than the one that had existed at Alma-Ata. A number of multilateral and bilateral agencies now believed that the goal of "Health for All" was far too idealistic. Also, the WHO had not established a clear source of funding for PHC, and the deadline "by the year 2000" was generally deemed to be vague and wildly unrealistic. Concerned about the identification of the most cost-effective and practical health strategies, in

---

[17] United States, Department of State, *United States Participation in the UN, Report by the President to the Congress for the Year 1987* (Washington, DC: US Government Printing Office, 1988), p. 204.

1979 the Rockefeller Foundation sponsored a small conference at its conference center in Bellagio, Italy. The inspiration for the meeting came from the physician John H. Knowles, president of the Foundation, a strong critic of the medical *status quo* and a believer in the need for more primary care clinical practitioners in the United States. The heads of other major agencies were also involved in the organization of the meeting: Robert S. McNamara, president of the World Bank; Maurice Strong, chairman of the Canadian International Development and Research Center; David Bell, vice president of the Ford Foundation; and John J. Gillian, administrator of the US Agency for International Development, among others. McNamara was trying to overcome the criticism that the Bank had ignored the social causes of poverty and in 1979 had convinced the executive board of the Bank to begin lending in health care.

The Bellagio conference was based on a paper published in the *New England Journal of Medicine* by Julia Walsh and Kenneth S. Warren, "Selective Primary Health Care, an Interim Strategy for Disease Control in Developing Countries."[18] The paper focused on specific causes of death, paying special attention to the most common diseases of infants in developing countries, such as diarrhea and diseases produced by lack of immunization. The authors did not openly criticize the Alma-Ata Declaration. Instead, they presented an "interim" strategy by identifying entry points through which basic health services could be developed. They also emphasized attainable goals and cost-effective planning. In the paper and at the meeting, "Selective Primary Health Care" (SPHC) was introduced as a new perspective and set of priorities. The term meant a package of low-cost technical interventions to tackle the main disease problems of poor countries. At first, the content of the package was not completely clear. For example, in the original paper a number of different interventions were recommended, including the administration of antimalarial drugs for children (something that later disappeared from all proposals). Interestingly, acute respiratory infections, a chief cause of infant mortality, were not included. These were thought to require the administration of antibiotics that nonmedical practitioners in many of the affected countries were not allowed to use. After the meeting, SPHC became for many health organizations the realistic alternative to trying to implement the Alma-Ata Declaration. For supporters of SPHC what was possible was to provide a minimum package of health care services to the poor.[19] The major

[18] J. A. Walsh & K. S. Warren, "Selective Primary Health Care, an Interim Strategy for Disease Control in Developing Countries," *New England Journal of Medicine* 301 (1979), 967–974.

[19] Kenneth S. Warren, "The Evolution of Selective Primary Health Care," *Social Science and Medicine* 26 (1988), 891–898.

proponent of this new version of PHC would be the new executive director of UNICEF, James P. Grant.

Grant was an American who was born and raised in China by a family for whom medicine and humanitarianism was in the blood. His grandfather was a medical missionary in China and his father a Rockefeller Foundation public health doctor who worked and lived in China and India. The younger Grant had worked for UNRRA in China at the end of World War II supplying food and provisions before the revolution of 1949. He later received a law degree from Harvard University and from 1954 to 1958 worked as a field officer of ICA in Ceylon and New Delhi and later as a deputy assistant secretary of the Department of State in charge of the Near East and South Asia. From 1964 to 1967 he was director of USAID in Turkey. He was also the author of articles on development and an expert witness in congressional hearings. In 1977, he became the president of the Overseas Development Corporation, a nonprofit organization established in 1969 to promote studies on development.[20]

According to Labouisse, Grant's predecessor at UNICEF, the appointment of Grant came after a competition with Europeans. Upon the announcement of Labouisse's retirement in 1978 and debate over his successor, the German government expressed its desire for a European in the position, complaining that too many other multilateral agencies either had or had had US nationals as leaders. The Swedish government and other "Nordic" European governments were eager to have the position go to Ernest Michanek, director of the Swedish bilateral agency, especially since Sweden was the second largest contributor to UNICEF and the second largest contributor to the UN system. After a conversation with Grant, Labouisse met with Cyrus Vance, US secretary of state, and convinced him to send "Jim's name over to the White House" for approval.[21] The official justification of Grant's candidacy emphasized that he was well-known to the senior officials of major multilateral and bilateral agencies and had broad contacts in a large number of developing countries. But above all, he had "an effective working relationship with the United States Congress which has consistently sustained the sizeable and increasing US contribution to UNICEF" and enjoyed "extensive contacts with leaders in the private sector in the United States."[22] In a Labouisse account of 1977, he quotes the secretary

[20] On Grant, see C. Bellamy, P. Adamson, S. B. Tacon et al. (eds.), *Jim Grant: UNICEF Visionary* (Florence, Italy: UNICEF, 2001).

[21] "Interview with H. R. Labouisse conducted by Jack Charnow at UNICEF Headquarters," February 21, 1985, Collection Henry R. Labouisse Papers MC199, Mudd Manuscript Library, Series 2 United Nations, Subseries 2C: United Nations Children's Fund (UNICEF), Box 26, Folder 1 (PUL).

[22] United States Mission to the United Nations, April 18, 1979, Collection Henry R. Labouisse Papers MC199, Mudd Manuscript Library, Series 2 United Nations, Subseries 2C: United Nations Children's Fund (UNICEF), Box 24, Folder 14 (PUL).

of state: "Mr. Vance said it was important for the United States to have this position. .... [I]f [the position] went to some other country, it would have an effect on congressional appropriations [for UNICEF]."[23]

Grant rapidly gained recognition as executive director, a position he retained until 1995. In one of the first interviews he gave as head of UNICEF, he reminisced that as a boy he had learned in China about "what we now call Primary Health Care, only then it was called community medicine." He also remembered LNHO officers working in China who stayed at his home (specifically Rajchman and Stampar) and who discussed with his father "how to bring the benefit of health services to the mass of people," even with limited available resources. He was convinced of the advantages of the agency he led over other UN agencies because of its focus on the local community. In his words: "It's the only UN agency that ... works up whereas most other institutions start at a much more macro level and work down."[24] He also believed that international agencies had to do their best with finite resources and short-lived local political opportunities. This meant translating general goals into time-bound specific actions, in this case actions showing affinity for SPHC rather than PHC.

Thanks to Grant, SPHC was associated with a set of specific, low-cost interventions captured by the acronym GOBI, derived from the four chief interventions: *Growth* monitoring to overcome subnormal growth because of inadequate nutrition (an intervention that meant the use of child growth charts by mothers in their homes), *Oral* rehydration techniques for diarrheal diseases, *Breastfeeding*, and *Immunization*. These four interventions seemed easy to monitor and evaluate, and funding appeared easier to obtain because indicators of success could be produced rapidly. In a few years, some agencies added FFF (Food supplementation, Female literacy, and Family planning) to the acronym GOBI, creating GOBI-FFF. Selective Primary Health Care attracted the support of significant donors and agencies, and in 1983 Grant announced that UNICEF was making GOBI the tool for a "Child Survival and Development Revolution" that would dramatically reduce childhood mortality and morbidity. Grant revealed his high hopes for the undertaking by comparing it to the Rockefeller Foundation's "'Green Revolution' for agriculture."[25] Two

---

[23] Henry R. Labouisse, "Conversation with Secretary of State Vance," March 26, 1977, Collection Henry R. Labouisse Papers MC199, Mudd Manuscript Library, Series 2 United Nations, Subseries 2C: United Nations Children's Fund (UNICEF), Box 24, Folder 14 (PUL).

[24] "Interview with James Grant," UNICEF Staff News 6, (no day) May–June 1979, pp. 4–5, Collection Henry R. Labouisse Papers MC199, Mudd Manuscript Library, Series 2 United Nations, Subseries 2C: United Nations Children's Fund (UNICEF), Box 24, Folder 13 (PUL).

[25] James P. Grant to Hugo Scheltema, November 16, 1982, Collection Henry R. Labouisse Papers MC199, Mudd Manuscript Library, Series 2 United Nations, Subseries 2C: United Nations Children's Fund (UNICEF), Box 16, Folder 16 (PUL).

years later his call was taken up by the US Congress when it established a Child Survival Fund of more than 150 million dollars, to be operated by USAID for mother and child health programs in developing countries.

Some supporters of comprehensive primary health care considered Selective Primary Health Care to be complementary to the Alma-Ata Declaration, while others thought it undermined the Declaration. Those who supported a wide-scale implementation of Alma-Ata tried to respond to the accusation that they had no clear targets. For example, a WHO working paper entitled "Indicators for Monitoring Progress Towards Health for All" was prepared at the Executive Board's request. Another publication provided specific "Health for All" sub-goals: 5 percent of gross national product devoted to health; more than 90 percent of newborn infants weighing 2,500 g; an infant mortality rate of less than 50 per 1,000 live births; a life expectancy of more than 60 years; and local health care units supplied with at least 20 essential drugs.[26] However, most supporters of SPHC argued that these indicators and sub-goals were unreliable.

A debate developed between the advocates of the original concept of PHC – sometimes called "Comprehensive PHC" – and the supporters of SPHC.[27] The former emphasized the incorporation of health programs into socioeconomic development, working in close intersectoral collaboration and sparking change from the bottom up. Moreover, the supporters of Comprehensive PHC saw health interventions as opportunities for using health as a means to empower under-privileged people in their struggle for lasting improvements in their living conditions. To supporters of comprehensive primary health care, oral rehydration solutions were Band-Aids in places where safe water and sewage systems did not exist. The more radical supporters believed that PHC should be an avenue to or an adjunct of social revolution. The radical advocates of PHC castigated SPHC as a narrow technocentric approach that diverted attention from basic health and socioeconomic development, did not address the social causes of disease, and resembled vertical programs. Newell, one of the architects of the Alma-Ata Declaration, harshly criticized Selective Primary Health Care as nothing less than a dangerous "counter-revolution."[28]

US bilateral agencies, the World Bank, and UNICEF began to prioritize some aspects of GOBI, such as immunization and oral rehydration. They believed that it was a grave error to promote something akin to revolution in developing countries but also naïve to expect changes from their conservative bureaucracies. It was more realistic to convince the governments of developing

---

[26] World Health Organization, "Primary Health: A First Assessment," in World Health Organization, *People Report on Primary Health Care* (Geneva: World Health Organization, 1985), 6–9.

[27] An example of the debate is Ben Wisner, "GOBI versus PHC? Some Dangers of Selective Primary Health Care," *Social Science and Medicine* 26:9 (1988), 963–969.

[28] Kenneth W. Newell, "Selective Primary Health Care: The Counter Revolution," *Social Science and Medicine* 26:9 (1988), 903–906.

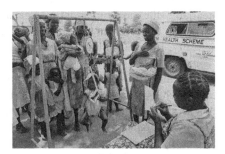

Figure 7.3 A routine weigh-in to improve nutrition programs conducted by a
mobile Primary Health Care team in Zimbabwe in the late 1970s.
Credit WHO/Liba Taylor. Courtesy: World Health Organization Photo Library.

countries of the advantages of SPHC. As a result, increasing tension and
acrimony developed between the PHC-supporting WHO and SPHC-
supporting UNICEF during the early 1980s. For example, WHO critics said
that GOBI did not work as expected because it implied the use of charts by
illiterate mothers (recording data was not an easy operation, weighing scales
were frequently deficient, and charts were subject to misinterpretation). The
use of anthropometry for the assessment of nutritional status was also difficult for mothers (as suggested by Figure 7.3). Moreover, studies demonstrated that although undernutrition in children was associated with an
increased risk of death, a decrease in infant mortality did not always follow
from a decrease in the prevalence of undernutrition. Research also demonstrated that proper nutrition was related to a family's income and the availability and cost of children's food.

Oral Rehydration Techniques (ORT) faced similar complications to those of
growth monitoring, even at a time when it was estimated that diarrhea took a
toll of millions of children annually (90 percent of children in developing
countries lived in areas without a safe water supply).[29] The technique could be
traced to the early 1970s, when oral rehydration solutions reduced cholera
death rates from 50 to 3 percent among refugees of the War between India and
Pakistan. In 1975, UNICEF and the WHO agreed to a standard packet for ORT
and promoted it all over the world. In the following years the WHO created a
Diarrheal Disease Control program that promoted the creation of national
diarrhea programs, and in 1979 USAID made a large donation to create the
International Center for Diarrheal Disease Research in Bangladesh. USAID
also provided millions of oral rehydration solution packets to developing
countries, representing about 40 percent of all packets distributed in the world.

---

[29] Grant to Scheltema, November 16, 1982 (PUL).

For *The Lancet*, ORT was "potentially" the most important medical advance of the twentieth century. During the first half of the 1980s, the annual production of ORT rose dramatically, from 60 million to 270 million one-liter equivalent packets.

Despite these developments, the technique could not solve structural problems that caused diarrheal diseases such as the lack of an adequate supply of potable water, deficient sanitation services, and unhealthy hygienic practices. These problems were aggravated by the rapid process of urbanization that together with the low priority given by governments to water, sewage, and sanitary infrastructure lessened many countries' abilities to keep up with the growing needs of people living in slums, shantytowns, and rural areas. ORT became a temporary fix in places where unsafe water systems persisted. Another wrinkle was that ORT use was restricted to medical personnel and did not become a tool for mothers and widespread home treatment, as originally designed. Inconsistent recommendations on the use of ORT, ranging from early and extensive to late and limited, caused additional confusion.[30]

Another GOBI intervention that encountered problems was breastfeeding (see Figure 7.4). The interest of the WHO in promoting breastfeeding can be traced to the 27th World Health Assembly in 1974, which approved a resolution urging member states to promote breast milk as part of the balanced nutritional requirements of infants and as the best form of prevention of early childhood infections. A resolution of the 1978 World Health Assembly called for the regulation of the sales promotion of artificial infant foods. These WHA decisions challenged a powerful industry. In 1979 it was estimated that global sales of artificial infant formula were USD 2 billion a year, with Third World nations accounting for 50 percent of the total. Companies such as Nestlé, the giant Swiss company, argued – incorrectly – that infant formula had to be used in developing countries because undernourished mothers could not produce proper milk and prolonged lactation would worsen their health.

In 1979, a joint WHO/UNICEF meeting on Infant and Young Child Feeding, attended by representatives of more than 130 WHO member states, international organizations, and NGOs as well as by nutritionists and pediatricians, began to prepare an "International Code for Marketing Breast-Milk Substitutes." The Code went through several drafts before being finally approved by the World Health Assembly in 1981, with the sole dissenting vote being that of the United States, which considered the Code an obstacle to trade. The Code placed restrictions on the unethical marketing of breast milk

---

[30] See Joshua Ruxin, "Magical Bullet: The History of Oral Rehydratation Therapy," *Medical History* 38 (1991), 363–397, and David Werner & David Sanders, *Questioning the Solution: The Politics of Primary Health Care and Child Survival, with an In-Depth Critique of Oral Rehydration Therapy* (Palo Alto: Health Rights, 1997).

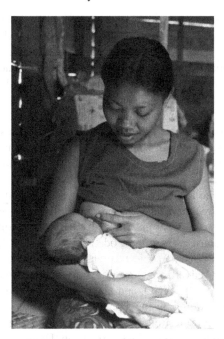

Figure 7.4 Breastfeeding a newborn in the fishing village of Rusila, on the East coast of peninsular Malaysia in the late 1970s. Colostrum, the yellowish, sticky breast milk produced at the end of pregnancy, was recommended by the WHO as the perfect food for the newborn and for babies up to six months of age.
Credit WHO/Jean Mohr. Courtesy: World Health Organization Photo Library.

substitutes (such as glamorizing infant formula), prohibited the distribution of free samples to doctors and hospitals, and condemned the practice of placing saleswomen wearing nurse-like uniforms in hospital waiting rooms in order to recruit young mothers.[31]

Behind the Code were medical missionaries, church activists, and grassroots organizations, most notably the International Baby Food Action Network (IBFAN), the Infant Feeding Action Coalition (INFACT), and the Baby Milk Coalition. Before Alma-Ata, these organizations accused baby food companies of seeking clients in Latin America, Asia, and Africa, which had high fertility rates and few regulations, because of declining birth rates in the United States and Western Europe. In 1971, several of these organizations launched a boycott against Nestlé. During the 1980s, Nestlé stopped its more

---

[31] S. Shubber, *The International Code of Marketing of Breast-Milk Substitutes: An International Measure to Protect and Promote Breastfeeding* (The Hague: Kluger Law International, 1983).

blatant marketing practices and agreed formally to implement the 1981 Code in developing countries. As a result, the boycott was suspended for a while but many NGOs and grassroots organizations believed that Nestlé would not keep its promises. The food companies and some US congressmen claimed that women from poor countries turned spontaneously to bottle-feeding because increasing numbers of them were working outside the home. These companies also argued that unsafe water, unsterilized bottles, improper refrigeration, and overdilution of the formula were the real problems and were not the responsibility of the companies. The confrontation with artificial infant food companies helped to change maternal practices in several countries but did little to excite the enthusiasm of donor agencies.

The International Code had no legal power because it was approved by the World Health Assembly as a recommendation and not a regulation and the governments of industrial countries were unwilling to follow the recommendation. Even in those few countries where the Code became national legislation, affected food companies were only subject to censure for failing to abide. The precise meaning of unfair "advertising" or "promotion" of artificial food was never clearly determined by the WHO, and a US congressman declared that most food industries were "doing business pretty much the way they did before voting the Code."[32] In 1980 testimony at a US Senate hearing, Nestlé and three US companies (Abbot Laboratories, American Home Products, and Bristol Meyers) admitted to not abiding by the International Code because they considered it restrictive of their business practices. Although formally accepting the Code, Nestlé lobbied heavily against it. After 1981, with Reagan as president, the US government openly opposed the Code, overriding the opinion of America's health experts. This was widely interpreted by other governments to mean that a strict enforcement of the Code was not required.

As the controversy around breastfeeding suggests, the "Comprehensive" and "Selective" versions of Primary Health Care were both difficult to implement because of general political factors and factors specific to the health sector. The latter included the need for the reeducation of health personnel, the challenges of engaging meaningful community participation, and the economic cost of PHC. The ideal professional participant in PHC and SPHC was a multipurpose health worker operating outside hospitals in small health centers. These health workers were supposed to collaborate with lay health workers and informal health practitioners, and these community-based workers were idealistically portrayed as parts of local cultures, channels for health education, and acceptable to all subgroups.

---

[32] Larry McDonald, "WHO Infant Formula Code," August 2, 1982, United States, Congressional Record, Proceedings and Debates of the 96th Congress, First Session, vol. 128, Part 14, July 29 to August 5, 1982 (Washington, DC: US Government Printing Office, 1982), p. 18928.

"Communities" were frequently regarded by health workers as single pyramidal structures whose members were willing to participate in health programs after their leaders received the necessary information. In point of fact, these communities were diverse and complex and many had local leaders for whom basic health imperatives such as sanitation were not priorities. Another critical and recurrent headache was the creation of new patterns of dependency because many of the health workers were used to receiving orders from above. In sum, community engagement was difficult to achieve. Besides, many professional health workers in industrial and developing countries had received an education in which prevention was subordinate to treatment and where the highest aspiration was to work in big hospitals or private offices. Many physicians perceived PHC as demanding too many personal sacrifices (few would consider moving to rural areas or shantytowns). Many doctors committed to PHC harbored paternalistic attitudes toward lay health workers whom they regarded as ignorant and as obstacles to health development. Those doctors who embraced PHC thought that it should be provided under the close supervision of qualified professional personnel and should become a first contact with the public health system, especially in rural and underserved areas. Even these doctors could not avoid considering PHC or SPHC as second-quality care or poor health care for the poor. The belief existed also among the poor. In many countries, basic health centers organized in shanty-towns and rural areas for common diseases were bypassed by people who preferred to be treated at the outpatient departments of the nearest hospitals.

A final challenge for PHC and SPHC was the lack of funds in a period of economic recession, growing foreign debt, structural adjustment policies, and increasing underemployment and poverty. During the 1980s, it became more difficult to invest resources in preventive care in developing countries facing inflation, recession, and economic adjustment policies that prioritized debt service payments. It was never clear just how and who would finance Comprehensive PHC. In contrast to other international campaigns, such as the global malaria eradication program of the 1950s where UNICEF and US bilateral assistance provided substantial funding, there were no significant resources in the WHO for training auxiliary personnel, improving nutrition and drinking water, or creating new health centers. A 1986 study examined several cost estimates of PHC in developing countries (amounting to some billions of US dollars) and concluded that "the wide range of costs ... is indicative of how little is known about this area."[33] The 1987 World Health Assembly tried to solve the PHC funding problem by suggesting increased tax

---

[33] M. Patel, "An Economic Evaluation of Health For All," *Health and Policy and Planning* 1 (1986), 37–47.

revenues and voluntary donations. However, there were few people in the governments of developing nations able to implement such measures.

Yet another obstacle to primary health care implementation was lack of effective political commitment. Some authoritarian regimes, such as the military regime in Argentina, formally endorsed the Alma-Ata Declaration but did not implement any tangible reforms. Many ministries of health in developing countries had few competent officers and created underfunded primary health care programs concentrated on one or two of the GOBI interventions. As a result, the ongoing tension between those who advocated vertical, disease-oriented programs and those who advocated community-oriented programs – with the notable exception of immunization discussed in the next section – was accepted as a normal state of affairs.

Immunization and Control under Adversity

Of all SPHC's interventions, immunization achieved the greatest success and prestige and, as a result, the control of some diseases in developing countries made significant progress. This occurred because immunization and disease eradication programs began to change. These programs had traditionally been short-term, independently-directed, and disease-oriented. After Alma-Ata and the success of smallpox eradication, there was a tendency to reject rigid top-down designs and to incorporate "horizontal" components by seeking the integration of public health systems, paying due attention to community participation and education, and integrating immunization into the regular activities of health services. Adaptation to local conditions meant gaining the cooperation of women (who usually took care of health in poor families), recruiting schoolchildren to be promoters of the immunization of their younger siblings, and working with a variety of private organizations and community leaders, thereby enlisting support outside the public health sector.

Immunization efforts built on the WHO's prior commitment to vaccination. In 1974 the WHO had launched an Expanded Program on Immunization (EPI) with the mandate to fight six diseases of infants – diphtheria, pertussis (whooping cough), neonatal tetanus, measles, poliomyelitis, and tuberculosis – and to improve planning, training, evaluation, and cold-chain system development. It was built on the progress of the global smallpox eradication program. Its head was the American Ralph Henderson, who formerly worked in smallpox eradication in Africa and went on to become assistant director-general of the WHO. The term "expanded" referred to the addition of measles and poliomyelitis vaccines to those traditionally used in infant immunization programs (promoted with posters such as the one shown in Figure 7.5). These were selected on the basis of the high incidence of these diseases and the availability of low-cost, reliable vaccines. "Expanded" also

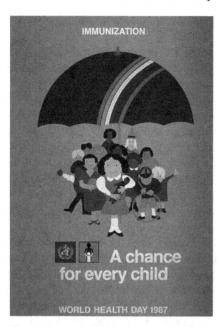

Figure 7.5 Poster used by the WHO in the late 1980s to raise awareness
of immunization as part of its Expanded Program on Immunization
created in 1974 to fight childhood diseases such as diphtheria, measles,
poliomyelitis, and tuberculosis.
Getty Images.

had a deeper connotation: It emphasized the need to increase the rate of
immunization in developing countries, train more health workers in immunization techniques, diminish dropout between first and last immunization,
and improve services in shantytowns and rural areas. Medical science had
made significant progress in the control and treatment of these illnesses and
had diminished adverse reactions following vaccine administration. In 1977,
when most developing countries still had immunization rates between 10 and
20 percent, the World Health Assembly adopted the target of universal
childhood immunization by 1990.[34] Immunization campaigns accelerated
in the developing world after the mid-1980s and added expanded systems
of surveillance and the celebration of National Vaccination Days. These
campaigns were pursued with special intensity when they targeted poliomyelitis, thanks to the help of philanthropies such as Rotary International and

---

[34] Maggie Black, *Children First: The Story of UNICEF, Past and Present* (New York, Oxford
University Press, 1996), 43.

Save the Children. Beginning in 1979, Rotary International provided the polio vaccine in developing countries.

Reinforcing EPI was the result of a negotiation process in which the WHO was a party. First, in 1982 the World Health Assembly recognized EPI as an essential component of Primary Health Care. Then in 1983 eminent medical scientist Jonas Salk, Robert McNamara of the World Bank, and Jim Grant from UNICEF joined forces to stress the urgency and feasibility of promoting control of the communicable diseases embraced by EPI. Third, in March 1984 the Rockefeller Foundation's Bellagio facility hosted another conference; this one was titled "To Protect the World's Children," and included D. A. Henderson and representatives of the WHO, the World Bank, and UNICEF. Some of the themes of the conference were how to cope with the reality of resource limitations and the need to accelerate immunization.[35] It was clear from then on that immunization was to spearhead PHC.

The WHO's newly charged immunization work now included the tackling of poliomyelitis, a highly contagious disease transmitted by a virus spread by fecal waste and contaminated food or water that paralyzes the muscles of the arms, legs, and respiratory system. The first polio vaccine had been developed by Salk and licensed in the United States in 1955. It was an injectable vaccine that contained a killed virus that produced immunity. In 1961, Albert Sabin had introduced an oral form of the vaccine known as OPV consisting of attenuated virus, which was cheap and easy to administer and became the tool of choice for international health agencies. The work against polio via immunization was reinforced in 1985 when the Universal Childhood Immunization Initiative was launched by UNICEF and the WHO. In the same year, the Pan American Health Organization (PAHO) launched a program to eradicate polio in the Americas by 1990. In 1988, when the disease was endemic in 125 countries on five continents, the WHO set a goal for the eradication of poliomyelitis worldwide by the year 2000. At the time, less than 50 percent of the world's children were receiving the recommended three doses of Oral Polio Vaccine. Together with Rotary International, the WHO and UNICEF set standard guidelines and uniform primary vaccination and revaccination schedules, organized national vaccination days to encourage the widest possible participation of local communities, and established the cold chain required for preserving the vaccine's potency, relying on both modern refrigeration and portable ice chests for vaccine storage.[36] Rotary contributed significant funds, provided a network of volunteers all over the world, and built political

---

[35] S. C. Joseph, *Bellagio Conference to Protect the World's Children: Rapporteur's Summary* (New York: Rockefeller Foundation, 1984).

[36] Bernard Seytre & Mary Shaffer, *The Death of a Disease: A History of the Eradication of Poliomyelitis* (New Brunswick: Rutgers University Press, 2005).

commitment through their "Polio Plus" initiative, launched in 1985. Polio Plus meant pressure on governments to commit themselves publicly to the goal of universal immunization and to provide complementary resources rather than depend wholly on donors and multilateral agencies.

Although in the mid-1970s there was no accurate global immunization information system, it was estimated at the time that most developing countries had immunization coverage among infants of five percent on average for the six most important diseases: measles, tetanus, diphtheria, tuberculosis, poliomyelitis, and whooping cough. Differential rates of coverage deepened the gaps between rich and poor nations. For example, measles, which in the mid-1980s killed about two per 10,000 cases in the United States, killed two per 100 cases in developing countries (the figure rose to about 10 per 100 cases in countries marked by malnutrition). In 1986, the WHO decided on the theme for the World Health Day for the following year: "Immunization: A Chance for Every Child," suggesting that every child in the world should have the right to a fair chance in life. ·

By the early 1990s, the WHO could boast progress: More than half of the children of the developing world received immunization each year. This meant the prevention of millions of infant deaths from polio, measles, and pertussis; and neonatal tetanus, while a severe filarial disease in Africa, was coming under control. Onchocerciasis is caused by the parasitic worm *Onchocerca volvulus* and is also known as "river blindness" because of its most extreme manifestation and because the female blackflies (the species *Simulium damnosum*) that transmit the disease concentrate in riverside areas. Onchocerciasis causes wrinkling and depigmentation of the skin, eye lesions, and blindness. Despite the fact that the illness is rarely life threatening, heavily infected individuals suffer from weight loss and a general state of weakness that makes them prone to other, deadlier diseases. Additionally, disease sufferers experience discrimination and depression. Common sights in affected villages were a line of blind adults linked together by poles being led around by a child and blind beggars on the streets. In the mid-1970s, it was estimated that the prevalence of the microfilariae in some towns was greater than 60 percent, and blindness affected more than 5 percent of the population on the West African Savanna (at the time the campaign was promoted by educational materials such as that shown in Figure 7.6). In 1974, it was estimated that more than 1 million individuals out of a total population of 10 million were suffering from onchocerciasis, and that at least 100,000 persons were blind. The disease was also an obstacle to the economic development of fertile areas near rivers since these areas were feared and abandoned. Small farming families living at a subsistence level moved to poorer lands that failed to provide adequate means of survival. The land "lost" to the disease was estimated to be between 65,000 and 80,000 square kilometers, and the mean

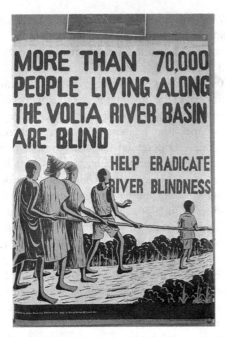

Figure 7.6 Onchocerciasis poster used in Ghana encouraging people to help in the fight against onchocerciasis. The poster depicts elder blind people attacked by the disease led by a child with the aid of a stick. The Onchocerciasis Control Programme (OCP) was launched in 1974 by the WHO in collaboration with other United Nation's agencies and private partners.
Courtesy: World Health Organization Photo Library.

age for blindness was 39 years, when individuals would otherwise be at the peak of their productive lives.[37]

Beginning with the post–World War II period, the disease was of grave concern to tropical medicine doctors, bilateral agencies working in Africa, and the WHO AFRO office. In 1974 the WHO implemented the Onchocerciasis Control Program (OCP) in West Africa, with headquarters in Ouagadougou, Upper Volta. OCP concentrated its work in seven countries of the savanna zone of the Volta River basin (Benin, Ghana, Ivory Coast, Mali, Niger, Togo, and Upper Volta), covering an area of 640,000 square kilometers. Partners in this venture were the United Nations Development Program (UNDP), the

[37] World Health Organization, The Onchocerciasis Control Programme, *Success in Africa: The Onchocerciasis Control Programme in West Africa, 1974–2002* (Geneva: World Health Organization, 2002).

World Bank, and the Food and Agricultural Organization (FAO). The interest of the Bank could be traced to 1972 when Robert McNamara visited West Africa to observe the impact of a drought, witnessed the devastation caused by onchocerciasis in the Upper Volta, and in the following year proposed to the Bank's Board of Executive Directors that they launch an international program targeting the disease.

Another member of the alliance was the Special Program for Research and Training in Tropical Diseases (TDR), created in 1976 by the WHO to improve investigation and control of major but neglected tropical diseases (malaria, filariasis including onchocerciasis, schistosomiasis, trypanosomiases, leishmaniasis, and leprosy). TDR was instrumental in bringing attention to the tragic fact that only a very small amount of financial resources was being used to study and design methods of control of diseases that affected millions of people. Initially, TDR emphasized the development of new medications and vector-control techniques and the training of researchers from disease-endemic countries. Progressively, however, attention shifted to the social and cultural dimensions of disease and the reframing of "tropical diseases" as illnesses linked to poverty and not to a specific region of the world. TDR was run efficiently by its first director Adetokunbo Lucas, a Nigerian medical scientist trained in public health at Harvard University, who held the position from 1976 to 1986.[38]

During OCP's first years, the primary aim of the program was to reduce the vector to a low density and prevent significant transmission. No suitable drugs without serious side effects existed for the treatment of onchocerciasis, but interruption of transmission through vector control seemed achievable. Yet one of the fundamental difficulties discovered in the implementation of the vector-control program was the unexpected reintroduction to riverside areas of adult flies from the forest. The adult blackfly populations could not be controlled because of their dispersal, ability to travel long distances, and their wide variety of resting places. One of OCP's techniques was spreading a larvicide using two fixed-wing aircraft and eight helicopters to destroy the *Similum* adults, combining this aerial attack with cheaper control methods on the ground. OCP also established entomological checkpoints, generally located in sites where transmission rates were very high, to capture adult blackflies for examinations of infectivity.

In 1980, when OCP was facing technical difficulties and had to renew the support of the agencies backing it, Dr. Ebrahim M. Samba of Gambia (see Figure 7.7) was appointed director (in 1995 he became the WHO's Africa regional director). An astute observer of the WHO summarized the role of

---

[38] C. Morel, "Reaching Maturity: 25 Years of TDR," *Parasitology Today* 16:12 (2000), 2–8.

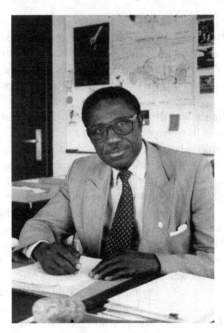

Figure 7.7 Ebrahim M. Samba, a Gambian physician, was appointed director of the WHO Onchocerciasis Control Program in West Africa in 1980 and would remain in that position until 1995. He was later director of the Regional Office for Africa of the World Health Organization between 1995 and 2005.
Courtesy: World Health Organization Photo Library.

Samba: He had turned an "ailing program ... into a success."[39] He developed a strategy that over ten years was designed to respond to the parasite's long lifespan while participating governments were asked to take over a number of activities. The charismatic Samba encouraged the creation of National Onchocerciasis Committees in each of the countries involved and requested an increase in the number of health workers in the program.

During the second half of the 1980s, new techniques and public health methods contributed to OCP's work. In 1987, ivermectin, traditionally used for deworming household pets, cattle, and race horses, was introduced as a new and effective microfilaricide drug with few side effects and as an adjunct to larviciding. Thanks to an agreement between the WHO and Merck, Sharpe & Dohme of New Jersey, which produced ivermectin for veterinary medicine, the

---

[39] Fionna Godlee, "The World Health Organization in Africa," *British Medical Journal* 309 (1994), 553–554.

drug was distributed free of charge. When administered orally, generally once a year, it killed the parasite microfilariae. Since transmission was still a problem, it was complementary to vector control measures. The director of TDR narrated the conversation with Merck's chief executive officer: "I was well prepared for tough negotiation about the pricing of the drug ... I had rehearsed my speech about the significance of the partnership between the WHO and TDR and the company ... Then came the bombshell! [He] told us ... of the corporate decision to donate the drug."[40] In 1987 the disease was controlled in eight countries in the sub-Saharan region. In the previous years, and not known to all medical researchers, Merck's investigator William Campbell demonstrated that ivermectin had an impact on onchocerciasis in humans and organized successful human trials in Dakar and other areas of Africa. Another precedent was that Merck made an unsuccessful effort to obtain financial resources from the US Congress to supply the drug at cost.

By the end of the 1980s, it was estimated that thanks to OCP, 27,000 individuals had been saved from going blind in the Upper Volta basin, around three million children born within the program area since the start of the operations were safe from onchocerciasis infection, and 70 percent of the patients originally suffering from eye infections had recovered.[41] The experience suggested that vector control could be accomplished by the community and successfully integrated into multi-tiered health programs. It also modeled collaboration between the private and public sectors and made internationally visible a previously "neglected disease."

By the late 1990s, the distribution of ivermectin, the control of the black-fly vector, and educational programs had treated and prevented thousands of cases of blindness and freed a million hectares of land for human use. Some years later, a beautiful and dramatic statue, "Sightless Among Miracles" by R. T. Wallen, unveiled in 1999 and depicting a child leading a blind man affected by the disease, graced the entrance of the WHO's building in Geneva.

OCP would be an example for other disease-control programs in Africa such as the campaigns against the parasitic dracunculiasis, better known as Guinea Worm Disease, begun in the early 1980s, and against leprosy, which had the help of the new Multidrug Therapy (MDT). It also attracted new donors such as the Carter Foundation, which served to increase the number of diseases it tackled from its initial commitment to eliminate Guinea Worm Disease. The lessons learned in OCP were applied against dracunuliasis, a disease

---

[40] Adetokunbo O. Lucas, *It was the Best of Times, from Local to Global Health: The Autobiography of Adetokunbo Olumide Lucas* (Ibadan: Bookbuilders, Editions Africa, 2010), p. 217.

[41] See Le Berre, R, J. F. Walsh, B. Philippon et al., "The WHO Onchocerciasis Control Programme: Retrospect and Prospects," *Philosophical Transactions of the Royal Society of London, Series B, Biological Sciences* 328:1251 (June 30, 1990), 721–727.

transmitted by drinking water contaminated with fleas carrying the larvae of the parasite, that affected overwhelmingly African countries, and against Leprosy, which had been a tragedy in more than fifty countries in the world, especially in Southeast Asia. In 1998, these diseases with five others (polio, measles, Onchocerciasis, Chagas disease, and lymphatic filariasis) were targeted for eradication. Progress in the case of polio was remarkable. By the end of 2001, the number of confirmed cases across 10 nations had fallen to a few hundred, and almost one-tenth of the world's population – 575 million children – received oral polio vaccine. Another achievement of the program was its legacy. After controlling the disease, the African Onchocerciasis Control Program closed in December 2015, only to become, the next year, the Expanded Special Project for Elimination of Neglected Tropical Diseases (ESPEN), which targeted other African Neglected Tropical Diseases where preventive chemotherapy was effective: lymphatic filariasis, trachoma, soil transmitted helminths, and schistosomiasis.

Health Promotion and the Persistence of PHC

Approximately ten years after the Alma-Ata Conference, the WHO organized a smaller meeting at Riga in the USSR. Officers of UNICEF and the WHO, including Mahler and more than 20 health experts, held a "midpoint meeting" on the goal of Health for All by 2000 in order to reflect on the progress of PHC and produce a report for the World Health Assembly of 1988. John Bryant, a veteran of Alma-Ata, prepared the background document and final report. The latter contained a definitely mixed review. The concept of Health for All was reported to have had a strong impact but practical commitments to Comprehensive PHC were few, especially in developing countries. Bryant reframed the goal of Alma-Ata by stating that the struggle for Health for All should go "up to and beyond the year 2000."[42]

More optimistic were officers of the WHO European Regional Office (EURO), who with Canadian health scholars had revised and transformed PHC by introducing a new concept: Health Promotion. This notion first appeared in studies conducted by the European regional office during the late 1970s and early 1980s. Initially, the concept was closely linked to the new emphasis in the 1970s on the need for changes in personal lifestyle and individual health behaviors, but in the 1980s Health Promotion broadened by emphasizing the participation of governments in tackling such issues as the rising costs of health care and the deterioration of the physical environment. A healthy environment was understood to concern not only sanitation and

---

[42] World Health Organization, *From Alma Ata to the Year 2000: Reflections at the Midpoint* (Geneva: World Health Organization, 1988).

waste disposal systems but also freedom from want, unemployment, and the threat of war. In 1984 a one-day workshop entitled "Beyond Health Care," held in Toronto, conceptualized and defined the field of Health Promotion policies. The main papers of the meeting appeared in a 1985 issue of the *Canadian Journal of Public Health.* At almost the exact same time, the WHO's regional office for Europe produced a report on *Concepts and Principles of Health Promotion,* which resulted from a meeting that had been held in Copenhagen in July 1984. This report clearly emphasized health-promoting changes in general social conditions over changes in individual lifestyles.[43] This approach was distinctly different from the one developed in the United States at the same time and suggested a subtle continuing influence of a broad social perspective and even of Mahler's "Nordic socialism."

In November 1986, Health Promotion achieved greater international recognition thanks to a meeting in Ottawa co-organized by the WHO, the Department of Health and Welfare of Canada, and the Canadian Public Health Association. Although the meeting organizers did not have the resources to secure the participation of all countries of the world, they gathered 200 participants from 38 countries, including scholars and government officials from industrialized countries who had experience in health promotion and preventive work. The leaders of the meeting were the Canadian Trevor Hancock, a public health physician, and the German political scientist Ilona Kickbusch, who directed the unit on health promotion in EURO that had been producing reports on the topic since 1981. She was appointed secretary of the conference in Ottawa and was credited with being "the key instigator" of the WHO's role in Health Promotion. Other prominent figures at the Ottawa meeting were Halfdan Mahler, Regional Director of EURO Jo Asvall, and Canadian Minister of National Health and Welfare Jake Epp. In a publication appearing after the Conference, Kickbusch explained that governments had the responsibility to ensure basic societal conditions for healthy life and to make healthy personal choices easier.[44]

The Ottawa meeting produced a seminal document that was infused with the spirit of Comprehensive PHC: the Ottawa Charter for Health Promotion. The two organizing principles of the Charter were that health was broad and multidimensional and that governments should work to control the socioeconomic and environmental factors affecting living conditions. The Charter proposed five areas of action: healthy public policies, supportive environments, community action, personal skills development, and preventive health

---

[43] World Health Organization, Regional Office for Europe, *Concepts and Principles of Health Promotion: Report on a WHO Meeting, Copenhagen, July 9–13, 1984* (Copenhagen: World Health Organization, 1984).

[44] Ilona Kickbusch, "Issues in Health Promotion," *Health Promotion* 1:4 (1987), 437–442.

care services.[45] The Ottawa Conference sparked a series of additional conferences that in the following years enriched the notion of Health Promotion (HP). In 1988, in Adelaide, Australia, the HP conference concentrated on healthy public policies to enable people to lead healthy lives. In 1991, the HP conference in Sundsvall, Sweden, had as its central theme supportive environments for health. The HP conference in Jakarta in 1997 emphasized community participation, health literacy, and social responsibility for health. The documents produced by these conferences were endorsed by the WHO, which also produced a number of documents and glossaries for HP.

In 1988, the WHA adopted the first global health promotion resolution and urged all member countries to implement the priorities set out in the Ottawa declaration. At the national level, the UK Royal College of Physicians used the Ottawa charter as the platform for policy development concerning alcohol and smoking control. At the same time, HP achieved recognition thanks to a project supported by the WHO known as "Healthy Cities," launched at a symposium that took place in Lisbon in April 1986 and attended by 56 participants from 21 cities and 17 countries. Two years later, 14 cities from Europe, Canada, and Australia participated in the project and a WHO Healthy Cities office was established in EURO headquarters in Copenhagen. In 1988 and 1989 other Healthy Cities symposia took place in Zagreb and in The Hague. These meetings proclaimed the need for equitable access to healthy environments and social services, for strengthening community involvement in health issues, and for establishing a strategy to cooperate with "non-aligned" and developing countries. The movement was supported by a working group on health promotion established by the WHO Regional Office for Europe in 1995 in cooperation with bilateral agencies and the US Centers for Disease Control (CDC). The working group organized workshops and conferences and commissioned several papers.

The rationale for the Health Cities was as follows: Municipal authorities were well positioned to marshal resources to develop and implement intersectoral policies and community participation. The initial group of European cities were expected to follow a set of parameters, collaborate in the implementation of intersectoral plans, and form a network. Healthy Cities became the model for other initiatives, such as healthy schools, healthy hospitals, and healthy workplaces but, unfortunately, this expansion was frequently confused with limited goals such as adequate disposal of garbage, reduction of traffic, control of pollution, and provision of shelter to the homeless. It became difficult to transform Healthy Cities into a true social movement because its activities were too constrained within the realm of local government. More

---

[45] *Ottawa Charter for Health Promotion* (Ottawa, Ontario: n.p., 1986).

ambitious goals, such as the reduction of urban poverty and the achievement of "social justice," were increasingly perceived as too political. Over time the Healthy Cities initiative increased the number of urban centers that participated but took on a life of its own that was not linked to a revival of PHC as its originators had hoped. A further difficulty was that HP was not a priority for the director-generals who succeeded Mahler after 1988. In 1998, Kickbusch left her position as director of the Division of Health Promotion, Education, and Communication in Geneva and took up an appointment as professor of public health at Yale University, where she remained until 2004. Meetings and academic activities devoted to HP have since taken place with a less-active participation and leadership of the WHO.

A New Director-General

During the 1980s, Mahler had crusaded for holistic primary health care in different forums and participated actively in the first Health Promotion meetings. Yet he did not have the full support of the WHO's bureaucracy, and his allies inside and outside the WHO were not always present to offer support in international forums. For example, Carl Taylor left Johns Hopkins University and was a UNICEF representative in China from 1984 to 1987. In 1985, Tejada-de-Rivero, one of Mahler's principal assistants in Geneva, moved permanently to Peru, where he became minister of health. The WHO also faced new financial challenges, although in 1987 it still had the second largest budget in the UN system (the United States still gave an important contribution of millions of dollars for the WHO's regular budget and for special programs).[46] The amounts pledged as voluntary contributions were growing – and becoming a menace to coherent governance in the agency – but were less than half of the regular budget.

In 1988, Mahler ended his third five-year term as director-general and after some hesitation decided not to launch another reelection campaign. No one else in the agency had sufficient stamina to keep promoting primary health care against all odds. The 41st World Health Assembly appointed Hiroshi Nakajima of Japan to the post of director-general for a five-year period starting in July 1988. Unfortunately, Nakajima did not live up to expectations and the generous financial support of Japan failed to compensate for his limitations as the new director-general. Under Nakajima, the WHO remedicalized, trimmed primary health care, and lost much of its worldwide credibility. Although a WHO team prepared an internal document in December 1997, "Health for All

---

[46] United States, Department of State, World Health Organization (Washington, DC: Department of States, 1987), pp. 2–3.

in the 21st Century," and had it positively reviewed in Geneva and the regional offices, it never really left the drawing board.[47] However, other WHO programs were beginning to take on a life of their own that did not depend on the initiative of the director-general's office. The response to AIDS was one of them.

[47] World Health Organization, *Health for All in the 21st Century* (Geneva: World Health Organization, 1998).

8   The Response to the HIV/AIDS Pandemic

The story of the WHO's response to the HIV/AIDS pandemic can be compared to a roller coaster ride. Initially, the multilateral agency underestimated the health issue and was indecisive; then, starting in 1986 it assumed a position as a key player in the fight against AIDS, before losing its leadership role during the 1990s; then in the early twenty-first century the agency regained its preeminence when it became clear that AIDS affected mainly the world's poor, especially in sub-Saharan African nations. It makes for an interesting story that is not without contradictions, although it is not one that exemplifies how best to respond to pandemic disease. The story in some ways demonstrates the peculiarity of HIV/AIDS as a highly stigmatized global disease that attacked rich and poor countries alike, but it also points to the contingencies of history, the often fruitless competition between powerful organizations, and the sometimes pivotal roles played by key individuals.

The international reckoning with AIDS demonstrated some of the recurrent problems of public health, including short-term and insufficient responses, blaming marginalized groups, emphasizing collective responsibility over individual rights, maintaining an artificial divide between prevention and treatment, and leaning on medical and scientific arguments at the expense of social and behavioral ones. An examination of the response to these challenges illuminates the struggle faced by the WHO in confronting a major disease in the twentieth century and in the early twenty-first century.

The Beginnings of a Pandemic

AIDS was first recognized in the United States in 1981 when doctors in Los Angeles and New York found clusters of unusual symptoms and infections among otherwise healthy young men.[1] These men died within a few months,

---

[1] On the early years of Aids, see: Elizabeth Fee & Daniel M. Fox (eds.), *AIDS: The Burdens of History* (Berkeley: University of California Press, 1988) and Virginia Berridge, *AIDS in the UK: The Making of Policy, 1981–1994* (New York: Oxford University Press, 1996).

after suffering from rare types of cancer and pneumonia. What the men had in common was that they were homosexual. Almost immediately, the media dubbed the disease the "gay cancer" or the "gay plague." Midway through 1982, the US Centers for Disease Control (CDC) had already reported 403 cases in 24 states, and at about the same time 200 AIDS cases had been identified in Europe, 42 of them in men of African origin. Early in 1984, two separate research groups, in Paris and Bethesda, Maryland, announced a breakthrough by identifying the disease's retroviral origin and later designed the first tests to identify the virus in the blood. This was at a time when most of the media was spreading stigma and panic about the risk of a disease that was almost always depicted as coming from an external threat or from "marginalized" individuals. Many developing country governments denied the problem, arguing that it only existed in industrial societies. Some medical scientists had doubts as to whether retroviruses could produce infectious diseases in human beings.

Not long after, cases of the newly recognized disease were diagnosed in people who had no history of homosexuality. IV drug users, hemophiliacs, and Haitians seemed to be heavily affected, leading to the epidemiological identification of various "risk groups." But the early identification of AIDS as a gay disease garnered both popular and scientific attention. It was therefore a considerable shock when cases of apparently heterosexual transmission were confirmed in Africa. Doctors in Kinshasa found that numbers of otherwise healthy young people were dying from a disease resembling AIDS and asked CDC to investigate. With support from the government of Zaire (now the Republic of Congo), the CDC, the National Institutes of Health, and the Belgian Institute of Tropical Medicine, Peter Piot, Thomas Quinn, and Jose McCormick traveled to Zaire and confirmed what the Kinshasa doctors had suspected, that certain central African countries seemed to be suffering from AIDS. To their considerable distress, they found that patients with AIDS were both women and men, in roughly equal proportions.[2] This implied that the disease was being transmitted heterosexually. It also suggested that there was a possibility the potential number of cases could increase massively; this disease was not going to be confined to a gay subculture. This important discovery went unnoticed by many experts. In the early 1980s, very few scientists and public health workers were concerned about AIDS. The scientific and medical worlds were in a state of denial.

AIDS posed a twofold challenge to scientists, physicians, health workers, policy makers, and the population at large. In the first place, nothing was

---

[2] The Belgian, Piot, was already famous for his co-discovery of the Ebola virus in 1976. See Thomas C. Quinn, "AIDS in Africa: A Retrospective," *Bulletin of the World Health Organization* 79:12 (2001), 1156–1158.

known about the disease. Initially, there were no methods for its diagnosis, treatment, or prevention. Secondly, the disease was closely linked to public debates about sexuality and national security, topics that are hardly ever linked or discussed. Furthermore, AIDS was related to certain types of sexuality that were considered deviant by conservatives and linked to the decline of body organs and tissues and fluids that are considered essential and private, including the skin, blood, and semen. Conservative political forces in both capitalist and communist nations reacted angrily to the discovery of cases of HIV infection, believing that the disease was to be limited to homosexuals, drug addicts, and other "deviants." The American politician Patrick Buchanan referred to AIDS as "nature's retribution" for gay individuals who had gone against nature, while many conservative religious leaders considered the disease to be divine punishment against immorality. It was therefore truly remarkable that individuals, groups, and organizations, both within and outside official agencies, overcame a limited resource base and considerable prejudice to throw their efforts into understanding and fighting AIDS with such speed. These efforts built on previous work by diverse organizations against homophobia and on the work of virologists.

In the first half of the 1980s, there was intense scientific debate and conflict over the diagnostic test for AIDS. Early in 1983, French virologist Luc Montaigner and other researchers from the Institut Pasteur published a paper in *Science* describing a new virus called lymphadenopathy (LAV). Robert Gallo, an American researcher at the NIH, claimed to have discovered the AIDS virus in an issue of the same journal the following year. In May 1985 the US Patent Office awarded the patent for the AIDS blood test to the American and the US Department of Health and Human Services. In the same year, the FDA approved the ELISA test (enzyme-linked immunosorbent assay) for detecting HIV antibodies in blood (two years later the more precise western blot test was approved). In December 1985, the Institut Pasteur sued the Department of Health and Human Services, contending that the French were the first to identify the virus and devise the test. In 1992, Gallo was accused of committing minor scientific misconduct by falsely reporting facts in his 1984 article, but he subsequently cleared his name. Although Gallo and Montaigner later reestablished a cordial relationship and even published a 2002 joint paper in *Science*, the primacy of the French was internationally recognized when Gallo and his colleague, Françoise Barré-Sinoussi, were awarded the 2008 Nobel Prize for the discovery of the human immunodeficiency virus. In any case, these investigations determined that the modes of transmission of the disease were blood and semen.

In the early 1980s, only a few cases of AIDS had been identified outside the United States and Europe, and the World Health Organization considered the disease to be a low priority. Halfdan Mahler, then director-general, thought that the disease was mainly found in the industrialized West, (although later he admitted that he had not taken the disease seriously enough). It seemed less important than malaria, tuberculosis, malnutrition, and a host of other problems that threatened the health of people in the developing world, and he feared responses to AIDS would divert attention from Primary Health Care work in Africa. Starting in 1982, the WHO did publish information on AIDS in the *Weekly Epidemiological Record* and called a meeting on AIDS at the end of 1983 to monitor the problem. The early activities of the agency were due in part to a growing concern of Fakhry Assad, an experienced Egyptian primary care physician with an interest in virology who had been in Geneva since the mid-1960s and became director of the Communicable Diseases Division. Initially, Assad believed that AIDS was a problem restricted to industrialized countries. However, thanks to his ties to the CDC, he led the fight to see AIDS more broadly and to make it a priority at the WHO. He participated in the organization in April 1985 of the first International AIDS Conference that took place at the CDC in Atlanta with sponsorship from the USPHS and the WHO. More than 2,000 participants attended the event, and papers were presented on all aspects of the disease, including diagnostic tests and psychosocial and behavioral issues. At that time, nearly 20 percent of cases documented worldwide had been reported outside the United States. After the conference, Assad began to set up Collaborating Centers on AIDS linked to the WHO, and in September of that year the agency organized a meeting of these Centers in order to arrive at a consensus on the mode of transmission and to identify practical control methods. One of Assad's most lasting contributions was a workshop with the CDC in Bangui in the Central African Republic that established a clinical case definition that was instrumental in developing countries because it could be used when laboratory confirmation was difficult. This definition, which would be used until 1994, was instrumental in developing countries where laboratory facilities for testing HIV antibodies were not available. It included clinically sound criteria and drew together a number of syndromes and diseases under an HIV umbrella: weight loss, continuous or repeated attacks of fever and diarrhea, herpes zoster, and generalized Kaposi's sarcoma. By 1986, 85 countries across all continents had reported several thousand cases of AIDS to the WHO.

Assad was decisive in making Mahler an advocate of the idea of a WHO program on AIDS. Another reason for Mahler's change of opinion is pointed out by Merson and Inrig: Mahler became aware of the uproar faced by diplomatic, political, and governmental inaction in late 1985. Assad was assisted by other European officers of the WHO. Once adequate testing and diagnostic equipment became available in the mid-1980s, some WHO officers, such as the Russian Boris Bytchenko, the regional officer for communicable diseases at EURO, began to take AIDS more seriously. The number of cases began to grow exponentially, and public health workers and NGOs came to put pressure on official health organizations. The identification of its etiological origin, description of clinical symptoms, and existence of laboratory tests convinced many skeptics that AIDS was a unique biological and clinical entity and required a political response. This was especially true in developing countries where the work of scientists, public health workers, and gay leaders was instrumental in overcoming government resistance.

In addition, AIDS became a public health concern because during the first years of the epidemic, prevention was the main response. The first medicine used to treat the disease was Zidovudine, marketed under the brand name Retrovir (AZT), which had been developed in the 1960s as an anticancer medication and was approved by the FDA in the late 1980s with the intention of using it against AIDS. However, AZT had serious toxic side effects, including anemia in many patients, and in the majority of cases it only provided temporary relief, leading to a more resistant virus. Thus, AIDS became a priority for public health rather than medical treatment.

The Origins of the WHO's Program on AIDS and Mann on Board

While origins of WHO interest and activities on AIDS can be traced to Fakhry Assad, its reputation would be linked to the American Jonathan Mann. Early in 1986, Assad still believed a specific program could be part of his Division of Communicable Diseases (he reached out to the CDC and got advice that the best individual to head a program devoted to AIDS would be Mann). In January 1986 both Assad and Mahler offered Mann the position (he would begin to work a few months later).[3] Mann was a charismatic young doctor from Boston with a master of public health degree from Harvard University who had, since 1984, been working on a project sponsored by the CDC and NIH in Kinshasa called Project SIDA (in that same year he met Assad in Geneva). Like Mahler, Mann was perceived as set apart from ordinary people, a gifted speaker and endowed with unique charisma. They both agreed that the disease was an unprecedented challenge not only to gay people but to global public health and the developing world. Upon being convinced of its urgency, Mahler devoted his energy to the issue: He and Mann flew to New York in November of 1986 and held a press conference at the UN headquarters (as seen in Figure 8.1) to announce that the WHO had underestimated AIDS, that

---

[3] Michael Merson & Stephen Inring, *The AIDS Pandemic: Searching for a Global Response* (Cham, Switzerland: Springer, 2018), pp. 25, 41.

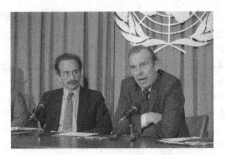

Figure 8.1 Jonathan Mann (left), who was in charge of the first WHO AIDS program, with Halfdan Mahler at UN Headquarters in New York City, addressing the first press conference in 1986 on the WHO's program to combat AIDS. Mann led the program until 1990.
Credit WHO /Milton Grant. Courtesy: World Health Organization Photo Library.

millions of people could soon be infected with the AIDS virus, and that the WHO would address AIDS prevention and control as a priority.[4]

After the ambivalence and denial of several representatives of developing countries, a compelling intervention of Uganda's minister of health at the 39th World Health Assembly in May 1986 recognized that his country faced a serious AIDS problem and requested urgent help from the WHO. The intervention was a turning point because it broke the official silence of AIDS in Africa. In May of 1986, the World Health Assembly unanimously approved a resolution giving full support to the WHO's strategy to combat AIDS. Initially the Program was part of Assad's Division of Communicable Diseases, but by the end of 1986 – because the program was growing so rapidly and because of the sickness and unfortunate death of Assad late in that year – it acquired substantial independence and autonomy. First it was called the "Control Program," and after a decisive January 1987 meeting of the Executive Board it became the Special Program on AIDS (although it would become known as the Global Program on AIDS, GPA). The GPA was similar to the Program for Research and Training in Tropical Diseases (TDR), the Special Program of Research in Human Reproduction, and the Expanded Program on Immunization, in that it fell outside of the WHO's regular bureaucratic structure and as a result had its own budget. Mann reported directly to Mahler and not to an assistant director-general like other programs. The GPA was built from scratch, starting with a single room, three epidemiologists, a secretary, and a typewriter. With Halfdan Mahler's enthusiastic support, Mann was able

---

[4] Lawrence K. Altman, "Global Program Aims to Combat AIDS Disaster," *The New York Times,* November 21, 1986.

to turn the GPA into the strongest, most influential, and best-financed program in the WHO. Within a matter of months, Mann had around 200 officers working with him. The GPA's first budget was made up of contributions of USD 5 million, but by the end of 1987 that had increased to USD 30 million, and USD 60 million in 1989. Funding came largely from donors and bilateral agencies from industrialized countries. Smaller donations came from protestant churches because the World Council of Churches, the same organization that inspired Primary Health Care, had, from 1986 onwards, agreed to a nonjudgmental position on AIDS. As a result, it called upon its supporters to provide care for the sick and promote education on HIV and sent representatives to the International Conferences on Aids.[5] Funding grew to such an extent that a WHO Trust Fund for the GPA was established to manage the donations.

Paradoxically, one of the reasons why the GPA enjoyed such financial success was that it allowed donor countries to avoid close identification with the disease and to fight the disease indirectly. Bilateral agencies were concerned enough to invest in AIDS, but for domestic political reasons they did not want to get involved in the details of dealing with "controversial" groups of people and themes such as gays, sex workers, and IV drug users, or condoms, genital ulcers and anal intercourse. Up until late 1985, USAID had no specific mandate related to AIDS or HIV infections, and in the years that followed it concentrated its support on grants for the WHO. The bilateral agency remained reluctant to fully confront the issues related to AIDS prevention, treatment, and research in the domestic sphere because President Reagan prohibited funding for the use of condoms, but it made general contributions to multilateral initiatives in order to avoid these restrictions. HIV/AIDS was not a foreign-policy priority for the Bush Administration but provided some needed financial resources to international agencies. Mann agreed with this tacit division of labor. He saw the advantages of having a technical organization like the GPA in the field and relying on the resources of bilateral organizations such as USAID. He also reinforced the autonomy and political support for his program.

Initially the goals of the program were to promote blood safety and biosecurity measures at hospitals, laboratory support and epidemiological surveillance, education to the public and health workers, and changes in lifestyles in "risk groups." These goals were part of an overall strategy that emphasized prevention, a reduction of the impact of the disease, and coordination of national and international responses. In time, GPA staff developed a

---

[5] Brigitta Rubenson, "What the World Council of Churches is Doing about AIDS," *Contact: A Bi-Monthly Publication of the Christian Medical Commission, World Council of Churches,* Geneva 117 December 1990, p. 7.

sophisticated human-rights approach and fought the discriminatory beliefs and behaviors that existed in society as well as regulations restricting travel. In 1987, Mann gave a briefing on AIDS to the United Nations General Assembly in which he underlined that health prevention and care was a human right. This was a historic moment that reflected the political significance of the emerging pandemic. Another indication that AIDS-related discrimination was a concern for some political authorities came at the World Summit of Ministers of Health on Programs for AIDS Prevention that took place in London in January 1988. The summit was organized by the British government and the WHO and was attended by representatives of more than 100 countries. Participation by ministers from developing countries was guaranteed through the support of Mann's program at the WHO. The meeting provided an update on the situation of AIDS globally, reviewed national policies for prevention and control, discussed guidelines for AIDS policies, and called upon the WHO to support establishing and strengthening national AIDS programs. At its close, a land-mark Declaration was issued, stating that in the absence of a vaccine or a cure the paramount intervention was prevention, with a focus on providing adequate information and education. Mahler was one of the speakers at the opening ceremony. A video was specially prepared for the meeting and referred to two long-standing themes in international health, that disease crosses borders and should be stopped everywhere: "The AIDS virus travels without respect for manmade boundaries. It cannot be stopped in one country until it is stopped in all countries."[6] According to one account, a leading theme throughout the whole meeting "was a strong plea from everyone – both WHO staff and country representatives – to fight bigotry and prejudice in dealing with persons infected by the AIDS virus."[7] This plea came in response to the initial reactions to AIDS that were based on ostracism and discrimination. Some governments prohibited entry to people with HIV and requested manda-tory testing for the military and even for marriage applicants. In the mid-1980s a quarantine program for AIDS patients was established in Cuba, and China made HIV testing mandatory for all foreigners who spent more than a year in the country. The Soviet Union did not fully recognize the extent of the epidemic. Initially, African governments also resorted to discriminatory prac-tices and were hesitant to be open about the HIV/AIDS problem because they felt that the rest of the world was blaming them for originating the epidemic. The GPA fought to convince many politicians and health workers that

---

[6] Overview for Video Presentation, World Summit of Ministries of Health on Programmes for Aids Prevention, London, January 25–28, 1988, Folder A20–87-23, Fourth Generation of Files, WHO.

[7] J. E. Asvall, Regional Director EURO, Visit to the United Kingdom, March 23, 1988, World Summit of Health Ministries on Programs for Aids Prevention, London, January 26–28, 1988, Folder A20–87-23, Second Generation of Files, WHO.

compulsory measures would not control the epidemic. Two influential events for the political recognition of AIDS occurred in 1988. First, the GPA and International Labour Organization (ILO) conference on AIDS in the workforce took place in Geneva, urging to protect the jobs and fight the discrimination of infected people. Secondly, the WHO and the London School of Hygiene and Tropical Medicine cosponsored an International Conference on the Global Impact of AIDS that provided a panorama of the world situation and the need for an interdisciplinary approach and protection of the rights of people living with HIV and AIDS.[8]

In April 1989, more than 146,000 cases of AIDS had been reported to the WHO by 148 countries, but because of underreporting, the GPA estimated the number of cases to be closer to 450,000, with most of them located in sub-Saharan Africa.[9] Between 1987 and 1989, Mann refined the human-rights approach that diverged from the traditional public-health view that the occasional infringement of individual rights, such as the isolation of the sick during an epidemic, was permissible. For him, the disease had given rise to the violation of basic human rights, including: the persistent scapegoating of the sick; their unequal treatment in medical services and unequal access to work and educational opportunities; and a lack of privacy about individual health status. Mann argued that the response was based on the misguided assumption that an epidemic could be controlled if "risk" groups were identified and risk reduction was enforced to change the behavior of individuals. In a context of fear, panic, and discrimination about AIDS, Mann argued that public health and individual human rights were perfectly compatible. For him, changes in the behavior of individuals could be better achieved by education and persuasion, while coercive and discriminatory policies such as travel prohibitions, quarantines, and mandatory HIV testing were counterproductive because they led individuals to disguise their HIV status and encouraged greater intolerance in societies.[10] Mann's view was that respect for individual rights was a precondition for HIV prevention and control. His right-based response aimed to address the multidimensional characteristics of AIDS.

The 1988 World Health Assembly proved to be fertile ground for sanctioning these ideas and approved a resolution entitled "Avoidance of discrimination in

---

[8] Alan F. Fleming, Manuel Carballo, David W. FitzSimons, Michael R. Bailey, & Jonathan Mann (eds.), *The Global Impact of AIDS* (New York: Liss, 1988).

[9] The figures were discussed in Public Hearing on Aids in other countries especially in countries of the Third World, Bonn Federal Republic of Germany, April 20, 1989. A20–86-1 1986 Third Generation of Files, WHO.

[10] James Chin & Jonathan Mann, "Global Surveillance and Forecasting of AIDS," *Bulletin of the World Health Organization* 67:1 (1989), 1–7. Mann's ideas would be later summarized and expanded in articles and books such as Jonathan Mann, "Global AIDS: Critical Issues for Prevention in the 1990s," *International Journal of Health Services* 21:3 (1991), 553–539.

relation to HIV-infected people and people with AIDS." Following this Assembly, the GPA organized two informal meetings in Geneva on human rights law, along with governmental agencies and NGOs. During the following months, Mann became a persuasive and tireless advocate of this public health approach to AIDS. At the IV International Conference on AIDS held in Stockholm in 1988, he delivered an address entitled "AIDS Discrimination and Public Health" that created a forum for people living with HIV. In October of the same year, Mann addressed a meeting of UN officers in charge of human rights at which it was agreed that December 1 would be World AIDS Day and a UN resolution was approved, entitled "Non-discrimination in the field of health."[11]

In addition to Mann, two outstanding GPA officers took forward this human rights approach: Daniel Tarantola, a French physician involved in the creation of *Medecins Sans Frontieres* who became an expert in setting national AIDS programs, and the sociologist from Gibraltar Manuel Carballo, head of the GPA's Social and Behavioral Research Unit, who had previously been responsible for leading the WHO's work on maternal health and breastfeeding. In a short space of time, dozens of requests for AIDS assistance were met. In 1986 and 1987, national AIDS programs were organized in 151 countries, thanks to the work of the program.[12] The GPA made direct contact with affected countries to organize national AIDS programs and help to design national policies and budgets, bypassing the bureaucracy of regional headquarters and frequently sending its own experts to organize these programs. It also produced guidelines and manuals that set out the GPA's human-rights approach in clear terms, involving anonymous testing, voluntary informed consent, confidentiality, and counseling. At the same time, the GPA staff was instructed to conduct country assessments to monitor the AIDS situation in given countries in order to review available national and bilateral resources and local politics, while leaving the running of programs to locals (avoiding the image of "foreign" experts parachuting into countries and dictating what should be done).[13] The programs were to be responsible for HIV surveillance (given problems that existed with unreliable data and significant underreporting of AIDS cases), blood screening in hospitals, the establishment of clinical

---

[11] Barbara Drew, "World AIDS Day, Essay Contest," *Canadian Medical Association Journal* 139 (1988), 1031.

[12] World Health Organization, *The Fourth Ten Years of the World Health Organization, 1978–1987* (Geneva: World Health Organization, 2011), p. 279.

[13] "Jonathan Mann Intervention," in Coping with Aids in Africa: Three Years into the WHO Program on AIDS, United States, House of Representatives, Hearings before the subcommittee on Africa of the Committee of Foreign Affairs, House of Representatives, One Hundred First Congress, First Session, June 14 and July 1989 (Washington, DC: US Government Printing Office, 1990), p. 32.

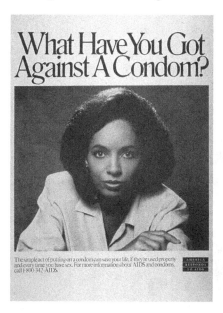

What Have You Got Against A Condom?

The simple act of putting on a condom can save your life, if they're used properly and every time you have sex. For more information about AIDS and condoms, call 1-800-342-AIDS.

AMERICA RESPONDS TO AIDS

Figure 8.2 HIV/AIDS poster promoting the use of condoms, 1990.
Image courtesy National Library of Medicine. Source: Smith Collection/Gado/
Getty Images.

programs, the collection of reliable epidemiological information, the creation of counseling units, the distribution of condoms, and public education. (Educational campaign posters are depicted in Figures 8.2 and 8.3.) Emphasis was placed on explaining to the public that the disease was only transmitted by unprotected sexual contact, contaminated blood transfusions and products, and needle sharing and on educating health workers about biosafety measures to reduce the risk of the occupational transmission of AIDS. The GPA gave grants to civil society groups and nongovernmental organizations that demonstrated a capacity to establish care and prevention efforts, diverging from the WHO custom of only working with governmental institutions. After a few years, there were significant increases in the number of countries reporting AIDS cases to the WHO and in countries with national AIDS programs.

Addressing the relationship between AIDS and breastfeeding proved to be a complex challenge because breastfeeding was part of long-standing tradition in public health. During the early 1990s, it was found that HIV could be passed from mother to child in the womb, during childbirth, and through breastfeeding. Moreover, it was estimated that avoiding breastfeeding by HIV-positive mothers could reduce significantly the risk of transmission to babies. Restricting and even prohibiting breastfeeding in some cases was difficult to accept by

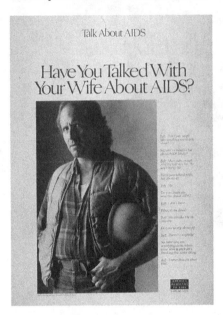

Figure 8.3 1990 AIDS health poster emphasizing the importance of a dialogue among couples.
Image courtesy National Library of Medicine. Source: Smith Collection/Gado/ Getty Images.

some agencies, such as UNICEF, and represented a challenge for international health. The Behavioral Research Unit had to address this and other difficult problems. The Unit was an innovation because until then much of the research done on AIDS was biomedical and little was known about the relationship between the disease and patterns of sexual behavior. Carballo worked under the assumption that behavioral change through information, counseling, and education helped to prevent AIDS and avoid discrimination and stigma.

In the meeting of ministers of health that took place in London in 1988 mentioned earlier, Mann portrayed the fight against AIDS as a universal humanitarian common cause: "AIDS has become a great and powerful symbol for a world threatened by its divisions, East and West, North and South. In a deep and remarkable way, the child with AIDS is the world's child; the man or woman dying of AIDS has become the world's image of our own mortality."[14] The statement was a reflection of the idealism that coexisted alongside tragedy during the initial years of the epidemic. After a few years, Mann could not

---

[14] Jonathan Mann "Intervention," in *A World Summit of Ministers of Health and Programmes for AIDS Prevention, London, January 26–28, 1988* (Geneva: Pergamon Press, 1988), p. 1.

understand the tendency of the WHO and many medical organizations to reestablish the response to AIDS within a biomedical framework.

Difficult Times for the GPA

In 1988, Halfdan Mahler retired as director-general and was succeeded by Hiroshi Nakajima. Nakajima disapproved of Mann's privileged position, his unorthodox style, what he perceived as publicity-seeking behavior, and the considerable freedom and financial resources he enjoyed and sided with the regional directors that considered that Mann disregarded regional offices and held a less expansive view of the importance of human rights for health.[15] There were clashing personalities too. Mann was a remarkable speaker and a compelling writer who could establish an easy dialogue with politicians and diplomats. In contrast, the low-key Nakajima, elected with the heavy burden of filling the shoes of the charismatic Mahler, was outperformed by Mann. According to one account, the GPA had become "like a state within a state."[16] Nakajima supporters inside the WHO argued that the AIDS program had too much autonomy and too many full-time employees and financial resources for the small number of confirmed AIDS cases. For them, the disease was less important than malaria or tuberculosis. Some complained that although extra-budgetary funding for the GPA had increased, other units in the WHO had not been so lucky. For instance, between 1990 and 1991, funding for primary health care programs fell by USD 5 million, training for human resources by USD 8 million, and maternal health/family planning by USD 20 million. A study of all WHO extrabudgetary funds in 1992 indicated that the GPA was by far the largest recipient, accounting for more than 25 percent of these resources.

Nakajima began to ignore, deny, or trim Mann's travel requests, vetoed Mann's choices for his own assistant, and restricted GPA operations. He also argued that the human rights of people with AIDS had to be balanced against the rights of society – a statement that Mann read as threatening a return to the kinds of restrictive public-health policy against which he had waged a successful campaign. According to an interview with Nakajima, in a last effort to keep the autonomy of his program Mann presented Nakajima with an "ultimatum": promote him to the level of an assistant director-general and guarantee the prerogatives he had had with Mahler, or he would resign. Nakajima

---

[15] Mann's feud with Nakajima is described in Joel E. Oestrich, *Power and Principle: Human Rights Programming in International Organizations* (Georgetown University Press, 2007), pp. 126–128.

[16] Peter Piot, *No Time to Lose: A Life in Pursuit of Deadly Viruses* (New York: W. W. Norton and Company, 2012), p. 181.

responded that the agency already had an American as one of the assistant director-generals and he could not upset that geographical balance.[17]

In March 1990, after a series of angry exchanges in European newspapers, Mann resigned his position at the WHO, citing disagreements with the director-general on a series of issues "which I consider critical for the global AIDS strategy."[18] Merson and Inring argue that the tension between Nakajima and Mann existed from the beginning of Nakajima's appointment. They recount a telling incident in 1988, shortly after Nakajima took office:

Nakajima gave an interview with the French newspaper *Le Monde* wherein he expressed some discomfort with the nondiscriminatory resolution that Mann had secured from the World Health Assembly earlier that year. Mann was shocked when he read a prepublication [copy] of the interview. ... Mann threatened to resign from GPA unless [Nakajima] allowed him to "fix" the interview to better reflect WHO's stance on nondiscrimination. Nakajima relented and Mann rewrote the piece, but the episode proved informative to both Mann and Nakajima. For Nakajima it must clearly have sent the signal that Mann had little concern about hierarchy. ... For Mann it plainly raised profound concerns about the support he felt he could expect from the new Director General.[19]

When Mann resigned, several members of the program left the WHO, and demoralization and fear set in among those who stayed. Mann resigned at a time when the budget for his program was still considerable but had started to decline. Donors were dissatisfied that there had been no immediate decrease in the number of people affected worldwide by the disease and were demanding more accountability on how the donations had been used. Bilateral agencies abandoned their earlier uneasiness about working against AIDS and began to fund their own programs instead of providing financial support to multinationals. A few European donors had announced that they would not increase the budgetary contributions for 1991, and the United States had announced that it was going to reduce its contributions to the GPA. But it still held true that after Mann's departure, the WHO received less funding for AIDS-related work, partly because the US and many governments from industrial countries distrusted Nakajima's decisions regarding AIDS.[20] In addition, several UN

---

[17] Merson & Inring, *The AIDS Pandemic*, p. 127.
[18] Cited in David Chandler, "Leader of Global Fight against AIDS Resigns," *The Boston Globe*, March 17, 1990, p. 21.
[19] Merson & Inring, *The AIDS Pandemic*, p. 118.
[20] In 1993, Mann became professor and director of the François-Xavier Bagnoud Center for Health and Human Rights at Harvard University's School of Public Health that published the journal *Health and Human Rights*. In January of 1998, Mann left Harvard to assume the position of dean of the new Allegheny University School of Public Health in Philadelphia. In September of 1998, he and his wife tragically died in an airplane crash while on their way to Geneva. "In Memoriam, Jonathan Mann 1947–1998," *Health and Human Rights, an International Journal* 3:2 (1998), 1–2.

agencies, such as UNICEF, the UNDP, and the World Bank, had already begun operating their own anti-AIDS programs.

Shortly after Mann's departure from the WHO, international experts were concerned that the organization's work against AIDS would come to be dominated by a biomedical approach and that the GPA's Social and Behavioral Research Unit would disappear. Richard Parker, a noted American medical anthropologist working in Rio de Janeiro, wrote to Nakajima demanding that the unit be maintained along with the GPS's social work.[21] The acting director of the GPA, Michael Merson, explained that the Program was being restructured but that it would maintain its support for social studies on AIDS.

Merson, a doctor from Brooklyn, New York (see Figure 8.4), had been at the WHO for 12 years and had solid managerial experience (he was former head of two programs at the WHO: the Control of Diarrheal Diseases Programme, CDD, and the Acute Respiratory Infections Control Programme, ARI). However, he had no experience in the field of AIDS with health activism. In May 1990, Merson was appointed director of the Global Program on AIDS. He was joined by Dorothy Blake from Jamaica as deputy director of the GPA, and he would remain in his new WHO position until 1995 when he left Geneva to become dean of public health at Yale University. More importantly, he had the support of the CDC, other UN agencies, several European donors, and the United States (the major donor of the program). At the time Mann left the GPA, it had a staff of about 400 people and an annual budget of USD 100 million.[22]

Where Mann had been a charismatic whirl of energy, passion, and conviction and regarded by his peers as a natural leader with a long-term vision, Merson was a methodical, hard-working, and meticulous manager concerned with tangible outcomes. Under Mann, funding had come in so quickly and in such large amounts that it sometimes went unspent. Initially, donors had required little in the way of budgetary reporting, but as time went on they demanded that careful attention be paid to monitoring and accounting for the disbursement of funds. It would be Merson's job to make sure all the accounts were in order, procedures were in place, and staff were supervised and evaluated. Mann's management style was horizontal and inclusive. Merson's was hierarchical and willing to shift more responsibilities of the GPA's main office to WHO Regional Offices. Mann worked in an environment of denial,

[21] Richard G. Parker to Hiroshi Nakajima, July 3, 1990, Global Program of AIDS, Psycho-Social and Behavioral Aspects of Aids, 1986–1990, Folder A20/370/8, Second Generation of Files, WHO Archives.

[22] "New Director for WHO Global AIDS Program Named," May 14, 1990, Press Release WHO/27, WHO Press Releases 1988–1990, WHO Library.

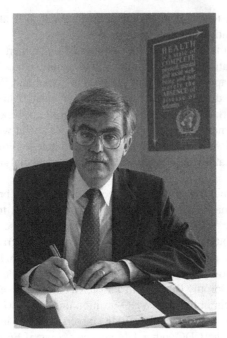

Figure 8.4 Michael H. Merson replaced Jonathan Mann as director of the Global Program on AIDS in 1990 and remained in this position until 1996. He had been director from 1980 to May 1990 of the Diarrheal Diseases Control Program of the WHO.
Credit WHO/Tibor Farkas. Courtesy: World Health Organization Photo Library.

panic, and emergency, whereas Merson took the helm when the sense of urgency about AIDS in wealthy nations had started to dissipate. Although Merson would never openly challenge the link between human rights and the fight against the epidemic, he emphasized protocols and guidelines that were particularly useful to clinicians. A test for Merson was the sixth International Conference on AIDS in San Francisco in 1990, organized with the theme "AIDS in the Nineties: From Science to Policy," and boycotted by several NGOs and governments because since 1987 the United States had forbidden entry to foreigners living with AIDS. Despite the fact that discrimination against people living with HIV had been criticized by the WHO, Merson took the controversial step to support the Conference after the American government declared it would accept infected foreigners if they requested a 10-day waiver that would permit them to attend the meeting. Mann's and Merson's styles came to a head at the 8th International Conference on AIDS held in Amsterdam in 1992. An indication that Mann was recognized as the leader of the AIDS movement was the fact that he was chairman of the Conference Secretariat. The meeting had been due to take place in Boston but was relocated in protest against US travel bans against people living with HIV. The focus of the conference was human rights, an issue about which Mann was considered to be a champion. Merson and his team were not always received warmly at international AIDS conferences, where long-time activists believed that Nakajima was trying to wreck the global fight against AIDS and Merson was perceived as a "Nakajima man." Nonetheless, the GPA kept participating in international AIDS meetings, and in 1994 the GPA and Nakajima helped to secure the presence of Prince Naruhito in the opening ceremony of the 10th International AIDS Conference that took place in Yokohama, Japan, at a time when Japan was one of the few Asian countries to admit it had HIV cases.

Merson joined the new global trend for "condom social marketing" (for example, packaging condoms with attractive names and using TV stars to teach how to use them). This was a meaningful effort to increase the visibility, availability, and demand for condoms, based on the well-founded assumption that information about condoms in developing countries was low. Under his direction, the GPA contributed to the budgets of different international conferences on HIV for children, women, and people living with AIDS and the AIDS virus. His programs received some support from the new administration in the United States. Early in 1993, President Clinton rescinded the restriction on population programs and agreed that USAID could support programs that promoted the use of condoms. Nonetheless, the Clinton administration did not take sufficient meaningful action on AIDS and later would confront activists demanding full access to drugs.

For Merson, the GPA's work in prevention should concentrate on improving surveillance and modernizing logistical facilities. The program also soundly reinforced harm reduction among injecting drug users, which was the predominant source of heterosexual transmission in Eastern Europe and in some middle-income nations.[23] "Needle-exchange" activities provided sterile syringes and needles, thereby lowering the rates of needle sharing among drug users without, it was shown, leading to an increase in drug use. These activities provided a space to provide information on safe behaviors. However, the program was considered controversial, as conservative politicians believed it implicitly condoned illicit drug use.

Merson maintained the GPA's negative stance on mandatory screening for HIV and refined evaluation indicators for the progress of programs. He also organized training courses for managers and promoted valuable new initiatives

---

[23] Michael Merson, "Global Status on HIV/AIDS," in *Global Challenge of AIDS: Ten Years of HIV/AIDS Research, Proceedings of the Tenth International Conference on AIDS/International Conference on STD, Yokohama, August 7–12, 1994* (Tokyo: Karger, 1991), pp. 3, 8.

such as on the relationship between AIDS and other sexually transmitted diseases. He likewise worked with women and promoted safe motherhood, components of the AIDS problem that had not fully been taken into account by the GPA under Mann (by 1990 it was estimated that one-third – or about two million women – of those with HIV infections around the world were women). He also refocused attention on the link between TB and HIV because about 80 percent of people with TB in poor countries were also HIV positive. Another contribution of the GPA under Merson was the revision of the definition of AIDS that had been established in Bangui in 1985. An expanded case definition was introduced in 1994 to incorporate HIV testing. In the new definition, AIDS is present when tests results are positive and one or more of the classic associated clinical conditions – weight loss, diarrhea, or fever – are found. The new definition reflected the increased availability of laboratory diagnostic methods and knowledge of the opportunistic infections that appear with AIDS. Nonetheless, Merson faced a number of obstacles including denial, under-recognition, and underreporting by the governments of many countries.

Another problematic area for the GPA under Merson was embracing a gender perspective (despite the appointment as regular consultant of Priscilla Alexander, who had helped to create the California Prostitutes Education Project, CAL-PEP, one of the first sex worker-organized HIV/AIDS prevention projects in the world). Furthermore, Merson was unable to maintain WHO leadership on AIDS because: "in the desire to improve management, reorganize ... momentum and motivation were lost."[24] A senior official in the American AIDS program suggested that Merson had put too much emphasis on efficiency, hated disloyalty, was distrustful of activities over which he had no control, and was very much different from Mann: "Mike's management style is 180 degrees around Jon's."[25] In the early 1990s, the GPA's relationship with NGOs had been so important in the initial response to the epidemic, and Mann accepted them as shock troops. The relationship of the WHO with AIDS health activists became more difficult because the latter were always considered too aggressive by some UN officers. One example of the deteriorating relationship between the UN and NGOs occurred in May 1991 when ACT UP (The AIDS Coalition to Unleash Power) and WHAM (Women Health Action Mobilization) organized a rally without a police permit in the United Nations Plaza, New York. UN AIDS officers agreed to participate by distributing a press release to participants but made it clear that they were unable to provide health care. In an undisclosed

[24] Gary Slutkin, "Global AIDS 1981–1999: The Response," *The International Journal of Tuberculosis and Lung Disease* 4:2 (2000), S24–S33, p. S30.
[25] Cited in Zeeshan A. Rana, "The Evolution of the World Health Organization's Policy Response to the HIV/AIDS Crisis," unpublished Master of Science thesis, University of Toronto (2006).

report, the liaison officer between the WHO and the UN office in New York complained that ACT UP had a low opinion of the WHO and that its aim was to get demonstrators arrested. According to the report, cooperation between the WHO and ACT UP was going to be difficult because the NGO liked to fight "in the trenches with unsheathed bayonets," a form of struggle that was inconceivable for international civil servants.[26]

Merson's work on AIDS should be seen in the context of the fight against AIDS during the mid-1990s. Industrial nations had lost some interest in the international aspects of AIDS as the AIDS-related mortality rates in these countries began to decline. AIDS began to be perceived as having reached a plateau, with patients suffering from a treatable, but not curable illness that could be managed with special clinical care and expensive daily medication. After the initial panic, complacency and inertia ensued. By the early 1990s, the cost of direct medical care for a person living with AIDS in an industrial country was estimated at about USD 25,000, and no leader of an international agency could imagine that such financial resources could be obtained for developing countries. Disappointment with the worldwide medical fight against AIDS also existed because the results of the search for a vaccine had proved inconclusive. In 1993, the "Concorde" trial of AZT, which consisted of studying the effects of the drug in more than 1,700 asymptomatic people living with HIV, suggested that the drug did reduce disease progression in the short-term but did not increase a person's chances of survival in the long-term.

In spite of Merson's best efforts and the financial support of the Sasakawa Foundation, an organization close to Nakajima, the GPA faced institutional and financial turmoil. It was too difficult for Merson to transition a program centered on human rights and Mann's charisma to a bureaucratic, mainly biomedical and technical organization. Some of these problems would have occurred even if Mann had stayed in the position. Bilateral agencies and donors had become disaffected, and contributions to the GPA had begun to decline. In 1991, the GPA budget was reduced, which resulted in a slowdown of activities and a scaling back of the budget. Some attributed it to "donor fatigue," meaning that many private and bilateral agencies were no longer willing to contribute to the international fight against AIDS because they had seen few results up until that point. Another reason for the decline of the GPA in the 1990s was that many governments, agencies, and donors did not agree that the fight against AIDS was also a political battle. Such a view had been introduced by Mann and sustained by the NGOs and still lingered in the GPA's activities under Merson.

---

[26] Jerry Kilker, Public Information and Liaison officer, WHO-UN, "Note for the Record: AIDS Rally at the United Nations, 19 June 1991," Global Program of AIDS: Collaboration with the United Nations System, Folder A20–371-30, Third Generation of Files, WHO archive.

By the mid-1990s, a lack of leadership, duplication of activities and rivalry among agencies, disorganization in the use of donations, and shrinking financial resources plagued the international response to AIDS. Troubles also existed at the local level. The support that came from the WHO, the UN, and bilateral and donor organizations was all provided in a piecemeal fashion to different national ministries and NGOs, which led to infighting between NGOs and governments and even among government officials. The need for a new and all-encompassing international organization had become clear.

Change from outside the WHO

In 1996, after complex negotiation, a new multilateral agency to coordinate all HIV and AIDS work globally was created: the Joint United Nations Programme on HIV and AIDS (UNAIDS). The other UN agencies that were to participate in UNAIDS were the WHO, UNDP, UNICEF, UNFPA, UNESCO, and the World Bank (additional cosponsors were included later). Although UNAIDS was intended to fall within the remit of the WHO and Nakajima hoped to have control of the new agency, it rapidly gained autonomy and took over the remaining budget of the GPA (by this time, Merson was no longer director of the GPA and had been replaced by acting director Stefano Bertozzi, who as of December 1995 closed the program). The biennial budget for the UNAIDS Secretariat in 1996 to 1997 was considerable: USD 120 million, of which the United States contributed USD 34 million, or about 28 percent.[27] In January 1995, Peter Piot from Belgium was appointed head of UNAIDS by Boutros-Ghali, UN secretary-general (he would remain head of the agency until 2008, when he was replaced by his deputy, the Malian national Michael Sidibe). Piot had a solid background in AIDS: He was the former chairman of the WHO steering committee on AIDS epidemiology during Mann's leadership of the GPA and in 1992 became associate director of the GPA's Unit for Sexually Transmitted Diseases, working with Merson. In 1994, Piot became the GPA's director of research and intervention development and had also been president of the International AIDS Society, the principal organizer of international and regional AIDS conferences. By 1996, UNAIDS had 38 professionals and 34 support personnel in Geneva and had established field operations in 40 countries (about 30 percent of its staff came from the GPA). Learning from the GPA's mistakes, national programs became more flexible and avoided the previous assumption that a "one-size-fits-all" model could be

---

[27] United States, General Accounting Office, Report to Congressional Requesters, July 1998, "HIV/AIDS, USAID and UN Response to the Epidemic in the Developing World," GAO/NSIAD-98–202 (Washington, DC: The Office, 1998), 3.

adopted by all countries. In contrast, UNAIDS's response was to adapt because it had learned that the pandemic was different in different population groups, including gays, women who were married to bisexual husbands, and injecting drug users.

A few years after its creation, the new agency began to publish updates on the epidemic to coincide with World AIDS Day. From 1998 onwards, UNAIDS published its invaluable annual *Report on the Global HIV/AIDS Epidemic* that became a reference source for data on the epidemic. UNAIDS' emphasis on improved surveillance and prevention was not similar to what the WHO advocated at the time. The difference between the two organizations was in the change of leadership at UNAIDS and its joined-up response to AIDS. Thus, UNAIDS became a reference hub for epidemiological information. UNAIDS also popularized a new technical language and acronyms to reduce discrimination. For example: "Men who have Sex with Men" (MSM) replaced "homosexuals," or even "gays," and "Commercial Sex Workers" (CSW) or "Sex Workers" (SW) replaced "prostitutes." The use of these terms also represented a strategy to confront discrimination and promote a more ethical response to AIDS. In addition, UNAIDS highlighted the fact that it was not enough to tell individuals to say no to sex or drugs. People's sexual and drug-related behaviors did not occur in a vacuum but in specific social and cultural environments, involving factors such as poverty or a lack of control over marital relationships, which could make it harder for individuals to have healthy behaviors.

Initially, the creation of UNAIDS was disruptive to the WHO's work since the latter felt that it symbolized a further decline of its authority. In fact, UNAIDS took responsibility for most of the Technical Service Agreements (TSA) signed by the WHO with national AIDS programs. Although Piot and Nakajima initially made commitments to collaborate, the competition between the two organizations often became unpleasant. From 1996 until the end of the decade, the WHO's work against AIDS was scaled back to a few officers working in an AIDS and Sexually Transmitted Diseases (ASD) unit. This unit and the WHO did not have a proactive role but just incorporated UNAIDS policies into the fabric of its global and country-level operations.

Within a few years of its formation, UNAIDS came to be one of the few multilateral organizations with NGO representatives on its governing body. This was a clear recognition of the crucial importance of activists, whose main weapon was moral outrage, to keep government accountable. The director of UNAIDS was also successful in getting different organizations to work together as reflected in a caustic comment made by a former UNAIDS officer: "Piot was like a nursery school teacher trying to get all children to play nicely together in the sand pit. It wasn't easy because the WHO, the biggest kid in the AIDS class, was still sulky about having its toys taken away and given to the other agencies to play with."[28] UNAIDS also maintained a good relationship with private donors and bilateral and multilateral funding organizations. A first example was the coordination of UNAIDS with the Gates and Rockefeller foundations that in 1996 sponsored the International AIDS Vaccine Initiative (IAVI) to conduct clinical trials and studies on possible HIV vaccines. Between 1996 and 1999, the World Bank increased its donations to AIDS projects from USD 65.9 million to 410.7 million. Most of these funds went to UNAIDS and to NGOs, not to the WHO.[29]

In 1995 and 1996, changes occurred in the international response to AIDS because of both science and politics. In 1995, a protease inhibitor or antiretroviral drug, saquinavir, was developed by the pharmaceutical company Roche and approved in record time by the FDA. In 1995 and 1996, the first generation of HIV protease inhibitors were developed. They demonstrated that combination therapies for HIV could reduce viral loads to undetectable levels, thus promising to turn AIDS into a chronic non-progressive or non-lethal condition. ARVs were not a cure but inhibited the replication of HIV and boosted the immune system's ability to fight infections. AIDS mortality dropped dramatically in developed countries, and the perception of the disease shifted from a death sentence to a treatable illness, leading to governmental complacency. As HAART (the term used for Highly Active Antiretroviral Therapy or effective drug combination therapies for HIV) looked more promising, attention gradually shifted from AIDS prevention to access to treatment. The telling term "Lazarus effect" came to be used to describe the rapid restoration of vitality in patients with advanced HIV infections. In 1996, ARV treatment was presented at the 11th International AIDS Conference that took place in Vancouver and became known as the "AIDS cocktail." The International AIDS Conferences, held every two years since 1994, had become key for alliances and debates among medical scientists, activists, members of pharmaceutical companies, and government representatives.

The World Bank, USAID, and the UK's Department for International Development raised serious reservations about promoting AIDS treatment in developing nations, given that the international price of AIDS drugs was far beyond what most citizens of developing and middle-income countries could afford (in the mid-1990s, about USD 10,000 to 15,000 per person per year). They questioned the wisdom of using ARVs in these countries, portrayed them as not being cost-effective, and suggested these countries concentrate on prevention. These agencies questioned the ability of poor people to adhere to

---

[28] Elizabeth Pisani, *The Wisdom of Whores, Bureaucrats, Brothels and the Business of Aids* (New York: W. W. Norton & Company 2008), p. 5.

[29] The World Bank published a landmark policy report entitled *Confronting AIDS: Public Priorities in a Global Epidemic* (New York: Oxford University Press, 1997).

strict treatments and argued that if they failed, it could lead to emerging resistant strains of the retrovirus. They expressed concerns about the availability of trained local personnel and a lack of medical infrastructure. There was some prejudice too. According to one USAID administrator, uneducated Africans would not be disciplined enough to take medications because their notion of time was vague and they did not use watches.[30]

The denial of treatment, when treatment existed, came at a time when the AIDS situation in Africa had become catastrophic. In a 1999 International Conference on AIDS and STDs in Africa held in Lusaka, the Executive Director of UNAIDS Peter Piot explained that in some parts of the continent life expectancy was being drastically reduced and that AIDS deaths were reversing gains in child health and survival. His agency estimated that a child born in a country with high HIV prevalence rates could expect to live on average to the age of 43 (without AIDS the expectation would have been 60). Piot also pointed out that a number of African countries had to face the fact that by 2005, AIDS-related medical costs would absorb two-thirds of government health spending.[31]

A change from prevention to treatment in developing countries began in November 1996 when the Brazilian President Fernando Enrique Cardoso took a landmark decision. He signed a law that made AIDS brand-name drugs and generic medication (drugs identical to a brand-name drug in safety and quality) universally available in the public health system of the country. The following year, a renewed National AIDS Program and new, ambitious Brazilian businesses that produced generic medicines for the drugs with expired patents established a target of producing half the drugs licensed in the United States in both public and private laboratories. The Brazilian decision was interpreted by powerful pharmaceutical companies as a challenge to their patent rights. The health minister of Brazil was successful in negotiating reduced drug prices with pharmaceutical companies for those medicines protected by a patent.[32] The decision was also instrumental in demonstrating that his government would offer the choice to patients to buy affordable brand-name drugs if they did not wish to use free generics. The Brazilian government strove to ensure the safety and efficacy of these drugs, and there was an almost immediate positive outcome: By June 1998, 58,000 Brazilian AIDS patients were taking ARVs. As a result, there was a decline in the number of AIDS deaths, a marked reduction in hospitalization rates for AIDS patients, and consequently

---

[30] Cited in Peter Piot, *AIDS between Science and Politics* (New York: Columbia University Press, 2015), p. 99.

[31] Peter Piot cited in Andrew Mutundwa, "International Partnerships in the Fight against AIDS," *AIDS Analysis Africa* 10:3 (1999), 15–16, p. 15.

[32] Amy Nunn, *The Politics and History of AIDS Treatment in Brazil* (New York: Springer, 2009).

significant savings for the Brazilian health system. Brazilian activists and the AIDS unit of the Ministry of Health established partnerships with the army, schoolteachers, makers of soap operas, and sex workers as well as with public companies to increase the production and use of condoms and drugs. A by-product of all this was a reduction in discrimination. More Brazilians were willing to take HIV tests and disclose and discuss their status because there was less stigma against Lesbian, Gay, Bisexual, and Transgender (LGBT) groups.

By the year 2000, initiatives similar to the Brazilian AIDS Program had launched in a number of developing countries and reinforced the demand of governments and NGOs for lower-cost, generic antiretroviral drugs as well as lower costs for brand-name medicines. By 2001, Brazil was producing a year's supply of antiretrovirals for USD 3,000, and in Senegal a year's supply could be purchased for USD 1,000. Shortly thereafter a large Indian generic drug maker, Cipla, announced that it could produce an annual course of combination therapy for as little as a few hundred dollars. From 2000 onwards, Thailand provided triple combination ART through its public health service. In South Africa, one of the most affected countries in the world with an HIV prevalence rate among 15–49 year-old individuals of about 25 percent, the government, led by Nelson Mandela, decided to produce and distribute generic antiretrovirals. Despite the fact that most generics produced were no longer protected by patents, some transnational pharmaceutical firms believed these countries and companies committed an act of piracy. In February 1998, the South African Pharmaceutical Manufacturers Association and several multi-national pharmaceutical manufacturers sued the government of South Africa, alleging that the Medicines and Related Substances Control Amendment Act, issued the year before, violated international patent agreements and the South African Constitution. At the same time, antiretrovirals were being delivered to specific locations by international NGOs and other organizations, such as Partners in Health, Oxfam, Doctors Without Borders, and Treatment Action Campaign (TAC) in South Africa; the Health GAP (Global Access Project) Coalition in the United States; Thai AIDS Treatment Action Group, the African Comprehensive HIV/AIDS, ACHAP, in Botswana; and several organizations of People Living with HIV/AIDS. These organizations questioned the limitations of strategies based solely on prevention and sought to empower people, but they did not have the financial resources to buy the drugs in large quantities from international companies and usually relied on Indian generic drugs. Even the WHO and UNAIDS led pilot programs in Côte d'Ivore and Uganda, providing HIV drugs with the aim of demonstrating that antiretrovirals could be used effectively in poor countries. Also important was that in the first months of 2001, the WHO and the World Bank negotiated with the largest pharmaceutical companies to reduce prices for antiretroviral drugs in five high-burden African countries.

The AIDS treatment movement had begun to take on a life of its own and it was to have an impact in the political sphere, in the face of opposition from pharmaceutical companies. The 13th International AIDS Conference in 2000, organized under the theme "Breaking the Silence" in Durban, South Africa (the first time it was held in the southern hemisphere), was a clear demonstration of the political influence held by the coalition of AIDS activists, scientists, and politicians that denounced the inequality in treatment access between the developed and developing countries. The meeting took place at a time when the disease was the primary cause of death in sub-Saharan Africa, killing men and women in their most productive years. The meeting has an important place in the history of AIDS because participants, including former President Mandela, took on President Thabo Mbeki – who had denied the epidemic and believed that antiretrovirals were toxic – and won. Equally significant were the activists' demands to provide drugs to developing nations.

The NGO movement also had an influence on multilaterals. In 2001, a landmark United Nations Special Session of the General Assembly (that began to be referred to as UNGASS) declared AIDS a threat to global security and approved a Declaration making a commitment to mobilize greater financial resources to facilitate access to drugs. To enhance the importance of UNGASS, the United Nations Secretariat Building was lit with a red ribbon, the symbol of the battle against HIV/AIDS. In the year 2001, a number of regional intergovernmental meetings took place and made similar commitments (for example, The Abuja Declaration and Framework for Action for the Fight against HIV/ AIDS, Tuberculosis and Other Related Infectious Diseases in Africa, on April 27, 2001; The Declaration of the Ibero-American Summit of Heads of State of November 2000 in Panama; and The Central Asian Declaration on HIV/AIDS of May 18, 2001, approved in Almaty, Kazakhstan). In 2002, the WHO listed Cipla products among the drugs that met its quality standards for AIDS treatment, generating criticism from the International Federation of Pharmaceutical Manufacturers.

Most pharmaceutical companies initially were annoyed by the growing conviction that the production and sale of antiretrovirals should be free since such a position challenged the traditional legal protection of drug sales with patents of 20 years' duration. In 1994, the World Trade Organization (WTO) had issued the Trade-Related Aspects of International Property Rights (TRIPS) agreement, which called for the standardization of intellectual property laws among all its members by January 2005. Since the late 1990s, pharmaceutical companies, with the support of the US government, denounced Brazil and other developing countries at the WTO (at the same time, some had their own charitable anti-AIDS drug initiatives, such as Bristol Myers Squibb's program "Secure the Future" in Africa). Brazil's legal position was strong because they argued that they could use to "compulsory license," a provision that existed in international law. Governments grant these licenses unilaterally in cases of emergency without seeking the rights-holder's consent. In 2000, pharmaceutical companies changed their strategy and decided to reduce the wholesale price of HIV medicines by 70 percent in an effort to undermine the so-called piracy movement initiated by Brazil. Even with this reduction, the lowest price for combination therapy was still beyond the reach of most poor African countries. In response to an "urgent" request from the WHO, five large AIDS drug manufacturers agreed to offer their drugs to African countries for little more than cost or to make donations on a case by case basis but asked that the principle of intellectual property should be recognized.[33] In a context of tension and negotiation and after pressure from some developing countries, late in 2001 a Ministerial Conference of WTO took place in Doha, Quatar, and approved a Declaration that made clear that nothing in the original TRIPS agreement impeded the use of generics drugs in case of emergencies and that health emergencies were declared by national governments. It is important to underline the transcendence of the Declaration. The 146 members of the World Trade Organization agreed that developing countries could waive patent laws in order to produce the drugs they needed by compulsory licenses. However, it was not completely clear if they had the right to import generic drugs from abroad and most did not have the domestic capabilities to produce the drugs.

The WHO tried to keep pace, and in 2000 a World Health Assembly resolution requested that member states increase access to treatments for HIV. Shortly thereafter, a new Department of HIV/AIDS in the Family and Community Health unit of the WHO was created with the mission of making the new antiretroviral treatments universal and affordable. In February 2001, Gro Harlem Brundtland, the WHO director-general, published a newspaper article stating that "popular outrage, political will, market forces and the best science" were enabling the pursuit of a fundamental public-health right: "the supply of medicines on the basis of need rather than on the ability to pay." She also mentioned the government of Brazil as an example of how developing country governments could commit their own resources in obtaining lower prices, and stressed the need for more financial resources to keep ARV prices down.[34] Later that year, at the launching of a new international alliance called

[33] Jonathan Engel, *The Epidemic: A Global History of AIDS* (New York: Harper and Collins, 2006), p. 309.
[34] The article was published in the *International Herald Tribune* and is quoted in World Health Organization, "Affordable AIDS Drugs Are within Reach," Note for the Press, February 14, 2001, Press Releases, Volume 2001, WHO Library.

the HIV Treatment Access Coalition, the WHO director-general stated: "Does anyone deserve to be sentenced to certain death because she or he cannot access care that costs less than $2 a day? Is anyone's life worth so little? Should any family become destitute as a result? Should children be orphaned? The answers must be no, no, no, and no."[35] In April 2001, the World Health Organization helped to organize a workshop of about 50 researchers and generic manufacturers in Norway that discussed how to improve poor countries' access to essential drugs as well as the issue of "differential pricing" or charging lower prices for medicines in developing nations. However, some lawyers and pharmaceutical companies argued that differential pricing was being used as a means for illicit re-export of lower-priced drugs into industrialized economies.

In 2003, the World Health Organization published a list of quality HIV and AIDS-related drugs that included both patented and generic versions. In 2002, Brazil reported about half the number of infections that the World Bank had predicted in the early 1990s (the prediction was 1.2 million). A year later, the Brazilian AIDS program received an award from the Gates Foundation of 1 million USD. The change was a boost to the central theme of the 15th International AIDS Conference that took place in Bangkok in 2004: "Access for All." By then, the World Bank, the governments of European industrialized countries, the US government, the WHO, and former President Clinton, (who, during his presidency, had sided with the pharmaceutical companies) had changed their position on treatment for developing countries and portrayed the AIDS programs of Brazil, India, South Africa, and other developing countries as examples to be followed.

If they were to save face, pharmaceutical companies would have to make further changes. A telling example was the dispute between Brazil and the pharmaceutical company Roche over drug pricing that ended in September 2001 when the Swiss company agreed to reduce the price of its antiretroviral drug (nelfinavir) by 40 percent.[36] This was a significant moment in the history of global health because the pharmaceutical industry accepted, at least on this occasion, that access to medicine was more important than profit. The novel concept of "global public goods" was applied to antiretrovirals. Whereas previously AIDS generic medicines had been defined at best as national public goods or small commercial enterprises and an option for the poor, the struggles made by developing countries to have free access to

---

[35] Cited in World Health Organization, "New International Coalition Aims to Expand Global Access to HIV/AIDS Treatment," Note for Press, December 11, 2002, Press Releases, Volume 2002, WHO Library.
[36] "Roche Gives in to Brazil over AIDS Drug," *The Lancet* 1:3 (October 2001), 138.

antiretrovirals meant that generics began to be seen as a priority for health systems and as a right of all citizens of the world.[37]

The use of generic ARVs was accompanied by a significant increase and diversification in funding for international health. In 2001, as a result of a proposal made by UN Secretary-General Kofi Annan for greater action from pharmaceutical companies, a Global Business Coalition on HIV/AIDS was established (with the participation of the CEOs of Abbott Laboratories, Bristol-Myers Squibb, Glaxo Smith Kline, and Pfizer, among others) and supported the WHO and other agencies working on AIDS. American private foundations became more active. Some of them, such as the Clinton and Gates foundations, were new and pledged millions of dollars for purchasing medicines for the fight against AIDS in Africa, India, and the Caribbean. This happened at a time when there was a fear that HIV would spread into the Russian Federation and China, countries in which the epidemic had initially been greeted with derision. There was also considerable anxiety that HIV/AIDS could destabilize political and economic systems in sub-Saharan Africa, contributing to economic crises, civil wars, and global insecurity. The US National Intelligence Council construed HIV/AIDS as an international security and humanitarian issue that went beyond public health.[38]

Collectively, these changes meant that the WHO was not the only institutional actor working on AIDS, nor was it even the most visible. At the same time, the WHO made an effort to assume a more prominent role in the global response to the epidemic. In May 2003, a draft resolution of the World Health Assembly made tentative reference to the WHO's work with other agencies in extending access to antiretroviral treatments to 3 million people by 2005. A bolder resolution by the Assembly mentioned the Doha Declaration of the WTO and requested that the director-general support the goal of providing effective antiretroviral treatment "within the context of strengthening national health systems" and maintaining a "proper balance between prevention, care and treatment" and to reach "at least three million people with HIV in developing countries by 2005."[39] The challenges of reaching these complex targets would make up the next phase of the multilateral agency's work on HIV.

---

[37] Inge Kaul & Michael Faust, "Global Public Goods and Health: Taking the Agenda Forward," *Bulletin of the World Health Organization* 79:9 (2001), 869–874.

[38] United States, National Intelligence Council, *The Global Infectious Disease Threat and Its Implications for the United States, No. NIED 99–17D* (Washington, DC: National Intelligence Council, 2000).

[39] World Health Organization, "Global Health-Sector Strategy for HIV/AIDS," 56th World Health Assembly, May 28, 2003, Agenda Item 14.4, WHA56.30, apps.who.int/iris/bitstream/10665/78339/1/ea56r30.pdf.

Recovering the Initiative

In 2003, Korean public health doctor Jong-wook Lee took over as director-general from Gro Harlem Brundtland (the next chapter will analyze the roles and backgrounds of both), and shortly after his appointment the WHO became a player in the promotion of global treatment for AIDS. Lee forged an alliance with UNAIDS to launch a program called the 3 by 5 initiative, which aimed to improve significantly the situation in developing countries, mainly in sub-Saharan Africa and Asia, where only about 400,000 people living with AIDS were receiving adequate HAART treatment (a small percentage of the people in the world living with AIDS). The goal of 3 by 5 had been previously proposed and discussed at the Barcelona International Conference on HIV/AIDS in 2002 by German epidemiologist Bernhard Schwartländer, who at the time was director of the WHO HIV/AIDS Department. The 3 by 5 initiative was portrayed as a major global effort to scale-up previous successful anti-retroviral experiences. Although the program had been running since early 2003, on December 1 of that year, taking advantage of the symbolism of World AIDS Day, Jong-wook Lee and Peter Piot, executive director of UNAIDS, officially launched the initiative. They declared the lack of access to antiretroviral therapy for HIV/AIDS in low- and middle-income countries to be a global health emergency. Although the program would only cover about half of those in need of the drugs because that was the figure that an article in *Science* had established as an achievable target, it was still considered a step forward compared with what had gone before, and in the years that followed, there was to be no discussion about the figure – whether it was too ambitious or not ambitious enough.[40]

The program was made possible on account of the global political and medical consensus about the level of urgency of the AIDS crisis and because antiretroviral drug prices had come down to less than USD 200 per person per annum. The 3 by 5 initiative simplified and reduced the number of first-line recommended regime treatments of drug combinations from 35 to 4. The most common drug was a single pill containing three drugs: lamivudine, stavudine, and nevirapine, which temporally suppressed replication of HIV (these generic drugs were mainly obtained from Indian generic companies). Thousands of professional and lay health workers in developing countries were trained to provide and monitor the use of fixed-dose combinations of ARVs (Indian

---

[40] The annual report of the agency discussed this program and provided the data mentioned in this paragraph, see World Health Organization, *The World Health Report 2004 – Changing History* (Geneva: The World Health Organization, 2004); Bernhard Schwartländer, John Stover, Neff Walker, L. Bollinger, Juan-Pablo Gutierrez, William McGreevey, Marjorie Opuni, Steve Forsythe, Lilani Kumaranayake, Charlotte Watts, & Stefano Bertozzi, "Resource Needs for HIV/AIDS," *Science* 292:3326 (June 29, 2001), 2434–2436.

generic companies were able to produce fixed-dose combination pills – essentially two or three pills in one – which was hugely influential in simplifying AIDS treatment in developing countries) that would suppress viral replication and improve symptoms in AIDS patients. The WHO became the scientific reference on ARV: approving, disapproving, and in some cases de-listing the various generic drugs that existed at the time.

Lee made use of an emergency clause in the WHO Constitution to make rapid decisions regarding staffing and funding for developing the initiative.[41] The initial director of the program was the American medical doctor and diplomat Jack Chow, who had been the WHO assistant director-general in charge of AIDS, Tuberculosis, and Malaria since the beginning of Lee's term. The Brazilian dermatologist Dr. Paulo Teixeira, the architect of Brazil's national program, was appointed director of the HIV/AIDS Department at the WHO for less than a year – replacing Schwartländer – and he assisted Chow until departing for health reasons. In March 2004, Jim Yong Kim, a Korean-American physician and founder of reputed American NGO Partners in Health, who was special adviser to the director-general, replaced Teixeira as director of the WHO's HIV/AIDS department. Shortly thereafter, Chow left the health agency. In 2004 and 2005, Kim became the head of the 3 by 5 initiative (and would later go on to be president of the World Bank). Bernhard Schwartländer, former director of the German AIDS program, consultant to the World Bank, and former director of the HIV/AIDS Department, moved to the Global Fund and supported the initiative. Kim played a decisive role in the elaboration of the biannual report of the health agency devoted to the 3 by 5 initiative, published in May of 2004 and entitled *The World Health Report 2004 – Changing History*.

In spite of all this, initially there was only a disappointingly modest increase in the number of people treated, which led the WHO to send experts to visit countries such as Brazil in September 2004 in order to learn how they had achieved such rapid results, with a view to replicating this knowledge in other countries. Progress was more notable during the second half of 2004, during which time 700,000 people in poor and middle-income countries received antiretroviral therapy.[42] It was also difficult to keep down the price of drugs because not all governments used the flexibility in international law to make medicines more affordable, and many generic drugs were not registered in many countries. In point of fact, the average price per person per year for the

---

[41] Jennifer Prah Ruger & Derek Yach, "The Global Role of the World Health Organization," *Global Health Governance* 1:2 (2009), 1–11, p. 5.

[42] Jong-wook Lee & Peter Piot, World Health Organization & UNAIDS, *"3 by 5" Progress Report, December 2004*, www.who.int/3by5/progressreport05/en/, last accessed October 18, 2017.

first-line treatment regime was USD 484, a figure above what was spent in more progressive developing countries.[43] In one of its final reports, published in mid-2005, the leaders of the 3 by 5 initiative sought, retrospectively, to give the campaign another meaning, stating that it had been intended as an "interim step" toward the goal of universal access to HIV treatment for those who needed it.[44]

As a strategy to bring effective therapy to 3 million people with HIV/AIDS in low- and middle-income countries, the 3 by 5 initiative fell short of its targets (in 2005, only about 1.6 million people were receiving HAART), and the epidemic was not contained. *The Lancet* lamented: "2005 is likely to be remembered more for the 3 million deaths and almost 5 million new infections it heralded than for the 300,000 lives saved through treatment for HIV."[45] The latter figure meant that more than 40 million people were living with the disease, or double the number of individuals infected in 1995. The regions of the world that already had advanced programs in providing therapy benefited the most. For example, in Latin America and the Caribbean coverage increased to almost two-thirds of the population in need of ARVs, but in sub-Saharan Africa and the Middle East, despite the accelerated growth, less than a fifth of those individuals needing the drugs had actually received them by June 2005.[46]

On the bright side, by mid-2005 the campaign had prevented an estimated 250,000 – 350,000 deaths, demonstrating that adherence rates to a prolonged drug regime were similar in developing countries to those obtained in industrialized societies. By the end of 2005, 81 drugs for HIV/AIDS had been prequalified by the WHO. The campaign had also emphasized the importance of universal access to antiretrovirals for all who needed them. After an epidemic peak in 2004, there was a marked increase in antiretroviral treatment in sub-Saharan Africa, a significant reduction of HIV infections and AIDS-related deaths, and the disease's prevalence – namely, the percentage of people living with HIV – began to level off. Another achievement of the program was the increase in the number of health workers trained to deliver antiretroviral therapy.

---

[43] The World Health Organization & UNAIDS, *3 by 5 December 2003 through June 2004 Progress Report* (Geneva: World Health Organization, 2004), pp. 8, 13, 19.

[44] World Health Organization & UNADIS, *Progress on Global Access to HIV Antiretroviral Therapy, an Update on "3 by 5" June 2005* (Geneva; the World Health Organization, 2005), www.who.int/3by5/publications/progressreport/en/, last accessed October 11, 2017.

[45] The phrase was taken from the Editorial, "Maintaining Anti-AIDS Commitment post "3 by 5," *The Lancet* 366:9500 (November 26, 2005), 1828.

[46] World Health Organization and UNADIS, *Progress on Global Access to HIV Antiretroviral Therapy, an Update on "3 by 5" June 2005* (Geneva: The World Health Organization, 2005), 13, www.who.int/3by5/publications/progressreport/en/, last accessed September 13, 2017.

The failure of the 3 by 5 initiative likely occurred due to a combination of technical and political reasons. In technical terms, the deadline was too short and unrealistic. Despite the initial resolution made at a World Health Assembly in 2003, the program did not prove to be an effective tool for achieving a balance between prevention and treatment, nor for strengthening national health systems. To make matters worse, many national treatment programs were not fully connected to TB and malaria programs. The endorsement by all 192 WHO member states – something only achieved in 2005 – was not sufficient. Many countries did not possess organized public health and activist communities, such as Brazil's, that could argue for greater government support and ensure that people were willing to come forward for testing. In addition, in Brazil and other developing countries with successful AIDS programs a network of health workers, clinics, and hospitals was crucial not only for treatment but for hosting open debates on sexuality. Another reason for the program's failure had to do with poor infrastructure and unanticipated expenses, particularly with regard to laboratory equipment, HIV test kits, and drugs to treat opportunistic infections – and a lack of health personnel, namely inadequate resources for counseling, surveillance, monitoring, and drug procurement and distribution. The original expectation was that around half of the costs would be covered by recipient countries, but governments that were dealing with external debt and a number of health emergencies could not raise the money needed in a short space of time. As a result, many country programs became fragmented and a comprehensive and sustainable program was difficult to maintain. Thirdly, second and third generation ARVs, with fewer side effects but much higher prices, were now available but were not an active part of the global program and were usually protected by more stringent intellectual property laws.

With regard to the political dimensions of the program, the WHO did not do enough to address the levels of denial and silence relating to AIDS that existed in many cultures, nor to fight discrimination against various groups and issues such as people living with AIDS, women and immigrants with low social status, and sexual minorities. Although a human-rights perspective appeared in the educational materials produced in Geneva, it did not clearly translate into practical activities in a program that basically focused on the drug distribution. The fact that in many developing countries violence against women and immigrants was tolerated and that homosexuality was a crime made testing, drug distribution, and prevention programs difficult.

Another political problem was that the program operated in a complex and sometimes adverse political context marked by the priorities of a new and well-funded bilateral agency created in 2003 by President George W. Bush: the President's Emergency Plan for Aids Relief, PEPFAR. President Bush announced his intention to create the program in his State of the Union address of January 2003, and in May of that year the Congress initiated an Act that stipulated a new bilateral commitment to fighting AIDS, Tuberculosis, and Malaria, meaning that the program became a reality in the budget for fiscal year 2004. PEPFAR, a reflection of the US governments' renewed distrust of multilateral institutions, emerged with a lot of money: USD 15 billion to be spent over the next five years in 15 selected countries in Africa, Asia, and the Caribbean. China, India, and Russia, where the AIDS situation was dramatic, were explicitly not part of the program because the US government believed that those countries had the resources to provide treatment for their people. The amounts were astronomical, while the reasons behind the creation of the program were ideological, economic, and political. In terms of ideology, the key term was "compassionate conservatism," supported by President Bush and many of his supporters, who considered the care of AIDS patients a Christian obligation.[47] Although the term itself was vague and pandered to the religious right, it came with the neoliberal assumption that it was not global economic policy that was to blame for misery and disease, but the poor themselves. It underlined the importance of traditional family values and charitable donations from the federal government, private companies, philanthropic organizations, and churches to solve social problems.[48] A difference with the conservatives' position in the 1980s at the start of the epidemic was that they did not condemn individuals living with HIV on moral grounds. It was the first time that a Republican administration in the United States had a major international program for HIV/AIDS. PEPFAR's economic motives became apparent when it was announced that it was not going to use generic drugs but more costly drugs produced by pharmaceutical companies. PEPFAR thus indirectly subsidized some of the very companies, located in the United States and industrialized countries, that had been the subject of criticism in the late 1990s. In terms of politics, the Bush administration was seeking to improve its foreign image in the same year that US troops were ordered to invade Iraq and were using billions of dollars in military operations in spite of a global wave of criticism.

Randall Tobias, a former CEO of the Eli Lilly pharmaceutical company, became head of PEPFAR and made sure that initially none and later only a small percentage of the drugs distributed were generic medicines (in line with transnational pharmaceutical companies that considered them unsafe and ineffective). One joke that did the rounds in UNAIDS corridors was that the new bilateral agency really stood for "Purchasing Expensive Pharmaceuticals From

---

[47] John Donnelly, "The President's Emergency Plan for AIDS Relief: How George W. Bush and Aides Came to 'Think Big' on Battling HIV," *Health Affairs* 31:7 (2012), 1389–1396.

[48] Discussed in Julian E. Zelizer (ed.), *The Presidency of George W. Bush: A First Historical Assessment* (Princeton: Princeton University Press, 2010).

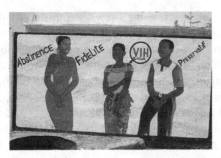

Figure 8.5 AIDS prevention message promoting the goals of "Abstinence, Be Faithful, and Condom Use," also known as ABC, on a wall outside a health center in Senegal, 2005. ABC was promoted by the President's Emergency Plan for AIDS Relief, PEPFAR, a well-funded US bilateral program created in 2003 under President George W. Bush.
Source: BSIP/UIG Via Getty Images.

American Retailers."[49] Furthermore, the PEPFAR funds earmarked for prevention were fewer than expected and favored governments and faith-based NGOs willing to follow the "ABC" guidelines (Abstinence, Be faithful – in mutually monogamous relationships – and use Condoms. The prominence of this campaign is suggested by Figure 8.5.) PEPFAR even allowed faith-based groups to drop the "C" in their prevention programs (because they considered the promotion of condoms to be an invitation to promiscuity). The program adhered to USAID policies that prohibited the funding of syringe and needle-exchange programs despite evidence that such programs prevented the spread of HIV among injection drug users (and feeding the false assumption that drug users were unable to adhere to ARTs). PEPFAR also required recipients to sign a pledge against "prostitution" and sex trafficking despite the fact that such discriminatory attitudes had proven to be counterproductive in the fight against AIDS. In several countries, these pledges undermined earlier work of AIDS programs with sex workers and contributed to the cultural prejudice that sex workers were not worthy of treatment.

In 2006, Mark Dybul, a physician from the National Institute of Allergy and Infectious Diseases, replaced Randall Tobias as head of PEPFAR, and this led to some changes in these restrictions (generics, for example, began to be used, which lowered the cost of treatment; and in 2008 the abstinence requirement was not enforced). While many AIDS activists around the world were irritated with the prevention policies of PEPFAR, leaders at the WHO and UNAIDS saw PEPFAR as an opportunity to raise funding for AIDS treatment. They

[49] Pisani, *The Wisdom of Whores*, p. 285.

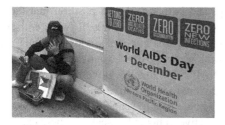

Figure 8.6 World AIDS Day 2011. A vendor sits next to a world AIDS day poster displayed in front of the WHO regional office in Manila. The poster identifies ambitious goals of "Zero New HIV Infections, Zero Discrimination, and Zero AIDS-Related Deaths."
Source: TED ALJIBE/AFP/Getty. Getty images.

even avoided criticizing PEPFAR because it prioritized bilateral aid over existing multilateral organizations. Thus, none of the major international agencies publicly criticized the ideological strings attached to the program (it is important to mention that in 2008 – and again in 2013 – PEPFAR was reauthorized by Congress for periods of five more years and received more funds).

In 2005, toward the end of the 3 by 5 initiative, the United Nations and the leaders of the G8 nations made a commitment to achieve universal access to antiretroviral treatment by 2010. When the World Health Assembly of 2006 took place, the initiative was already dissolved and the Assembly approved a resolution on the need for improving coordination among donors for integrated work against AIDS. However, an assessment of what had gone wrong before was absent.[50] Later, the goal was to reach 15 million people living with HIV with antiretroviral drugs in 2015. (A goal of reaching zero infections also emerged; see Figure 8.6.) With the adoption of the Sustainable Development Goals (SDGs) by UN agencies and other organizations in that year, the target is ending the HIV/AIDS epidemic by 2030.

Final Remarks

Although the WHO was a late entrant to discussions about AIDS and how to control it, and the organization had mixed experiences in addressing the crisis, it did have global influence during the second half of the 1980s, particularly thanks to Jonathan Mann. The WHO was a leader in establishing a close link

---

[50] World Health Organization, 59th World Health Assembly, "Resolution: Implementation by WHO of the Recommendations of the Global Task Team on Improving AIDS Coordination among Multilateral Institutions and International Donors," May 27, 2006, WHA59.12, http://apps.who.int/iris/bitstream/10665/21437/1/A59_R12-en.pdf.

between AIDS, public health, and human rights, a position that the agency insisted upon despite the economic crisis of the 1980s. Its work with burgeoning movements of NGOs and associations of people living with HIV was also an innovation for the multilateral agency. After a troubled period at the end of the twentieth century when UNAIDS became the global leader in the response to the epidemic, the WHO recovered the initiative by adopting the examples set by developing and middle-income countries and embracing universal ARV treatment through the 3 by 5 initiative. It helped to scale-up these examples and moved the AIDS discussion away from debates about whether treatment should be for everyone. It was an effective strategy for reasserting the political and medical role of the World Health Organization in the struggle against HIV/ AIDS and a demonstration of its ability to scale-up interventions. After losing much of its momentum and most of its staff and budget during the 1990s, the WHO once again became a key player in the fight against HIV/AIDS and placed people living with the disease high in the international political agenda. However, despite the efforts of some of its officers, the WHO was unable to establish a balance between research, prevention, treatment, and political advocacy, areas that are interdependent and mutually reinforcing, and it compromised its leadership by not questioning PEPFAR, which represented a form of bilateral aid that carried strong ideological and religious conditions.

An important change in the WHO's response to AIDS was that the agency accepted, with some reluctance, the notion that it had to find partners to pool significant human and financial resources and galvanize action to confront the challenges posed by the disease and by new medical and political realities. The lasting impact of this change will be examined in the last chapters of this book.

9   An Embattled Director-General and the Persistence of the WHO

The period from the late 1980s through most of the 1990s proved to be one of the most difficult times in the WHO's history. A decline in income, challenges to organizational coherence and operational capacity, increasing competition with new international organizations, and confrontation with governments that were critical of the UN all served to erode the agency's once unassailable leadership. The relationship between these organizations and the American administrations of Ronald Reagan and George H. W. Bush reached a low point. These problems and challenges occurred at a time of significant political and economic transformation, often called "globalization," although it was a term that was subject to different interpretations: Many saw it as an opportunity to advance the rules of a liberal economy. During this period, the WHO found it difficult to convey its mission. While the international political and economic order was being remodeled by neoliberal governments, the World Bank, and transnational corporations, the WHO was perceived – or portrayed – as obsolete, befuddled, and misled.

Most of this period covers Dr. Hiroshi Nakajima's two terms as director-general of the WHO (1988–1997), a leadership that was subject to criticism from both inside and outside the organization. His critics would blame him for not doing enough to defend the goals of Primary Health Care, for failing to adapt the agency to new political realities, for sheltering the organization in the face of external criticism, and for slowing the pace of institutional reform. One problem was the growth of a heavy and dysfunctional bureaucracy. Under Nakajima, the number of top-ranking posts almost doubled, and management was top-down. Criticism was frequently personal and involved accusations of corruption, the questioning of his ability to command a multinational organization, and the avoidance of much needed internal restructuring.

Neoliberal Politics

As neoliberal governments and policies in industrialized countries became more entrenched during the mid-1980s, the standing and relevance of the UN and the WHO were increasingly undermined. Neoliberal economic policies advocated for a reduction in public services, such as international health, and for restrictions on the funding of multilateral agencies. The foreign policies of these countries concentrated on assertive unilateral actions in which agencies such as the UN had little importance. Neoliberalism undermined one of the original assumptions of the UN and the WHO. These agencies had been created when nobody questioned the role played by Nation States, and very few Non-State Actors played a role at all. Neoliberalism created a perception that would carry into the twenty-first century, namely that nation states and multilateral organizations were dysfunctional. But, it was not only an ideological or geopolitical issue: The United States and industrialized European countries that had championed the creation of the UN no longer held sway in the assemblies of multilateral institutions. The Reagan administration complained that developing country representatives dominated UN assemblies and took every opportunity to contradict and criticize American foreign policy.

Discussions about the WHO budget proved to be another contentious arena. Since the mid-1980s, the US delegations to the World Health Assembly had put pressure on the WHO to be more cost-effective and reign in its budget. The pressure could be traced to a 1964 meeting in Geneva of the 11 donors to the UN that decided to restrain the growth of the budget of multilateral agencies. During the 1980s, the United States cut its allocations to the regular budget or slowed payment. It is worth remembering that in the mid-1980s the United States' assessed annual dues to the WHO (of USD 73 million) represented 25 percent of the organization's total budget, so this budgetary shortfall represented a severe constraint. As a result of pressure from the United States and other industrialized countries, the World Health Assembly froze the WHO budget. In 1985, the United States refused to pay its assessed dues to the WHO on the grounds that a revised version of the "Essential Medicines" list was contrary to the interests of the United States' pharmaceutical corporations. A list of 200 drugs and vaccines had been established in 1977 and updated every two years. In the spirit of Alma-Ata, this list represented an attempt to convey the notion that some drugs were more essential than others and should be available at reduced prices. A conference took place in Nairobi in 1985, under the auspices of the WHO, at which the relevance of the list was confirmed and participants discussed the best means to procure and distribute safe and good-quality medicines for the poor. Moreover, behind the list was the notion that commercially driven drug development was dysfunctional with respect to the medical needs of the poor.

Since the late 1980s, US government officials criticized the WHO's "inappropriate" interference in the pharmaceuticals, arguing that the list was an attempt to regulate the production and distribution of pharmaceutical products. The American Congress took a more radical stance by signing off on fewer funds to specialized UN agencies than the federal government had requested. At the same time, the WHO was also receiving less money because of the economic crisis and structural adjustment programs that had been imposed by the International Monetary Fund and the World Bank.

All of these developments occurred prior to 1988, the year in which Mahler was replaced as director-general. During his final two years in office, Mahler communicated with US leaders to express his concern about the damage caused to WHO programs as a result of slow payments. Mahler argued that the WHO was being "unfairly victimized" because it belonged to the UN system. Mahler's diplomatic skills meant he was able to maintain a fluent dialogue with American and European political and health authorities to ensure a courteous tone in political discussions and, behind the scenes, to persuade representatives to avoid controversial themes in official meetings. All of these elements were instrumental in guaranteeing temporary funding for the health agency.

The WHO's tense relationship with the United States was to worsen after Mahler left his position in 1988, at a time when he had no second-in-command. One indication that the WHO was divided was that whereas in the past, Mahler had run alone for reelection as the undisputed leader, in 1988 campaigns for the position of director-general were launched by candidates representing Africa, the Middle East, Europe, Latin America, and Asia (including four of the six WHO regional directors). Successive votes eliminated all but Nakajima of Japan and Carlyle Guerra de Macedo of Brazil. The United States and a number of European countries – and even Mahler – supported Macedo, but Nakajima went on to win a close election. At the 41st World Health Assembly meeting, Nakajima was appointed to the post of director-general for a five-year period beginning in July 1988. A brief biographical sketch of the fourth director-general will follow.

Nakajima was awarded his degree in medicine in 1955 in Tokyo and later specialized in neuropsychiatry and pharmacology at the University of Paris, a city in which he worked for some years.[1] In 1967, he returned to Japan to take up the position of director of the research unit of the Nippon Roche Research Center in Tokyo, where he remained until 1973. The following year, he joined the WHO as the director of the WHO Regional Office for the Western Pacific in Manila (where he replaced Francisco J. Dy), and in the early 1980s he became chief of the WHO program on Drug Policies and Management in Geneva. He contributed to the WHO essential drug list, a significant but underfunded component of Primary Health Care. Nakajima appeared to have all the experience required for the new position in the WHO: a successful

---

[1] "Hiroshi Nakajima," *World Health Forum* 19 (1998), 444.

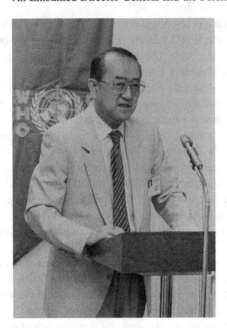

Figure 9.1 Hiroshi Nakajima from Japan became director-general at the 41st World Health Assembly in 1988. He was previously chief of drug policies and management at the WHO and regional director of the WHO's Office for the Western Pacific Region. His tenure was marked by controversy – in part generated by his conflict with Jonathan Mann, head of the WHO's AIDS program. He supported the proposal for essential medicines and the fight against polio, tuberculosis, and other diseases. He served for two consecutive terms until 1998.
Credit: WHO/Tibor Farkas. Courtesy: World Health Organization Photo Library.

career as a medical investigator and administrator, expertise about drugs in public health programs, and a record of authored publications on psychopharmacology in mainstream journals. In addition, he was appreciated in Japanese academic circles: In 1984 he received the Kojma Prize, the highest award given for achievements in public health in Japan.

Nakajima (see Figure 9.1) received the full support of Japan, a factor that was important during difficult times for UN agencies as a result of US foreign aid policy. In the late 1990s, many believed that Japan would replace the United States as the most industrialized nation in the world: It already manufactured nearly a quarter of the world's cars, and Japanese corporations conquered global markets with sophisticated high-tech goods including computers, cameras, and electrical appliances. From 1975 onwards, Japan began to participate in the annual summits of the most industrialized nations. As a major funder of the World Bank and other UN specialized agencies, providing millions of USD in assessments and voluntary contributions, in the mid-1980s Japan sought a permanent seat in the UN Security Council. Officials from the country believed that a Japanese citizen should be given a position of international responsibility in line with the nation's economic power, techno-logical leadership, and contribution to multilateral agencies. Japanese nationals had been appointed to lead UN units of secondary importance, such as the UN Transnational Authority in Cambodia, but Nakajima was the first to be elected as head of a major UN agency, an election sought and supported by the Japanese government and Ministry of Foreign Affairs. His appointment was framed in the context of the United States' loss of influence within the WHO: "The Japanese have been anxious to secure one of the top United Nations posts for some time ... The United States has lost its influence through its refusal to pay assessed contributions, and the United Kingdom ... has found their traditional power ... reduced."[2]

However, although Nakajima's reputation was that of a well-traveled leader who was fluent in both English and French, the two languages used in Geneva, in reality his command of these languages and his communication skills were poor. Several controversies marred Nakajima's administration. Some of them were anecdotal but suggested poor judgment and a growing dissatisfaction inside and outside the WHO. Other controversies suggested that some govern-ments expected that the agency would keep a low profile as a technical body or that it would be willing to welcome the growing role of the World Bank in the international health arena. Two examples of anecdotal interventions that compromised Nakajima's leadership are: Contrary to UN tradition, he signifi-cantly increased his salary as director-general, and in a probable attempt to secure votes, he unsuccessfully tried to pass a resolution to upgrade air travel from economy to business class for World Health Assembly delegates and members of the WHO Executive Board, whose travel expenses were paid for by the WHO. Another anecdotal, ineffectual decision made in 1990 was an award given to the little-known Princess Somdet Phra Srinagarindra Bor-omarajajonani, a member of the Thai Royal Family, for her contributions to Health for All.[3] He was also criticized for the growing influence of the entrepreneur Ryoichi Sasakawa, who was suspected of corruption and was head of a Memorial Health Foundation that supported the WHO's work. Sasakawa made significant donations during the tenure of Nakajima, who

---

[2] Fiona Godlee, "WHO in Retreat: Is It Losing Its Influence?" *British Medical Journal* 309 (1994), 1493.

[3] Cited in United States Department of State, *United States Participation in the UN, Report by the President to the Congress for the Year 1989* (Washington, DC: US Government Printing Office, 1990), p. 220.

established a Sasakawa prize at the WHO for outstanding work in health development. Nakajima was also accused of trying to smuggle valuable icons out of Russia. More serious were the rumors that he traded favors for votes and had no remorse in suspending or arbitrarily transferring anyone daring to disagree. In his defense, his supporters pointed out that charges never were brought. In 1995, there was calls for his resignation after he made a racist remark for which he later apologized. Moreover, his supporters argued that severe structural weaknesses within and outside the agency were responsible for threatening the legitimacy, prestige, and effectiveness of the institution, irrespective of these scandals.

In the political sphere, Nakajima identified with developing countries, arguing that he had been born and raised amidst the tragic legacies of post–World War II Japan. He was unable to moderate discussions inside the WHO and his positions on certain initiatives were unclear, which irritated some WHO members. For example, he initially agreed that the WHO would admit the Palestine Liberation Organization (PLO) as a member "state"; the PLO had formed in 1988 in occupied West Bank and Gaza and applied for WHO membership a year later. The Reagan administration warned that if that were to happen, the United States was likely to leave the WHO. A 1983 US bill obliged the United States to deny funding to any UN program that supported the Palestine Liberation Organization or SWAPO, the independence movement in Namibia.[4] Nakajima eventually conceded and deferred the PLO's application for membership until 1990, when the World Health Assembly also failed to approve it, meaning it was postponed indefinitely. This incident was an embarrassment to the new director-general. Other political issues that were discussed by the Health Assembly and resented by the United States included the debate of the medical consequences of nuclear war and Israeli policies in Gaza.

From the late 1980s onwards, Arab countries regularly began to propose contentious resolutions to WHO bodies. Although very few were approved, the proposals included condemning Israel for health conditions in "occupied Palestine territories," for waging war against its neighbors, and for denying the WHO health workers from entering these territories. Some of these proposals were tolerated by Nakajima and went before World Health Assemblies, thereby antagonizing Israel. In 1991, for example, a World Health Assembly resolution criticized Israel for its poor handling of health issues in occupied Palestinian territories. Israel announced that it would withdraw from the WHO (but fortunately never did).[5]

---

[4] "The WHO's Health, and the PLO," *The New York Times,* May 8, 1989.
[5] United States Department of State, *United States Participation in the UN, Report by the President to the Congress for the Year 1991* (Washington, DC: US Government Printing Office, 1992), p. 262.

Another complication for the WHO was that the global political environment meant there was less funding for the UN during this period. The
collapse of the Soviet Union and the political transformations in Eastern
Europe meant that a significant number of countries stopped paying their
annual assessments. With the end of the Cold War, the WHO faced a
troubled system of finances. In spite of the WHO's sizeable reputation and
even greater responsibilities, its USD 800 million budget in 1990 was
roughly comparable to that of the Helsinki University Hospital in Finland.[6]
In 1991, the WHO depleted its working capital fund and borrowed USD
56 million against internal funds, namely the budget earmarked for other
programs.[7] For the next biennial budget, the WHO had to freeze the implementation of 10 percent of its budget (amounting to USD 36 million a year)
because of nonpayment of dues by several countries. In the following years,
the Secretariat allowed extensive borrowing of funds within the agency. By
1996, the WHO's deficit was USD 206 million. As a result, the WHO began
to depend more and more on borrowing and on unpredictable extrabudgetary
resources that came from voluntary contributions. This dependency
increased the risk of transforming the agency into a tool for donors and
bilateral agencies, increased the competition among WHO programs for
funding from outside the organization, and undermined any coherent and
comprehensive planning.

As Gill Walt of the London School of Hygiene and Tropical Medicine has
noted, in the early 1990s there was a shift from predominantly relying on the
WHO's "regular budget"– drawn from member states' contributions and based
on population size and GNP – to greatly increasing dependence on "extrabudgetary" funding coming from "donor" nations and private philanthropies.[8]
In 1971, the regular budget was USD 75 million and the extrabudgetary
portion, 25 million. By 1986–1987, the amount of extrabudgetary funding –
USD 437 million – was almost the equivalent of the regular budget of USD
543 million. In 1989, a remarkable event occurred in the history of the agency,
anticipated budgetary resources for the two-year period of 1990–1991 would
exceed the regular budget, and, by the beginning of the 1990s, extrabudgetary
funding had overtaken the regular budget by USD 21 million, representing

---

[6] Meri Koivusalo & Eeva Ollila, *Making a Healthy World: Agencies, Actors and Policies in
International Health* (London: Zed Books, 1997), p. 9.

[7] This section is based on Brown, Cueto, & Fee, "The World Health Organization and the
Transition from 'International' to 'Global' Public Health," American Journal of Public Health
96:1 (2006), 62–72.

[8] Gill Walt, "WHO under Stress: Implications for Health Policy," *Health Policy* 24 (1993),
125–144.

54 percent of the WHO's overall budget. These changes led to enormous challenges for the organization.

Extrabudgetary contributions created an unequal distribution of resources inside the WHO. By the late 1980s, 9 out of 60 WHO programs received about two-thirds of all extrabudgetary funds (plus 10 percent, on average, of the regular budget). As another by-product of voluntary contributions, donors began to demand higher "standards" of accountability, rapid and transparent financial reporting, and better management practices, all of which suggested that the financial and administrative practices within the WHO were open to criticism. These private donors and government aid programs criticized the decision to borrow against internal funds as being unwise.

Although extrabudgetary funding rescued the WHO's finances in the short term, it led to coordination and continuity problems because of changing donor interests and short-term financial commitments. By the early 1990s, ten countries provided 90 percent of all extrabudgetary funds and the same countries provided more than half of the regular budget through assessed contributions. A study with a telling subtitle: "Is the Organization Donor Driven?" examined the role played by these contributors and concluded by answering the question with a cautious affirmation.[9]

Nakajima was unable to present a coherent response to these problems. In his first meetings with the Executive Board and Health Assemblies in 1991 and 1992, the director-general announced his interest in drawing up a new "WHO paradigm for health" that would be a new philosophical rationale for the WHO to attract new funds for the agency. However, several delegates raised questions about the content, coherence, and ultimate goal of his proposal, and the Executive Board requested that the paradigm be fleshed out, but this never occurred.

In 1991, the United States and the WHO clashed over the Gulf War. The WHO Executive Board was in session at the outbreak of the American offensive against Iraqi forces in Kuwait, and the Iraqi member requested an urgent discussion on the health impact of the UN Security Council's resolution to place an embargo on Iraq. The US delegate objected to a discussion on the grounds that it was a matter for the Security Council. After a debate, the Board eventually rejected the Iraqi request by a vote of 11 to 3 with 8 abstentions. Around a year later, Nakajima upset the Americans by accepting a unique payment of contribution arrears from Iraq (which temporarily restored the country's voting privileges at the Health Assembly). The Americans argued that the check sent to Geneva was worthless because it was drawn on an Iraqi

---

[9] See J. Patrick Vaughan, Sigrun Møgedal, Gill Walt, Stein-Erik Kruse, Kelley Lee, & Koen de Wilde, "WHO and the Effects of Extrabudgetary Funds: Is the Organization Donor Driven?" *Health Policy and Planning* 11:3 (1996), 253–264.

account based in the United States that had been blocked by the UN Security Council. For the US federal agency, Iraq was purchasing arms with hard currency and sending a phony check to Geneva only for "having propaganda" at the WHO's expense.[10]

Many of the complaints against the WHO and Nakajima referred to his lack of understanding of the economic forces of globalization, his tendency to overemphasize the biomedical dimension of health issues, and his reluctance to acknowledge the emergence of new actors and stakeholders in international health. In the past, the WHO had been the sole leader of international health policies, but from about 1990, new institutional actors came to occupy leading positions in global health. Among these were the World Bank and US bilateral assistance programs. They shared the assumptions that the world was rapidly changing and that the traditional governmental and intergovernmental agencies, such as the WHO, were ill-equipped for the new challenges because of cumbersome bureaucratic procedures, insufficient resources, and an outdated organizational structure. In contrast to the WHO, the World Bank's influence had begun to burgeon during the late 1980s and 1990s.

The World Bank and Globalization

From the 1980s, the WHO not only had to deal with a new political world order but with the growing influence of the World Bank, which between 1986 and 1991 was led by its talented president, the lawyer Barber B. Conable, Jr., a former Republican congressional representative nominated by President Reagan and the first politician to hold the post, who managed to convince his former colleagues to double US Congress appropriations to the Bank. He combined the promotion of liberal economic policies with the fight against extreme poverty around the world. He was succeeded as president by Wall Street banker Lewis Preston, who held the post from 1991 to 1995, and by the Australian-American economist James D. Wolfensohn (1995–2005).

The Bank, which had been established in 1946 to assist in the reconstruction of Europe after World War II, soon expanded its mandate to provide loans, grants, and technical assistance to developing countries. At first, it funded large investments in physical capital and infrastructure, but in the 1970s under the leadership of McNamara it began to invest in population control, health, and education.[11] In 1979, the Bank had created a Population, Health, and Nutrition

---

[10] United States Department of State, *United States Participation in the UN, Report by the President to the Congress for the Year 1992* (Washington, DC: US Government Printing Office, 1993), 260.

[11] Jennifer P. Ruger, "The Changing Role of the World Bank in Global Health," *American Journal of Public Health* 95:1 (2005), 60–70.

Department, directed by John R. Evans, a Canadian pediatrician and business-man, who merged and bolstered different units in the Bank that worked in these areas. The Department adopted a policy of funding both stand-alone health programs and health components of other projects. Where the Bank had previously viewed health expenditures as unproductive drains on public finances, it now began to see health expenditures as potentially productive investments.

In its 1980 World Development Report, the Bank argued that malnutrition and ill health could be addressed by direct government action. It suggested that improving health and nutrition could accelerate economic growth, thus pro-viding an argument in favor of social-sector spending. Throughout the 1980s, the Bank awarded loans and grants for food and nutrition, family planning, maternal and child health, and basic health services. As the Bank began to make direct loans for health services, it called for the more efficient use of available resources and for competition between public and private organiza-tions in the delivery of health services. As a result, trade liberalization led to greater foreign private investment in the health sector of some developing countries, in an area that had previously been quite restricted.

In the mid-1980s, the World Bank enforced strict structural adjustment policies on poor nations that were burdened by massive foreign debt. These economic policies placed a precedent on the free market for financing health care. A 1987 World Bank report on "Financing Health Services" advocated user fees or copayments for public hospitals and government-run health services in developing nations.[12] According to the report's recommendations, patients and their families should begin to pay for part of the costs of public services and facilities that in the past had been free, at least for the poor via state subsidies. The rationale behind user fees was that communities had to participate in the financing of health services and subsidize health facilities for additional revenue for the public health sector, reduce frivolous demand that some people made of public health services, and make people prefer low-cost primary care instead of expensive specialized medical services. Critics of these reforms argued that a commitment to the notion of cost-effectiveness had now become the single greatest rationale behind health work. Services came to be viewed as "commodities," and patients became "consumers" of health ser-vices – suggesting that the humanitarian side of medical care was being lost.[13]

In the context of widespread developing country indebtedness and increas-ingly scarce resources for health expenditures, the World Bank's promotion of structural adjustment measures and cuts in social and health spending drew

---

[12] John S. Akin, *Financing Health Services in Developing Countries: An Agenda for Reform* (Washington, DC: World Bank, 1987).
[13] Koivusalo & Ollila, *Making a Healthy World*, p. 139.

criticism. There was a close, almost symbiotic relationship between debt management policy and macroeconomic and social reforms. Debt management ensured that individual debtor countries continued to abide by their financial obligations. Through debt refinancing, repayment of the principal could be deferred, while interest payments were enforced. Creditors agreed to reschedule only if debtor nations agreed to "conditionalities" attached to the loan agreements. By the mid-1980s, World Bank loan agreements included stringent conditionalities, and loans were granted only if governments complied with demands for structural adjustment. The Bank oversaw "reforms" in health, education, industry, agriculture, and the environment. It also supervised the privatization of state enterprises and revised the structure of public investment and the composition of public expenditures. Debt restructuring demanded cuts in social programs such as health and education and often led to the leaders of these programs requesting funding from outside their governments.

The World Bank attempted to show that it was not indifferent to this situation and began to elaborate on the developmental utility of social, educational, and health projects. In 1993, the World Bank published a landmark report, *Investing in Health,* which had been prepared by a team headed by the health economist Dean Jamison.[14] This was the first annual report devoted to a specific sector and it clearly announced the Bank's entry as a player into the field of international health. The report noted an increase in health assistance in the early 1990s after a period of stagnation during the early 1980s. It also argued that good population health was a prerequisite for a sound economic model, that a more rational selection process for health interventions could be developed, and that the "global burden of disease" should be measured.[15] This measure was the "Disability Adjusted Life Year," or DALY. In simple terms, the DALY was an individual composite measure (which took gender and age into account) that calculated items including the time lost to different illnesses and disabilities, lost wages and productivity, medical expenses, savings produced by cost-effective medical interventions, and productive time lost to premature mortality.

The Bank advocated for health spending on cost-effective programs (such as immunization) and decentralizing and reforming health services to promote quality and competition. This was the beginning of a growing consensus among health economists that health interventions should denote

---

[14] World Bank, *World Development Report 1993, Investing in Health,* (New York: Oxford University Press, 1993).

[15] For a discussion of DALY, see Christopher J. L. Murray & Alan D. Lopez (eds.), *The Global Burden of Disease: A Comprehensive Assessment of Mortality and Disability from Diseases, Injuries, and Risk Factors in 1990 and Projected to 2020* (Cambridge: Harvard University Press, 1996).

evidence-based decision-making for the allocation of financial and human resources and should have clear expected outcomes. Health reform came at a time of financial crisis marked by recession, indebtedness, and disillusionment with the state. As a result, the focus of many health policies shifted from the attainment of PHC to concerns about good management, cost-effective interventions, and financing health systems. This focus was not without its critics because it created a trade-off between equity and efficiency and paid little attention to the former.

By 1996, the Bank held a USD 8 billion portfolio in health programs and was the largest single financier of health activities in low- and middle-income countries.[16] It created a special program in International Health Policy and by the end of the decade had become a leading voice in national and international debates on health policy. Health systems around the world came under increasing pressure to make radical reforms along the lines recommended by the World Bank. "Health reform," "quality assessment," "cost containment," "accountability," and "cost-effectiveness" became the code words used by many health workers, health ministries, and health agencies around the world. Even patients came to be known as "clients" or "consumers" who had to pay part of the cost of health services. The aim of the reforms was to improve the performance of and access to quality health services. A common component of these reforms was that providers and purchasers of health care came to be separated by third-party payment mechanisms. Managed care companies that found themselves facing a largely saturated US market were happy to extend their reach into Third World countries. Health sector reforms resulted in reduced access to health services for the poorest sectors of societies, both because of reductions in public expenditures and the increasing free market costs of medical materials and technologies. This was part of a wider neoliberal movement toward downsizing the state and transforming it into a sort of steward of society, promoting a laissez faire culture and facilitating private investments.

The WHO's response to the neoliberal economics that underlined the restructuring of health systems was a timid one. In 1990, the director-general complained to the Executive Board about the fact that "economics" was distorting the aim of "free access to health care for all."[17] However, the WHO never managed to launch a genuinely alternative proposal for health reform that would be different from the one proposed by the Bank.

---

[16] Marian Claeson, Joy de Beyer, Prabhat Jha, & Richard G. Feachem, "The World Bank's Perspective on Global Health," *Current Issues in Public Health* 2:5–6 (1996), 264–269.

[17] Statement by the Director-General to the Executive Board at its Eighty-Fifth Session, February 15, 1990, Box 1, Hiroshi Nakajima Papers (WHO).

Criticism against the World Bank was more acute outside of the WHO. Some public health scholars and practitioners saw the World Bank Report of 1993 as an attempt to take over the health sector by neoliberal actors who were determined to insert the market into social security and health services. Critics found shortcomings in the DALY methodology and denounced the dual discourse of the Bank, on the one hand, advocating to slash government spending in the social sectors of health and education and, on the other, glamorizing specific disease-control programs.[18] For both the Bank's critics and supporters, the publication of the 1993 report, *Investing in Health*, was viewed as the Bank's assertion of a leadership role in international health. In 1995, the Bank appointed Richard Feachem, who was dean of the London School of Hygiene and Tropical Medicine, as director of the Bank's Health, Nutrition, and Population unit. He would remain in that position until 1999, becoming an influential figure in global health.

The inauguration of the World Trade Organization (WTO) in 1995 marked a new phase in the evolution of the international economic system, as a triangular division of authority among the IMF, the World Bank, and the WTO began to unfold. Henceforth, many of the mainstays of the structural adjustment program (trade liberalization, privatization, and foreign investment) became permanently entrenched in the WTO's articles of agreement. The deregulation of trade under WTO rules and new clauses pertaining to intellectual property rights enabled multinational corporations to penetrate local markets and extend their control over many new areas of domestic manufacturing, agriculture, and the service economy. In particular, the WTO's intellectual property rules provided obstacles to supplying low cost pharmaceuticals to developing countries. The WTO's dominance was soon resented and its meetings generated anti-globalization protests around the world. But what was globalization?

In economic terms, globalization, at least initially, meant the dominance of the world economy by multinational banks and corporations under the economic leadership of the United States, the superpower that "won" the Cold War. Financial capital was now relatively free to flow across borders unhampered by national governments, while multinational firms produced for a global market. The internationalization of macroeconomic policy transformed countries into open economic territories and "reserves" of cheap labor and natural resources. But even as trade liberalization and the deregulation of domestic commodity markets increasingly brought the price of food staples up to world market levels, wages and labor costs in the Third World and Eastern Europe remained much lower than in the OECD countries.

---

[18] A. C. Laurell & O. L. Arellano, "Market Commodities and Poor Relief: The World Bank Proposal for Health," *International Journal of Health Services* 26:1 (1996), 1–18.

Income disparities between nations were now found alongside extremely high-income disparities within nations.

One illustration of the global extension of neoliberal ideas was the 1992 endorsement of free market forces as key for economic growth by China's leader, Deng Xiaoping. Globalization was also associated with the speed of international communications, brought about by advances in technology. It was also marked by accelerated urbanization in the developing world, where poor people flocked to overcrowded and unsanitary city slums. Globalization produced and was reflected in the remarkable growth of international travel: By the end of the 1990s, 1 million individuals worldwide traveled by air every day, and 2 million people crossed national borders.[19] These figures would increase further in the years that followed.

Beyond the first George Bush administration, the ideas that globalization was good for America and that the UN should be reformed persisted. During Bill Clinton's administration, although a more cordial tone was adopted, the notion of a UN reform and similar neoliberal economic policies at home and abroad also endured.[20] After Clinton's failed attempts to reform the US health system, the Clinton administration acted in much the same way as the previous Republican administrations with regard to the welfare state: It was a burden and an obstacle to economic growth. Clinton's foreign policy, which he only developed fully during his second term, was largely concerned with the opening of foreign markets for American investors and unilateral interventions in international emergencies. The belief in American economic progress persisted despite apparently isolated tragedies, such as Rwanda, elsewhere in the world. "Failed states," civil wars, growing social disparities, social turmoil, natural disasters, and new epidemics plagued the globe and were frequently portrayed as the regrettable collateral effects of liberal economics.

Emerging and Reemerging Diseases

On the heels of the AIDS epidemic, a changing international epidemiological period emerged, marked by newly "emerging" and "reemerging" infectious diseases. This reinforced the perception that the world had entered a globalized era and it attracted the attention of scientists, health leaders, journalists, politicians, and science-fiction writers. Although there was no precise definition for emerging disease, the term was usually applied to diseases that appeared in a population for the first time or, where it had existed previously,

[19] David Satcher, "Global Health at the Crossroads: Surgeon General's Report on the 50th World Health Assembly," *Journal of the American Medical Association* 281 (1999), 942–943.

[20] See William G. Hayland, *Clinton's World: Remaking American Foreign Policy* (Westport, CT: Praeger, 1999).

it was marked by an increase in incidence or geographic range. The term "reemerging" was ascribed to communicable diseases that reappeared after a period of absence. For many experts, these diseases were a natural component of "globalization." Infections that arose in any part of the world could rapidly spread to any other part due to the ease and speed of transportation of people, goods, livestock, and food supplies. Other causes of these diseases were the dissemination of unhealthy lifestyles, such as smoking; global warming and population growth; the proliferation of overcrowded cities with poor sanitation; deforestation; and the reckless use of natural resources. Such transmissions could also grow as a result of refugees fleeing civil wars. The existence of such diseases pointed to a newly hostile environment containing unknown and unpredictable dangers that could undermine the stability of rich and poor countries alike. Most studies agreed that the globalization of diseases was also due to the breakdown of public health infrastructure and a deterioration of infectious disease surveillance systems, particularly in poor and former socialist countries, that occurred in the 1990s after a series of drastic changes in their health and economic policies. For some experts, the globalization of disease was not a new or completely natural phenomenon and shed light on both old and new social injustices.[21]

The World Health Organization was initially slow to respond to the new global epidemiological landscape, but after a few years, and in spite of its internal issues, it assumed a leading role and designed a new set of international regulations for the control of pandemics with humanitarian and protective responses. The new centrality of infectious diseases stood in contrast to the assertions of those medical experts in the 1960s and 1970s who had predicted that industrial countries would eliminate major infectious diseases thanks to vaccines, antibiotics, and sulfas and would focus their attentions on chronic illnesses resulting from sedentary lifestyles. Nevertheless, emerging diseases and reemerging bacterial, fungal, viral, and parasitic diseases appeared everywhere in the 1990s. This marked the end of the belief in two distinct epidemiological processes that were supposed to distinguish rich countries from poor ones. The first was the progressive tendency of industrial nations to overcome the respiratory and diarrheal infections that had predominated until the early twentieth century and, with longer life expectancies, to confront heart disease and cancer as the major new causes of mortality. The second was the slower progress in poor countries, where communicable infections and short life expectancies persisted but where the health situation was beginning to mirror that of more developed countries with a new prevalence of chronic diseases.

---

[21] Paul Farmer, "Social Inequalities and Emerging Infectious Diseases," *Emerging Infectious Diseases* 2:4 (1996), 259–269.

Some examples illustrate the growing trend toward globalized infections. One that became a concern was a new strain of TB called multidrug-resistant tuberculosis (because it was resistant to most of the existing tuberculosis therapies) that was found in at least 10 percent of TB cases across the globe. In the years leading up to 1985, the United States had experienced 6 percent annual declines in the rate of tuberculosis, but the incidence of the infection started to increase from 1986. By 1992, rates of new cases of TB in the United States showed a 12 percent rise versus those from 1985.[22] The problem would acquire dramatic proportions in the following years. Between 2000 and 2009, an estimated 5 million people were infected with multidrug-resistant tuberculosis.

Other new menaces included Legionnaires' disease, Campylobacteriosis, tick-transmitted Lyme disease, Hantavirus, Spongiform Encephalitis, West Nile Virus, and food-borne illness caused by Escherichia coli. In 1997, the WHO identified more than 60 "significant infectious diseases outbreaks of both 'classic' diseases and new unfamiliar diseases."[23] These conditions were increasing in both developed and developing countries. In the 1990s, epidemics believed to be on the verge of extinction appeared in unexpected places and took health workers by surprise. Some examples were: diphtheria in the Russian Federation in 1990; cholera in Peru in 1991; yellow fever in Kenya in 1992; bubonic plague in India in 1994, Ebola in Zaire in 1995; human cases of Creutzfeldt-Jacob Disease, CJD (related to "mad cow" disease) in the UK in 1996; and "avian" influenza, H5N1, in Hong Kong in 1997. In 1996, dengue hemorrhagic fever, a viral disease with dramatic clinical symptoms (high fever, vomiting, and bleeding from capillaries) that was considered to be restricted to the Caribbean, began to invade South America and threaten other parts of the world. For many of these diseases, there was no good scientific explanation for their transmission, no specific treatment, or no vaccine. Medical scientists were faced with a greater challenge in that new strains of bacteria, viruses, and parasites were becoming resistant to standard antibiotics and other antimicrobial drugs, making treatment extremely difficult and sometimes impossible. In hindsight, it became clear that human antibacterial resistance had come about as a result of the trend among clinicians to over-prescribe antibiotics, along with poor compliance with medical regimes on the part of patients and unregulated sales of medicines. In addition, the traditional separation between infectious and chronic diseases began to blur during the 1990s. Scientists found that some forms of cancer had infectious etiologies. Cervical cancer,

---

[22] World Health Organization, "World Health Assembly Emphasized Tuberculosis Crisis," May 14, 1993, Press Release WHA/14, WHO Press Releases 1992–1999.

[23] World Health Organization, Division of Emerging and other Communicable Diseases Surveillance and Control, *EMC Annual Report 1997* (Geneva: World Health Organization, 1997), p. 7.

for example, could result from the human Papilloma virus, liver cancer could be produced by both Hepatitis B and Hepatitis C virus, and stomach cancer could be caused by Helicobacter pylori.

The first responses to these diseases came from American and European medical scientists. Stephen Morse and Joshua Lederberg, two prominent American researchers, demanded political action to address the threat of "emerging" infectious diseases. Morse was a virologist at the Rockefeller University, New York, and Lederberg was a prestigious microbiologist who had won the Nobel Prize in 1958 for his discoveries on genetic material of bacteria and was president emeritus of the Rockefeller University (and both were advisors to the WHO). Morse and Lederberg's insistence on a new global epidemiological profile was supported by leading health experts and researchers such as Donald A. Henderson, the former head of the WHO's smallpox eradication campaign, and by Yale University epidemiologist Robert E. Shope. They participated in a landmark 1989 conference, sponsored by the National Institutes of Health, entitled "Emerging Viruses: The Evolution of Viruses and Viral Diseases." The conference was attended by more than 200 participants and covered by the journals of the time. There, the "new" diseases were framed as the unanticipated result of economic progress achieved by a global society, contact with diseases whose animal reservoirs had been forced out of the jungle, the uncontrolled growth of megacities with poor sanitation, and an increase in global travel.

The themes of the meeting were taken up by the US's Institute of Medicine and the National Academy of Sciences which, along with Morse, Lederberg and Shope, produced a milestone report in 1992 on new epidemic diseases portrayed as serious threats to the United States.[24] The report traced the origins of the new illnesses, stressing the impact of genetic, environmental, and social changes linked to globalization. The report warned that no location was so remote that it was immune from global health risks; an epidemic starting in any one village could rapidly spread out of control. In addition, developing countries were now enduring the negative impacts of unhealthy lifestyles as a result of tobacco, alcohol, and drug abuse and poor nutritional habits linked to obesity. Finally, global warming and the breakdown of health systems added to the urgent need to respond to infectious disease pandemics. According to the report, old and new infectious diseases needed to be controlled in order to protect both trade and people: Novel measures were proposed, including a new global surveillance network; the reinforcement of food-supply safety measures; closer collaboration between scientific disciplines, from genetics to the

---

[24] Joshua Lederberg, Robert E. Shope, & Stanley C. Oaks, Jr. (eds.), *Emerging Infections: Microbial Threats to Health in the United States* (Washington, DC: National Academy Press, 1992).

social sciences; the promotion of behavioral changes; and more funds for research on new drugs and vaccines.

In 1994, the CDC produced its own report that basically followed the ideas of the Institute of Medicine's report. Throughout the 1990s, following the lead set by these two reports, organizations and individuals produced articles and books, organized meetings, provided grants, published special issues of mainstream medical journals, and launched the CDC journal *Emerging Infectious Diseases*. Some WHO officers were also convinced that the globe was facing new menaces and that it was essential to establish new surveillance systems and medical and preventive programs and to develop dialogue and organize meetings and activities with other organizations.

In 1994 and 1995, for example, the WHO organized meetings on Emerging Infectious Diseases in Geneva that included representatives from Europe, India, Japan, Africa, and the United States (including Morse, Lederberg, Shope, and other American members of the CDC and NIH) that recognized that a global approach should be spearheaded by the World Health Organization. The main recommendations of these meetings was to rebuild the human and laboratory capacities for surveillance of infectious diseases, strengthen the international infrastructure to respond to disease emergencies, and promote applied research on new infections.[25] The meetings were also an opportunity to reinforce the relevance of a number of programs including GASP (or Gonococcal resistance to penicillin and tetracycline) and WHONET, a computer program developed by the WHO that assisted hospital laboratories around the world in addressing antibiotic resistance.

In 1995, the New York Academy of Medicine and the New York State Department of Health convened the Conference "Emerging Infectious Diseases: Meeting the Challenge," which was attended by James LeDuc, the WHO officer in charge of arboviruses and viral hemorrhagic fevers during the period 1992–1996. Participants discussed several cases of pathogens that were rapidly and without warning able to cross oceans and continents in apparently healthy individuals. In the same year, the National Institutes of Health sponsored an International Conference on Pandemic Influenza that focused on the need for preparedness against a threatened influenza pandemic. At the same time that these meetings were taking place, a study conducted by the WHO on several virology laboratories used as reference centers revealed that about half of these centers lacked the ability to diagnose diseases such as yellow fever, hantavirus, dengue, and other diseases because they did not have the necessary diagnostic reagents. Politicians and governments also came on board to respond to emergent diseases.

---

[25] World Health Organization, "Emerging Infectious Diseases: Memorandum from a WHO meeting," *Bulletin of the World Health Organization* 72:8 (1994), 845–850.

In 1996, for example, President Bill Clinton issued a Presidential Decision Directive that identified infectious diseases as a threat to domestic and international security and requested about USD 100 million from Congress. A 1997 publication from the Institute of Medicine, which used the term "protection" in its subtitle, was telling, entitled *America's Vital Interest in Global Health.*[26] The following year, the CDC and a further 60 sponsoring institutions organized an International Conference on Emerging Infectious Diseases, attended by 2,500 researchers, clinicians, and public health professionals. The meeting attempted to define the precise needs and demands for surveillance, prevention, and control. A parallel development was that in the G-8 meetings, beginning in Denver, Colorado, in 1997, heads of industrialized countries requested effective coordination in the response to international outbreaks of communicable diseases and the development of a global surveillance network. During the year, a number of epidemic outbreaks, such as cholera in Mozambique and Kenya, Dengue in Malaysia, and yellow fever in Bolivia, raised the concern of international agencies and the public.

Scientists, writers, and movie producers sparked in the public imagination the fear of uncontrolled infectious epidemics crossing between poor and rich countries. Two prominent science journalists who had built their reputations working on global emerging diseases were Richard Preston from the *New Yorker* and Laurie Garrett from *Newsday*. Preston's bestselling book *The Hot Zone*, published in 1994, brought Ebola from a remote African village to a backyard in the United States through an African monkey that escaped from a laboratory. Garrett was a fellow at the School of Public Health at Harvard University when she published her acclaimed book *The Coming Plague: Newly Emerging Diseases in a World Out of Balance* (1994). In the preface, she warned that AIDS was only one of many new infections stemming from ecological imbalances, social inequalities, and the dramatic decline in public health systems. She would elaborate on the latter theme in her next book, *Betrayal of Trust*, adding that the public-health trust between government and society was broken.[27] In 1995, the film industry followed suit, releasing *Outbreak,* which became a box office success. It blamed a frightening new epidemic on a sick African monkey that had entered undetected into the United States.

Around the world, politicians shared in the growing concern about epidemic disease and, in turn, began to participate in dialogue with medical scientists

---

[26] Institute of Medicine, *America's Vital Interest in Global Health: Protecting Our People, Enhancing Our Economy, and Advancing Our International Interests* (Washington, DC: National Academy Press, 1997).

[27] Laurie Garrett, *The Coming Plague: Newly Emerging Diseases in a World out of Balance* (New York: Farrar, Straus and Giroux, 1994), p. 15, and Garrett, *Betrayal of Trust: The Collapse of Global Public Health* (New York: Hyperion, 2000).

and health leaders. In one of the hearings on the subject organized by the US Congress, a US representative recalled an international health theme by making clear that infectious diseases "honor no national boundaries ... affect citizens of all countries [and] are clearly a global health issue." Moreover, it was not possible to protect the health of US citizens without addressing problems occurring elsewhere in the world.[28] He also insisted that industrial nations had to abandon their complacency about infectious diseases and to design modern methods of surveillance, and that whatever criticisms there might be of the WHO, the multilateral agency had to be a partner in these efforts. In 2001, the CIA produced its own report on global infectious diseases that were portrayed as major factors contributing toward social and economic crises around the world. The CIA warned about the high economic costs of infectious diseases and their threat to the United States.[29] American political concern with global diseases was further fueled by the fear of bioterrorism and the use of anthrax in the mail after September 11, 2001.

Public health institutions in Canada and Europe made similar political commitments to the control of international infectious diseases. In 1998, for example, Canada's Center for Disease Control, in collaboration with the WHO, created a Global Public Health Intelligence Network (GPHIN) as a fee-based electronic reporting service for reports that were considered important to public health. The following year, the European Union created a global Communicable Diseases Network that would go on to become the European Center for Disease Prevention and Control.

The combined impact of the concerns of leading US scientists and American medical institutions, the work of popular writers, the involvement of the US Congress and politicians from industrial nations, and the work of WHO underlined the argument that in a borderless world, epidemic outbreaks had to be controlled at their source. For some, this new awareness formed part of a wider process that sought to redefine the role and scope of multilateral and bilateral health agencies such as the WHO. For most official institutions in the West, AIDS, emergent diseases, and global health were in sum a domestic-security issue and an opportunity for global humanitarian intervention, which did not necessarily imply that a human rights approach was required, as Mann had proposed in the 1980s. This led to revamping traditional international health goals and attaching them to the notion of global health security as a

---

[28] "Senator Bill Frist, Opening Statement" in United States Congress, Senate, Committee on Labor and Human Resources, Subcommittee on Public Health and Safety, Global health: US Response to Infectious Diseases: Hearing before the Subcommittee on Public Health and Safety of the Committee on Labor and Human Resources (Washington, DC: US Government Printing Office, 1988), pp. 1–3, p. 2.

[29] United States, Central Intelligence Agency, *Global Infectious Disease Threat and Its Implications for the United States* (Washington, DC: Central Intelligence Agency, 2000).

response to challenges that transcended national borders and to framing infectious diseases as exogenous threats in need of a renewed legal instrument to protect developed countries from epidemic outbreaks.

The Renewal of Epidemiological Surveillance

The WHO did respond to some of the unique disease challenges during this period. During Nakajima's first year as head of the agency in 1989, he created a new assistant director-general position to oversee communicable diseases. The American Ralph Henderson, a CDC officer who previously was deputy director of the West African Smallpox Program and had directed the WHO's Expanded Program on Immunization, was appointed to the new position. During the years that followed, the agency began to improve the international surveillance system to monitor and rapidly inform on epidemic outbreaks and to coordinate a coherent international response. In November 1994, the WHO's Division of Communicable Diseases convened a Scientific Working Group to examine drug-resistant bacterial infections, a growing clinical and public health problem inside and outside hospitals for which there were often no effective drugs. Experts from more than 20 countries and a number of pharmaceutical industries analyzed the nature and costs of drug resistance, the best way to limit its spread, and the financial burden posed to health care systems around the world.[30]

In May 1995, the 48th World Health Assembly passed a resolution to identify rapidly emerging and reemerging diseases, created a new unit, the Division of Emerging Viral and Bacterial Disease Surveillance (EMC, later renamed the Division on Emerging and other Communicable Diseases and Control), and began a process of updating its International Health Regulations. The EMC absorbed a former unit known as the Division of Communicable Diseases (CDS) and recruited staff from a number of WHO Divisions, including Health Situation and Trend Assessment (HST) and Diarrhoeal and Acute Respiratory Diseases Control (CDR) as well as from some of the personnel who worked on surveillance at the Global Program on AIDS (GPA). An indication of EMC's relevance within the agency was that by 1997 it had a staff of 63 professionals. The Division's mission was to strengthen national and international surveillance networks, expand the WHONET computer program to analyze microbiology laboratory data, and modernize the WHO's *Weekly Epidemiological Record* and its *International Travel and Health* handbook (both published in English and French). Although the WHO's financial

---

[30] Fred C. Tenover & James M. Hughes, "WHO Scientific Working Group on Monitoring and Management of Bacterial Resistance to Antimicrobial Agents," *Emerging Infectious Diseases* 1:1 (1995), 37.

constraints meant that only 6 percent of the new Division's budget came from the agency's regular budget, the EMC secured extrabudgetary funds to support its activities in the succeeding years. David L. Heymann, an American epidemiologist trained at the London School of Hygiene and Tropical Medicine who had worked for 13 years with CDC, was appointed as director of the new division.

Under Heymann's stewardship, the EMC built the capacity to mobilize onsite a team of experts to anywhere in the world within 24 hours' notification of an outbreak in order to begin epidemic control measures. One of the most important activities of the EMC was to rebuild the scientific and surveillance capacity of middle-income and poor countries and make their laboratories part of a network of WHO collaborating centers. Heymann also emphasized the study of antibiotic resistance-monitoring networks and the modernization of international health regulations to transform them into a real global alert system. As a result, it became obligatory to report any event that may constitute a public health emergency of international concern. The new IHR helped to deploy active surveillance systems, including a novel "WHO Rumor/outbreak list." The list contained unconfirmed rumors of communicable and zoonotic disease outbreaks that were made available to government officials. It was estimated that in the late 1990s, up to five rumors were received each week at the WHO from sources which ranged from the international press to NGOs and WHO collaborating centers. When a rumor was received, the relevant science staff and WHO country representatives investigated it. Only when a rumor was confirmed was it made public, via the EMC website. However, the implementation of the IHR was regarded as the responsibility of ministries of health, with little participation of finance and agriculture ministries, a flaw that would be more visible in the epidemic outbreaks of the following years. Another goal of the IHR was to discourage the unscientific behavior, by states and organizations of the early 1990s, consisting of imposing excessive, counterproductive, and irrational barriers against travel and commerce from countries that were considered the origin of disease outbreaks.

These scientific responses were published by the WHO in its annual report for 1995, *Bridging the Gaps*, which placed much less emphasis on the biological dimensions of emergent diseases and opened with a dramatic, and for many, dissonant statement underlining the social causes of illnesses that evoked Alma-Ata:

The world's biggest killer and the greatest cause of ill-health and suffering across the globe is listed almost at the end of the International Classification of Diseases. It is given the code Z59.5 - extreme poverty. Poverty is the main reason why babies are not vaccinated, why clean water and sanitation are not provided, why curative drugs and other treatments are unavailable and why mothers die in childbirth. It is the underlying cause of reduced life expectancy, handicap, disability and starvation. Poverty is a major contributor to mental illness, stress, suicide, family disintegration and substance abuse.[31]

This social interpretation came as something of a surprise in a period when most officers of the agency emphasized responses based on science and technology. The following year, the WHO's annual report for 1996 entitled *Fighting Disease, Fostering Development* and devoted to emergent infections, emphasized the need for a rapid response to infectious diseases that were killing about 17 million people a year.[32] To ensure better surveillance and faster responses to epidemic outbreaks, the report also announced that the WHO's *Weekly Epidemiological Record* would be made available for free in electronic format. The emphasis on emergent infections continued into the following year, 1997, when the theme "Emerging Infectious Diseases: Global Alert, Global Response," was selected for the World Health Day celebrations on April 7, to draw attention to an urgent problem.

The WHO's first test in responding effectively to an emergent disease came in 1996 when Ebola, a viral hemorrhagic fever, first appeared in the Zairian city of Kikwit. The city of around 400,000 inhabitants was located 240 miles east of the country's capital of Kinshasa, near the Ebola river in one of the poorest and most corrupt countries in Africa (today the Democratic Republic of Congo). The virus produced frightening symptoms: sudden high fever, chills, severe abdominal pain, vomiting, and diarrhea. The disease had a short incubation period – about three days – and an extremely high fatality rate. In a given outbreak, 50 – 90 percent of people died within two weeks of becoming infected. Personal contact with an infected person was the main route of transmission and the disease frequently struck down health workers who were caring for the sick. The virus' natural reservoir was unknown. The outbreak in Zaire ended with 315 confirmed cases, of which 244 resulted in fatalities. At the WHO headquarters, a Task Force headed by Heymann was set up and different units, including EMC and the Division of Emergency and Humanitarian Action (EHA), worked with AFRO in mobilizing resources and personnel to the affected area. CDC and WHO officers arrived at the site of the epidemic within a few hours of being notified, establishing a disease detection system and palliative measures and training local health workers on how to use them. The international teams used astronaut-like protective suits, and the CDC scientists treated samples with the highest level of biosafety protection against infection. This collaborative effort meant that Ebola's spread

---

[31] World Health Organization, *The World Health Report 1995 – Bridging the Gaps* (Geneva: World Health Organization, 1995).
[32] World Health Organization, *The World Health Report 1996 – Fighting Disease, Fostering Development* (Geneva: World Health Organization, 1996).

to Kinshasa, a city of 2 million people, and to the rest of the world was successfully prevented.[33]

In another part of the globe, a new pandemic threatened in 1997: avian influenza. This new disease, which originated in the crowded live poultry markets of Hong Kong and Southeast Asia, again put the WHO to the test. Medical scientists identified it as a new version of the influenza virus that had shaken the world in 1918, producing at least 20 million deaths (smaller influenza pandemics swept parts of the world again in 1957 and 1968).[34] In 1997, Hong Kong medical reports confirmed that, after massive numbers of chicken deaths in farms, 18 people had become unwell and six had died of the Influenza H5N1 viral subtype. The real number of sick may have been much higher. By the end of the year, Chinese veterinary authorities decided to slaughter 1.6 million chickens belonging to vendors located in or near Hong Kong. Shortly thereafter the WHO confronted the Chinese authorities who had originally denied early cases of the disease and mounted control programs around the world. In Canada, a small number of cases – carried by air passengers from Hong Kong – produced considerable anxiety. The response to the disease was accompanied by an abrupt change at the WHO.

Shortly after avian influenza hit China and threatened to spread to the rest of the world, EMC was transformed into a more powerful Program on Communicable Diseases (CDS), with Heymann as its head. The CDS aimed to become the focal point for global information exchange on infectious diseases and reinforced the agency's role as the coordinator of information on pandemics. This did not represent a completely new departure for the WHO, but it was an approach that had become blurred during the 1980s. With the exception of influenza surveillance (a WHO network of virus laboratories had been in operation since 1948, and the organization annually agreed on the composition of the following season's influenza vaccine), little change had occurred in this area since 1951 when the WHO standardized former agreements and approved the International Sanitary Regulations that covered the "quarantinable diseases" (bubonic plague, cholera, yellow fever, smallpox, louse-born typhus, and louse-born fever). It promoted the sanitation of ports and airports, made obligatory immunizations against yellow fever, smallpox, and cholera, and emphasized disinfection of people and goods to protect against the spread of louse-borne and flea-borne diseases (such as typhus and plague); in addition, the controversial and ineffective bills of health for ships,

[33] World Health Organization, "Rapid Response to Emerging Disease," World Health Forum 17 (1996), 99.

[34] Reneé Shack, Alan P. Kendal, Lars R. Haaheiim, & John Wood, "The Next Influenza Pandemic: Lessons from Hong Kong, 1997," Emerging Infectious Diseases 5:2 (1999), 195–203.

aircraft, and isolation hospitals were abolished as well as the irksome practice of taking rectal swabbings from those arriving from cholera endemic areas. However, these regulations were not fully enforced because between the 1950s and the 1970s, disease surveillance was not considered a priority by industrial countries (indeed, few amendments were made in the mid-1950s to the 1951 Regulations), which felt safe from infectious diseases stemming from poor nations. In addition, few developing countries applied the Regulations which were perceived as an interference with world trade. Some change occurred in 1969 when the WHO regulations were revised and renamed the International Health Regulations (IHR). In 1973 and 1981, the IHR were themselves revised to include cholera in the first year and to exclude smallpox in the second in view of its eradication. Nonetheless, by the mid-1990s, these changes were clearly insufficient. But providing protection from disease while maintaining the free flow of people and goods would prove a difficult task.

In the 1990s, the IHR came under severe criticism because it only considered it obligatory to report on classic infectious diseases and failed to address other infections – especially the new and reemergent diseases – because governments repeatedly violated these regulations during epidemics, and because many WHO regional and country offices could only resort to persuasion and non-mandatory recommendations. Another complication relating to the IHR that tested the nature of the WHO as an intergovernmental agency was the fact that formally the health agency had to rely solely on information provided voluntarily by the governments of member states. Government authorities concealed epidemics and did not comply with the IHR because they were concerned about the potentially disastrous economic consequences. In 1992, for example, the government of Peru changed the system for cholera testing (from clinical stools to laboratory tests) to reduce the number of cases and minimize the economic impact of an epidemic that in 1991 alone attacked 1 percent of the population and meant the loss of more than USD 700 million in trade. Other Latin American governments followed this example. Legally, the WHO could not force Peruvian or Latin American officials to provide the real numbers of cholera cases.

In 1995, change began to occur. The World Health Assembly instructed the director-general to revise the IHR and create mechanisms for making governments adhere to technical decisions. The means deployed in order to achieve these goals were to increase links between local, national, and international epidemiologists. A series of meetings organized by the WHO resulted in the establishment of a network of old and new collaborating centers across the world that was later called the Global Outbreak Alert and Response Network, GOARN. The network included governmental and nongovernmental centers, ran reliable field tests, worked in real time using electronic, telephone, and video communications, and shared a common terminology on emerging infections that facilitated the comparison of epidemiological data.

The process of revising the WHO's IHR was accelerated by the sudden outbreak of Severe Acute Respiratory Syndrome (SARS) in China in early 2003, that eventually infected more than 5,300 people and killed 349 nationwide, extending to more than 30 countries. The Chinese government concealed SARS cases, suppressed information about the outbreak until after the disease had spread to Hong Kong, and was slow to allow WHO officials to visit affected areas (a position that was criticized by the WHO and other medical experts). SARS was a coronavirus that was similar to the viruses that cause the common cold but had never been seen before in humans, with a high case-fatality rate and alarming ease of transmission. Initially, no diagnosis, vaccine, or treatment existed. The disease was the result of a pattern of rapid urbanization without sanitation in the developing world, the massive and unsafe farming of poultry, and the collapse of health systems that followed neoliberal economic reforms. The disease spread in a matter of days from Guangdong province in mainland China to Hong Kong, Singapore, and Hanoi, generating panic everywhere. Many countries issued strict infection-control travel advisory guidelines (including for customs officials to wear masks at airports and interrogate passengers coming from Asia as well as the isolation of people with symptoms). The fear was real because China was becoming the world's fastest-growing economy and was directly involved in an enormous volume of global commerce with many nations around the world. Canada was also affected and there was a fear that the disease would spread rapidly outside Asia. For a WHO officer: "SARS challenged the assumption that wealthy nations, with their well-equipped hospitals and rigorous standards of hygiene, would be shielded from its spread."[35] Above all, the response to SARS reestablished the WHO as a coordinator for disease outbreaks.[36]

In March 2003, the WHO and the CDC issued the first global alerts, putting pressure on the Chinese government to provide full information on the outbreak and to allow WHO teams to inspect infected areas, helping to identify the best means of prevention, establishing contact-tracing methods, and implementing rational measures for isolating the sick. WHO officers were in Beijing in early April but only received permission to visit the affected province a week after their arrival. Prevention initiatives included isolating patients,

[35] David L. Heymann, Mary Kay Kindhauser, & Guénaël Rodier, "Coordinating the Global Reponse," in World Health Organization, Western Pacific Region, *SARS: How a Global Epidemic Was Stopped* (Geneva: World Health Organization, 2006), pp. 49–55.

[36] Jon Lidén, "The World Health Organization and Global Health Governance: Post-1990," *Public Health* 128 (2014), 141–147, p. 144.

quarantining their contacts, and a strict control of the animal market. All of these actions led to the containment of the pandemic in four months, by which time SARS had killed fewer than two thousand individuals. The health emergency had turned the WHO into a "supranational" authority, breaking with the tradition of cooperating only with governments upon request and instead establishing ties directly with local virologists, clinical doctors, epidemiologists, and public health workers; declaring international and national levels of emergency; and dictating the technical decisions that were to be implemented. This occurred not only in Asian countries: At the height of the epidemic, WHO authorities advised travelers to avoid Toronto, a decision that was questioned by Canadian authorities. The WHO exercised its power to issue travel alerts without the permission of any government, something that was unprecedented because it had traditionally relied on soft power or consensus.[37]

A by-product of the response to the epidemic was that it justified the need for a supranational role for the agency, challenging the tradition of noninterference with governments. A tragic event enhanced the WHO's authority and prestige: SARS killed the WHO officer Carlo Urbani, an Italian microbiologist who was working for the agency in Cambodia, Laos, and Vietnam. He was the first WHO officer to identify SARS, in an American businessman who had been admitted to a hospital in Hanoi, and had emphasized the need for strict infection control and sent throat swabs of the patient he was looking after to laboratories in Tokyo, Atlanta, and Hanoi. His work had helped to improve global surveillance, meaning that many new cases were identified before they infected hospital staff and other patients. In May 2003, Toronto was removed from the WHO's list of areas affected by SARS, and in June the agency lifted its advisory against travel to Beijing after it was clear that the epidemic was in control, and on August 16 the last two SARS patients were discharged from a Beijing Hospital. An article in the *New York Times* declared: "The WHO has earned accolades for its quick and decisive response in detecting and stopping the spread of SARS in many countries and for continuing the surveillance needed to ferret out the disease's possible return."[38]

From 2004, the WHO sought to respond to new epidemiological challenges by applying new, revised, and more powerful International Health Regulations (IHR) that emphasized alerts and security in health emergencies, the establishment of national focal medical centers, and synergies between

---

[37] David A. Scales, "The World Health Organization and the Dynamics of International Disease Control: Exit, Voice, and Trojan Loyalty," unpublished PhD dissertation, Yale University (2009).

[38] Lawrence K. Altman, "The Doctor's World: Rising from the Ranks to Lead the WHO," *The New York Times*, July 22, 2003.

these centers and political institutions.[39] A year later, the 61st World Health Assembly unanimously adopted the new IHR text that incorporated new and ambitious goals such as giving power to the WHO director-general to determine when an event was a Health Emergency of International Concern. Approved in 2005 and officially entered into force in June 2007, the IHR allowed the WHO's director-general and Secretariat capable of declaring a "Public Health Emergency of International Concern," or PHEIC, and denouncing countries that attempted to conceal epidemics. Another important decision of these Regulations – that would be tested in the following years – was that it called governments to develop and strengthen as soon as possible (but no later than 2012) the human, laboratory and institutional capacities to detect, assess, collect, and notify accurately the WHO "within 24 hours" of epidemic outbreaks and to maintain a national public health emergency response plan, including the creation of multidisciplinary teams. In 2007, the IHR was upheld in the WHO's annual report: *A Safer Future: Global Public Health Security in the Twenty-First Century.*

Other outbreaks of emergent diseases occurred in the wake of SARS. In 2005, the WHO predicted that an influenza virus known as H5N1, which had already ruined poultry farming in Vietnam and South Korea, could affect millions of people. In 2009, another epidemic produced by the H1N1 virus, known as "swine flu," hit India, China, Turkey, Thailand, Sri Lanka, South Korea, Mexico, and other countries. Both epidemic events created panic. In both cases, the disease was spread by human contact (usually through respiratory droplets) and caused by unhealthy farming practices (in the case of Mexico, the disease's origins were traced to Granjas Caroll in Veracruz, unhealthy pig farms that were part owned by the multinational Smithfield Foods). By late April 2009, there were more than 1,614 cases all over the country. The Mexican government recommended frequent hand-washing, isolated the sick, promoted "social distancing measures" (such as eschewing kisses when greeting), used soldiers to distribute protective masks, and, to its credit, was quick in providing information to its citizens (see Figure 9.2). The Mexican President Felipe Calderon also took the unprecedented steps of asking citizens to stay home for part of a week in May and for an almost complete shutdown of schools, restaurants, public events, and many economic activities to try to stop the disease from spreading. The fear of an explosion in the number of cases resonated with stories of the 1918 "Spanish" pandemic that killed millions of people. In April, the World Health Organization announced that H1N1 was a new virus that could sweep around the globe,

---

[39] Lawrence O. Gostin, "International Infectious Disease Law: Revision of the World Health Organization's International Health Regulations," *Journal of the American Medical Association* 291:21(2004), 2623–2627.

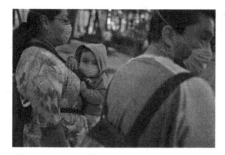

Figure 9.2 A family wearing face masks to prevent contagion by a new strain of the influenza virus known as H1N1 or "swine flu" walks in Mexico City on April 30, 2009. Earlier that month, several organizations, including the WHO and the Centers for Disease Control and Prevention, warned of a widespread influenza pandemic. The World Health Organization raised its flu alert to phase five out of six and recommended countries to stockpile the medication Tamiflu. The WHO was accused of overreacting. In August of 2009, the WHO officially declared the pandemic over but called for worldwide surveillance.
Credit: EITAN ABRAMOVICH/AFP/Getty Images.

and the UN called on governments to prepare for a global epidemic. The WHO also raised its flu pandemic alert level twice in a few days from after April 27 and raised it again in June to phase six, the highest level of alert. The United States, Canada, and some European countries advised against all non-essential travel to Mexico, and tourists hurried to leave the country.

The agency took the controversial decisions of asking pharmaceuticals who make the drugs that treat the disease to ramp up production and urging governments to purchase Tamiflu, a patented antiviral drug. Thankfully, although H1N1 was reported in several countries and unfortunately killed more than 18,000 people, the virus did not turn into an unpredictable monster as had been anticipated (in the second week of August of 2009, the WHO declared that the new virus had largely run its course). However, medical experts criticized the WHO for its haste in declaring an emergency and accused it of corruption in the sale of Tamiflu. More precisely, the organization came under criticism for not being able to manage the conflict of interest between the scientists, who worked with the WHO and advised on pandemic planning, and the financial ties of those very same scientists with pharmaceutical firms that profited from the sale of Tamiflu. The WHO was also criticized by some countries that believed it had exaggerated the need for drugs and vaccination materials, making them sign unnecessary advance-purchase contracts to stockpile these medical materials only to give billions to the manufacturers. According to director general Chan, there was no conflict of interest at the WHO, as she had relied only on the advice of reputed influenza experts, virologists, and public health officials.[40]

As a response to the epidemic outbreaks previously described, the approval of the IHR per se was not enough. The WHO needed to forge its role as a leader in the response to global health threats. This meant helping to build the necessary manpower, infrastructure, and equipment in developing countries to detect epidemic outbreaks, reinforcing the supranational role of the health agency, and establishing clear ethical criteria in the relationship between epidemiologists and pharmaceutical companies. Another challenge related to the incipient supranational role taken by the agency appeared in another health campaign.

Toward a Framework on Tobacco

The WHO was responsible for establishing the first World No Tobacco Day on April 7, 1988 (a date changed to May 31 in subsequent years), aimed at reducing the 2 million plus premature deaths per year linked to tobacco worldwide. This took place after several decades of scientific studies that demonstrated an association between smoking and lung cancer, cardiovascular diseases, and other adverse health effects such as chronic bronchitis and emphysema. The landmark moments during this period included the 1962 British report of the Royal College of Physicians, the 1964 US Surgeon General's Report, the organization of pressure groups of health activists, such as the British Action on Smoking and Health (ASH), set up in 1971 after the second report on smoking by the Royal College of Physicians, and the World Conferences on Tobacco or Health of the late 1960s and early 1970s.[41] In 1984, the International Union against Tuberculosis became the International Union against TB and Lung Disease and created a special committee on smoking. The following year, as part of the WHO strategy of Health for All, the 32 member states comprising the WHO European Region launched a pilot program against tobacco. The region organized a first regional meeting in Madrid in November 1988 and approved a "charter" that asserted that "fresh air free from tobacco smoke" was an essential component of the right to a

---

[40] See Deborah Cohen & Philip Carter, "WHO and the Pandemic Flu "Conspiracies," *British Medical Journal* 340 (2010), 1274–1279, and Margaret Chan, "WHO Director-General's Letter to British Medical Journal Editors, 8 June 2010," www.who.int/mediacentre/news/statements/2010/letter_bmj_20100608/en/, last accessed February 22, 2018.

[41] See Allan M. Brandt, *The Cigarette Century: The Rise, Fall and Deadly Persistence of the Product that Defined America* (New York: Basic Books, 2006), and Virginia Berridge, *Marketing Health: Smoking and the Discourse of Public Health in Britain, 1945–2000* (Oxford: Oxford University Press, 2007).

healthy and unpolluted environment and called for the formation of alliances in society to promote good health and the fight against tobacco.[42]

In 1986, the World Health Assembly passed a resolution against tobacco consumption on account of its link with fatal and disabling diseases and condemned passive and involuntary secondhand smoking, which was considered to be particularly harmful to the health of children throughout the world, most of whom were exposed involuntarily at home. An important decision was taken the following year when smoking was banned on all WHO premises (a decision that came with Mahler smashing an astray!). The problem was no longer only a concern of industrialized nations, but from the early 1980s had also become particularly acute in the developing world. As soon as restrictions were placed on companies in developed countries, the focus was shifted to emerging markets in developing countries. Initially, the companies used a vast array of defenses such as arguing that tobacco control increased the illicit trade of tobacco in developing countries, which in turn encouraged the trafficking of illegal drugs, and that tobacco control was not a health priority in developing countries.

In 1990, with the support of extrabudgetary funds, the WHO created the Program on Tobacco or Health, directed by the American physiologist Roberto Masironi. (These efforts paralleled US campaigns, as illustrated by Figures 9.3 and 9.4.) A multidisciplinary Technical Advisory Group formed by experts from around the world assisted him and prepared relevant publications that provided a panorama on the extensive use of tobacco worldwide. In the late 1990s, Masironi's unit formed the basis of a more ambitious WHO program called the Tobacco Free Initiative that had a larger but still insufficient budget, representing less than one percent of the agency's overall budget. During the 1980s and most of the 1990s, tobacco companies infiltrated the WHO to discredit the agency's work against tobacco, to keep anti-smoking resolutions embroiled in red tape, and to bribe some officials and scientists. The US Lawyer Paul Dietrich wrote articles in US newspapers questioning why tobacco was a priority for the WHO, arguing that too little was being done to control infectious diseases in backward countries. In 1990, without revealing that he had been paid by the tobacco industry, Dietrich became an advisor to PAHO and began to promote the idea that the regional agency should focus its efforts on immunization and cholera. His attempts at misleading PAHO formed part of a wider effort: Tobacco companies sought to cast doubts about the risks of secondhand smoke, supported governmental

---

[42] Cited in World Health Organization, Regional Office for Europe, "The Charter against Tobacco, 1988," www.euro.who.int/data/assets/pdf_file/0003/115338/E93946.pdf, last accessed January 12, 2018.

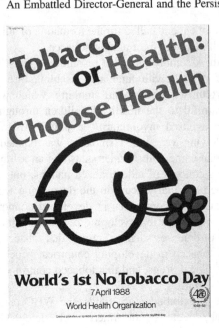

Figure 9.3 A 1988 poster of the World Health Organization used by the Norwegian Ministry of Health to raise awareness about the dangers of smoking cigarettes.
Source: Universal History Archive/UIG via Getty Images.

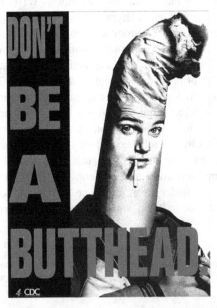

Figure 9.4 "Don't Be A Butthead," a 1998 American poster to raise awareness against smoking cigarettes.
Source: Universal History Archive/UIG via Getty Images.

charities, tried to water down any regulations, and used an insidious strategy in relation to the WHO as they aimed to discredit its policies.

In January 1991, support for the fight against tobacco grew as a result of a consultation convened by the WHO in Geneva that gathered experts from developed and developing countries to address the relationship between tobacco and trade liberalization in poor nations. The meeting denounced the neoliberal economic policies that put pressure on countries to open their markets to foreign products, including products from tobacco companies. At the same time, the World Bank and a number of governments from industrialized nations donated to the WHO's anti-tobacco campaign, thereby supporting a consensus on the harmful effects of tobacco. These donations meant an important change since governments, corporations, and multilateral agencies had traditionally remained silent on the relationship between health and tobacco for fear of confronting the powerful tobacco industry.

During the 1990s, the WHO was supported in its fight against tobacco by outstanding health leaders such as Ruth Roemer, professor at the University of California, Los Angeles. Roemer was the author of a book commissioned by the WHO that was first published in 1982 and reviewed tobacco legislation around the world.[43] In 1993, Roemer began a collaboration with the lawyer Allyn L. Taylor, a University of Maryland professor who had studied the possibility of creating a legal framework for the WHO. Roemer and Taylor worked on the possibility of a specific international regulatory mechanism for tobacco control. Also in 1993, Roemer attended the first All Africa Conference on Tobacco or Health, held in Harare, Zimbabwe, and discussed the issue with the co-chair of the meeting, South African public health expert Derek Yach, who later became a force for the anti-tobacco work at the WHO. In the same year, she visited the WHO and discussed the novel idea of a UN-style convention on tobacco that utilized international law to advance public health.[44] As a result, in 1995, the World Health Assembly approved a resolution requesting the director-general to examine the feasibility of developing a legal instrument on tobacco control, despite the resistance of some officers and country representatives. Shortly thereafter, the WHO invited Roemer and Taylor to work on a legal strategy to curb tobacco consumption. In 1996, they published a WHO technical document entitled the *International Strategy for Tobacco Control* that became the basis for a legally binding protocol or

---

[43] Ruth Roemer, *Legislative Action to Combat the World Tobacco Epidemic* (Geneva: World Health Organization, 1993).

[44] L. A. Reynolds & E. M. Tansey (eds.), *WHO Framework Convention On Tobacco Control: The Transcript of a Witness Seminar Organized by the Wellcome Trust Centre for the History of Medicine at UCL, in Collaboration with the Department of Knowledge Management and Sharing, WHO, Held in Geneva, on 26 February 2010* (London: The Wellcome Trust, 2012), p. 24.

Framework Convention on Tobacco Control.[45] Members of the agency that disliked Roemer and Taylor's proposal presented a code of conduct on tobacco as an alternative (similar to the WHO International Code of Marketing of Breast-milk Substitutes), a nonbinding legal international instrument. Other opponents of the idea of a WHO Framework suggested transferring any decision on tobacco to the UN. The supporters of the idea of a protocol argued that a nonbinding code of conduct would be ineffective and that the WHO, not the UN, was the right agency for the negotiation of this global health treaty. At its January 1996 meeting, the WHO Executive Board, with the support of Nakajima but with opposition from the WHO Secretariat, adopted the resolution "An International Framework Convention for Tobacco Control" that reflected the ideas of Roemer and Taylor. In May 1996, the World Health Assembly approved a resolution for the development of the Framework. The main objectives of the treaty were: more taxes and higher prices on tobacco products to reduce consumption, bans on tobacco advertising, mandatory dramatic warning messages on tobacco products, educational programs to raise public awareness, and support for economically viable alternatives for tobacco growers. The Framework also urged governments to persecute and punish sales to minors and increase the number of public spaces where smoking was forbidden. It was hoped that the Framework would be instrumental in neutralizing the persistent counter-tactics used by tobacco companies that included discrediting science, creating controversies between financial and health ministries (by exaggerating the economic contribution of tobacco in terms of taxes), and intimidating governments with litigation.

A number of meetings supporting a legal international instrument for tobacco control were held toward the end of the twentieth century, including: the ninth World Conference on Tobacco or Health, held in Paris in October 1994; the 1996 meeting of the International Civil Aviation Organization that resulted in the decision to ban smoking on flights; the WHO's International Conference on Tobacco and Health that took place in November 1999, in Kobe, Japan; and the WHO's International Conference on Global Tobacco Control Law, held in New Delhi in January 2000. These meetings were instrumental in changing policies in the United States and other industrialized countries, which began to ban the use of tobacco in different spaces. Some also prohibited elected officials from lobbying on the industry's behalf, something that had occurred prior to the 1990s.

During the late 1990s, the implementation of the 1996 WHA resolution began in earnest, and the negotiation of the WHO's FCTC gained political momentum and turned into a worldwide public health movement. In 1999, the

---

[45] Judith Mackay, "The Making of a Convention on Tobacco Control," *Bulletin of the World Health Organization* 81:8 (2003), 551–551.

World Health Assembly approved a Tobacco Free Initiative, TFI, for which a new senior management position was created. The South African epidemiologist Derek Yach was recruited as head of the TFI, having previously worked as the WHO's executive director for noncommunicable diseases and mental health. Before joining the WHO, Yach directed the South African Center for Epidemiological Research, which focused on health inequalities and chronic diseases. During the second half of the 1990s, the WHO worked with world athletes and artists to eliminate tobacco advertising from sporting and artistic events across the world. This move went against tradition because tobacco companies had pumped millions of dollars into sponsoring sporting, film, and musical events in order to glamorize their products.

In 1999, 30 organizations from 100 countries set up a Framework Convention Alliance that sought support from outside the realm of government. At that time, millions of people smoked worldwide, and smoking caused thousands of deaths annually. The WHO's annual report for 2002 underlined tobacco consumption as one of the 10 leading risk factors affecting the global population.[46] In March 2001, representatives from African governments held a high-level meeting in Johannesburg to affirm their full support for the Framework Convention. Similar meetings occurred in other regions of the world and served to support the WHO's negotiation process.

The Framework opened for signature in Geneva in June 2003 after its approval at the 56th World Health Assembly and was later deposited at the UN Headquarters in New York. By June 2004 it had already been signed by 168 of the 192 WHO member states. After some difficult negotiations when the governments of some countries – including Germany, China, and the United States – expressed reservations or opposed the treaty, the Convention entered into effect in February 2005, 90 days after the 40th country had approved it, and it remained open to further adherence at the UN. Even during the final stages of this process, the US government pushed for a fundamental change, namely the right of a government to opt out of any provisions of the treaty with which they disagreed. Governments in favor of the convention complained, and under pressure President Bush signed the Framework. At a time when the agency seemed to be struggling to find its way, the Framework demonstrated that a group of able officers in alliance with public health experts and health activists could reach a milestone in the history of international health. The Framework was an unprecedented, mandatory, global legal instrument and was a decisive factor in supporting the anticipated global transition from communicable to noncommunicable diseases. The new legal instrument was dynamic and flexible because it allowed for the possible creation of

[46] World Health Organization, *The World Health Report 2002 – Reducing Risks, Promoting Healthy Life* (Geneva: World Health Organization, 2002).

tougher compulsory protocols. Its full implementation entailed the daunting challenge of reducing the billions of people in developing countries that use tobacco and the death of millions of people around the world because of tobacco. Despite becoming signatories to the Framework, many countries, such as China where the production of tobacco is a state monopoly and millions of farmers depend on tobacco cultivation, have adopted its recommendations at a very slow pace.

The section that follows will discuss the contextual and institutional developments that surrounded a contradictory WHO during the final years of the Cold War and the early post–Cold War period.

A Troubled Command

The World Bank's reforms and the neoliberal interpretation of globalization meant that health agencies were forced to undergo a process of reform and become accountable for their activities. The WHO was no exception and formally accepted the idea, appointing a committee to identify financial problems, establishing priority targets and undergoing reform internally.[47] These changes took place in 1992 as the WHO was in the process of electing a new director-general. Many medical experts and governments from industrial nations strongly believed that reform would only occur under a new director-general since Nakajima's leadership had been found wanting.

Nakajima and the government of Japan thought quite differently (in 1992, using the resources of the organization, the incumbent visited 35 countries in 11 months to seek votes). He launched a bitter – and for some, corrupt – campaign to be reelected that left a sour legacy and criticism of the election process. Candidates subsequently agreed to discuss their ideas publicly, responding to questions posed by the Executive Board that were published in *The Lancet*. Also, after having previously no limit on the number of five-year terms that the director-general could serve, because of Nakajima an important change was made: a limit of two terms (i.e., renewable once) for this post was introduced. He insisted on running for reelection despite a series of editorials in the *British Medical Journal* in which donors were reported to be considering moving their extrabudgetary funds to other agencies if Nakajima were reelected.[48] In a last-ditch effort, France, the United States, Canada,

---

[47] United States Department of State, *United States Participation in the United Nations, Report by the President to the Congress for the Year 1993* (Washington, DC: US Government Printing Office, 1994), 70.

[48] Fiona Godlee, "WHO at the Crossroads," *British Medical Journal* 306 (1993), 1143–1144, and Lawrence K. Altman, "Embattled Japanese Doctor Retains WHO Post," *The New York Times*, May 6, 1993. Other articles by Godlee were "WHO's Election Throws Agency into Bitter Turmoil, British Medical Journal 306 (1992), 161; "The Regions – Too Much Power, Too Little

the European Community, and Arab countries attempted to block Nakajima's reelection and supported the candidacy of a 55-year-old Algerian neurologist, Mohammed Abdelmoumene – former dean of the Algiers Faculty of Medicine – who had been Nakajima's deputy director-general since his appointment in 1988. He was ousted from his post by Nakajima as soon as he made his candidacy known. Nakajima won the election against his challenger by a vote of 18 to 13 at a 1992 meeting of the Executive Board and was appointed director-general by the World Health Assembly the following year.

After Nakajima's reelection, the relationship between WHO headquarters, on the one hand, and the United States and other Western European powers, on the other, deteriorated. Nakajima believed there was nothing wrong with the election process. He only noted the paradox of "Western donors" who supported a candidate from a developing country "which is not at all successful with its health service, while I come from a developed country and was supported by developing countries."[49] These comments suggest the fear of poor nations of having to agree to an imposed candidate who was portrayed as disloyal to his former chief and their use of an opportunity to express their anti-Western sentiments.

It is interesting to note that the incumbent Nakajima was reappointed at a time when the United States had elected President Bill Clinton, who did not oppose the UN but at the same time did not show interest in developing a specific policy toward the multilateral body. The Japanese government believed that Nakajima's faults could be overcome, the polarization legacy left by his election diminished, and considered his reappointment a matter of national pride, applying considerable pressure to secure it. The editorial of one medical journal argued that what was at stake was not simply a choice of leader for the WHO but a matter of "face to be saved for the Japanese … Government," which had initially been lukewarm in view of the harsh criticism directed at Nakajima, but then "flung itself wholeheartedly behind him as he campaigned to save his job."[50]

After Nakajima's reelection, WHO headquarters discussed – but failed to fully implement – the reform envisioned by the World Bank. The WHO formed a working group on Global Policy that included regional directors and assistant directors-general. Its aims were to transform the WHO's top-down management system and rigid set of rules – that were deemed to suffocate creativity – and, instead, to enhance collective management, propose

Effect," *British Medical Journal* 309 (1994), 1566–1570; and "WHO in Crisis," *British Medical Journal* 309 (1994), 1424–1428.

[49] The response of Nakajima appeared in Fiona Godlee, "The World Health Organization: Interview with the Director-General," *British Medical Journal* 310 (1995), 583–588, p. 586.

[50] J. Cohen, "Editorial: WHO: Power and Inglory," *The Lancet* 341:8840 (January 30, 1993), 762–763.

reforms in the organization's administrative structure and program priorities, and update the WHO's policies and priorities. Many critics of the WHO believed that the dynamics of regional offices impeded any centralized control of the organization. The regional directors of these offices, elected by their constituent countries rather than appointed from Geneva, could hire and fire staff within their regions and appoint country representatives who supervised the implementation of programs. It was envisioned that in the working group the functions and responsibilities of the assistant director-general would be expanded and that of regional directors limited. After one year of discussions, the working group submitted 47 specific recommendations, including limits on the number of tasks the WHO would attempt to achieve, a closer relationship between the regional offices and headquarters, a single unified budget, checks on the recruitment of new staff, and the mobilization of new financial resources.

Under Nakajima, the Secretariat took these recommendations merely as suggestions and sent them to the six regional committees for further study. This decision made the possibility of reform less likely since the regional offices were thought to want to guard their independence and not to care much about the global coherence of the agency. Consequently, the attempt failed. Nakajima's supporters argued that the agency had to manage as best it could just to survive, faced with the zero-growth policy of its regular budget, the arrears in assessed contributions, and the increasing cost of operations. In 1993, the Japanese addressed the World Health Assembly, complaining that the WHO was completing its "fifth biennium under a policy of zero growth in terms of its regular budget." And it had to do it again for the 1994–1995 period.[51]

In 1996, Nakajima faced the WHO Executive Board with an argument that was difficult to refute: For more than 10 years, the WHO had had to work with a zero-growth budget, insufficient coverage for cost increases, and uncertainty about receipts of assessed contributions, all of which had produced a considerable reduction in all programs. In a contradictory move, the following year Nakajima told the World Health Assembly that the ongoing reform process was beginning to be implemented and was creating a more streamlined, flexible, accountable, effective, and more focused organization with better communication with the regions. In 1996 and 1997, the Board held a series of meetings that emphasized that work should be concentrated on coordination, development of health policies, setting of norms, promoting health globally, and providing advice and technical cooperation. These recommendations were echoed by other scholars and practitioners in a 1997 meeting

---

[51] World Health Organization, "WHO Director-General Calls for a New Partnership on Health," May 4, 1993, Press Release WHA/4, WHO Press Releases 1992–1999.

entitled "Enhancing the Performance of International Health Institutions," organized by the Rockefeller Foundation in Pocantico, New York, that argued that the WHO should be the "conscience" of global health and that it had wrongly overemphasized technical assistance over its normative functions.[52] The assumption was that other institutions were already addressing operational functions, including funding health programs and technical cooperation, and that the WHO should stick to a normative role.

Despite the WHO's best efforts, criticisms of Nakajima's confusing leadership continued throughout 1995, 1996, and 1997. Critics of the agency argued that it needed to undergo real, palpable reform to overcome its weak operational capacity and to acknowledge that it was no longer *the* single global health organization. As has been described before, the World Bank, which had expanded its influence by taking on an independent role in a number of health campaigns and cooperating more readily with nongovernmental organizations, was emerging as a competitor to the WHO's leadership in international health.

In 1995, the World Health Assembly rejected the director-general's budget proposal (and approved a "working budget of USD 824.7 million for 1996–1997"). In the same meeting, African representatives from Namibia and Zambia introduced (and later withdrew) a resolution calling on Nakajima to step down because of "racist" comments on the "low capabilities" of African people as the reason for the scarcity of Africans in executive positions at WHO headquarters (he later apologized).[53] At the same time, Sir John Bourn, the British WHO external auditor, resigned on the grounds that he did not have access to essential information to assess the allegations that the director-general's reelection for a second term was connected with contracts to ensure him a majority vote.[54] Sweden, one of the biggest contributors to the WHO, drastically reduced its allocations, and Denmark – another chief donor – cut its subsidy to the agency entirely. By the end of Nakajima's term, opposition to his regime was out in the open. Rumors of misused funds during his reelection, irregular donations from the Japanese millionaire Ryoichi Sasakawa, and low morale among staff because of an absence of meritocratic criteria for promotion became overwhelming. Nakajima's discourses on the reorganization and revitalization of the agency were not taken seriously. An indication of the state of mind of the officers is that in 1993 the Staff Association conducted a survey of the 1,507 headquarters staffers, of whom only 513 responded. It revealed that 55 percent of respondents rated the

---

[52] Retreat, Pocantico, Enhancing the Performance of International Health Institutions, February 1–3, 1996.

[53] United States, Department of State, *United States Participation in the United Nations, A Report to the President for the Year 1995* (Washington, DC: US Government Printing Office, 1995), p. 86.

[54] Lee, *Historical Dictionary*, p. 102.

organization's effectiveness as "worse" than before, and that for 73 percent the staff's morale was "worse."[55] A Japanese doctor critical of Nakajima warned that the WHO was in danger of becoming "the next UNESCO" (In 1984 and 1995, the governments of the United States and the UK withdrew from UNESCO for its allegedly anti-Western political decisions).[56]

By the end of 1997, it was clear that Nakajima was going to leave his post the following year and had lost the favor of Japan (who ceded to the pressure from other industrial countries). He decided to bid farewell with the 1998 annual report, *Life in the 21st Century: A Vision for All*. The report is a panoramic and valuable source of what had been achieved by the WHO since its inception in 1948. The publication celebrated Nakajima's "contributions": the promotion of generic drugs, the campaign to eradicate polio, assistance to civilians in troubled countries such as Yugoslavia, Somalia, and Rwanda, and the fact that the WHO was becoming a truly global agency (its members increased from 166 in 1988 to 191 in 1998, and a democratic South Africa was integrated into the agency in 1994 after an absence of 30 years).

Final Remarks

Although Nakajima is generally regarded outside the WHO as the main reason for the agency's decline during the late 1980s and 1990s, it is very likely that other factors, including the hegemony of neoliberalism, the prominent role of the World Bank, and the struggles faced by multilateral agencies at the end of the Cold War were going to tarnish the WHO anyway. During the 1980s and early 1990s, bilateral support took an upturn. Among the most significant bilateral agencies were: the Canadian International Development Agency (CIDA), the Danish International Development Agency (DANIDA), the Finnish International Development Agency (FINNIDA), the German bilateral agency, the French Ministère de la Coopération et du Développement, the Japan International Cooperation Agency (JICA), the Swedish International Development Authority (SIDA), the Swedish Agency for Research Cooperation with Developing Countries (SAREC), the British Overseas Development Administration (ODA), and USAID. There was a tension between these agencies, on the one hand, and the world health assemblies, on the other, which were dominated by developing countries and frequently outvoted the proposals of industrialized nations. At the same

---

[55] Alen McGregor, "WHO: New Look Fails to Impress," *The Lancet* 341:8854 (May 08, 1993), 1205.

[56] Alan McGregor, "Round the World: WHO: Continuing Unease," *The Lancet* 341:8852 (24 April 1993), 1082.

time, the leaders of the WHO took some time to accept the fact that they now had to share leadership in international health.

Other political developments outside the control of any health authority complicated the WHO's finances, functions, and legitimacy, such as genocidal wars in Central Europe and Africa and the Gulf War. Nakajima's legitimacy was compromised because Japan did not become a new superpower in the post–Cold War years, it failed to establish a coherent policy toward multilateral agencies, its significant donations to the WHO were not used for internal reform of the agency, and it did not provide unwavering support to Nakajima. Thus, Nakajima's limitations as a leader may have appeared greater than they probably were because they provided a convenient explanation for the troubles of an agency that for political reasons several major actors wanted to present as backward. And last but not least, exaggerating Nakajima's faults served the purposes of those governments that did not wish to see Japan lead international politics, nor to see a multilateral agency articulating a socio-medical perspective.

Nonetheless, despite the WHO's troubles described in this chapter, some programs adapted to the imperatives of globalization and developed entirely new activities almost on their own, as demonstrated by the cases of the modernization of the international health regulations and the tobacco program. In these cases, WHO staff learned to collaborate with other organizations based on the assumption that the WHO could no longer be the sole leader of international health affairs and worked patiently for restoring the credibility of the agency in the post–Cold War period. Toward the end of the twentieth century, several WHO officers began a process of self-examination and reassertion in the rapidly changing context marked by the end of the Cold War and the emergence of a new global order.

The following chapter will describe these processes.

10 The Competitive World of Global Health

At the turn of the twenty-first century and in the early years of the new millennium, directors-general Gro Harlem Brundtland, Jong-wook Lee, and Margaret Chan reestablished the WHO's prestige but made the agency more dependent on extrabudgetary funds. These changes occurred at a time when Western European governments and the US presidency, under Bill Clinton, George W. Bush, and Barack Obama, developed a friendlier relationship with the UN, new bilateral programs involved collaboration with the WHO, and new donors and organizations entered the global health arena.

The Radical Reforms of a Director-General

In July 1998, Gro Harlem Brundtland (see Figure 10.1) began her tenure as the fifth WHO director-general. Several prominent members of the WHO and the UN had stood for election in the World Health Assembly in May of that year, including George Alleyne from Barbados, director of PAHO; Nafis Sadik, executive director of the United Nations Population Fund (UNFPA); Ebrahim Samba, regional director of AFRO; and Uton M. Rafei, regional director of SEARO, but the members of the Executive Board sought a radical change. Brundtland was the first outsider and the first woman ever elected to head the agency. She was a physician, with a medical degree from Oslo University and a master's degree in public health from Harvard, and had a distinguished political career. Brundtland was minister of the environment, and at the age of 41 became prime mister of Norway; she was the youngest prime minister ever elected and the first woman; her cabinet, consisting of eight women and nine men, represented the highest level of gender equality in political history. Brundtland served as prime minister three times (1981–1984; 1986–1989; and 1989–1992). As head of the UN's World Commission on the Environment and Development, she popularized the concept of "sustainable development" and was responsible for the landmark

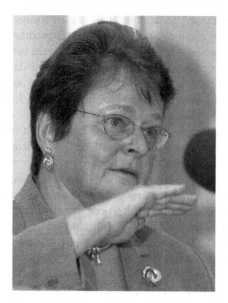

Figure 10.1 Norwegian Gro Harlem Brundtland, director-general of the
World Health Organization between 1998 and 2003. Formerly, she was prime
minister of Norway and chaired the UN World Commission on Environment
and Development. She established the WHO's Commission on
Macroeconomics and Health, made quitting smoking a condition of
employment at the agency, and promoted public health partnerships to
control major diseases. In the photograph she addresses correspondents at the
UN headquarters in New York City in the late 1990s at a briefing to launch
the "Roll Back Malaria" campaign, a campaign supported by leaders of
malaria-endemic countries, bilateral and multilateral organizations,
philanthropic foundations and private companies, nongovernmental
organizations, and academic institutions.
Photo by Alain Nogues/Sygma/Sygma via Getty Images.

report, *Our Common Future*; her recommendations provided momentum for
the United Nations Earth Summit in Rio de Janeiro in 1992.[1]

Many saw Brundtland's election to head the WHO – at one of the lowest
points in the history of the health agency – as an opportunity for real reform
within the beleaguered organization, which had been roundly criticized as
being politicized, underfunded, and overcommitted. For many, she represented
an opportunity to raise the WHO's profile in the global arena, to establish some

---

[1] Gro Harlem Brundtland, *Madam Prime Minister: A Life in Power and Politics* (New York:
Farrar, Straus and Giroux, 2002).

priorities in international health, and to demonstrate a model for institutional reform that other UN agencies could follow. Furthermore, Brundtland raised hopes that fresh and sizeable financial resources could be obtained because her arrival came at a time when neoliberal policies were in the ascendancy. She could count on the support of the governments of the United Kingdom (Tony Blair), the United States (Bill Clinton), France (Jacques Chirac), Japan, and Canada, which all had cordial relationships with multilaterals, subscribed to the idea of world's poverty reduction, understood the fight against infectious diseases in terms of security, and were willing to work on the social and health disparities created by economic globalization. In her favor was also the line of thought and action pursued by UN Secretary-General Boutros-Ghali and his 1995 report *An Agenda for Development* that supported the ideas of economic growth as the engine for development and the need for new partnerships. Richard Feacham, the former director of health, nutrition and population at the World Bank, declared: "WHO just elected the best possible leader that it could elect. Dr. Gro Harlem Brundtland is fantastic; and her leadership heralds an era when WHO can be a truly powerful and influential agency."[2] An American representative at the WHO declared that Brundtland was "superbly qualified to lead the WHO into the next century."[3]

As soon as she was elected, Brundtland addressed all WHO staff in Geneva and in the regional offices by means of a teleconference and announced her firm intention to "make a difference ... change the course of things," restore the credibility of the agency, and reassert the WHO's standing in the world. She also added that it was paramount to have an impact "on the ground" but that the WHO was not going to become a "field agency."[4] Brundtland made it clear that she expected to make the agency more effective, efficient, transparent, and accountable, with clearly defined deadlines and distribution of responsibilities. Some inspiration may have come from the UN, where Kofi Annan, shortly after he was appointed secretary-general in 1997, launched a much-demanded, comprehensive reform of the UN. In any case, Brundtland stated that the WHO should not be primarily engaged in operating programs but should become recognized as a normative agency – setting standards, developing guidelines, and providing information to be used by governments and agencies. She set herself two complex tasks: internal management reform and direct engagement with donors, such as the Gates Foundation, and

---

[2] Kamran Abbassi, "Education and Debate. The World Bank and World Health: Interview with Richard Feachem," *British Medical Journal* 318 (1999), 1206.

[3] Elizabeth Olson, "Ex-Prime Minister of Norway Wins Top Job at WHO," *The New York Times*, January 28, 1998, p. 12.

[4] World Health Organization, "Dr. Gro Harlem Brundtland Takes Up Office and Confirms Her Intention to 'Make a Difference,'" July 21, 1998, Press Release WHO/54, WHO Press Releases 1997–1998.

"globalization" agencies, particularly the World Bank. From her point of view, these two tasks were interrelated.

Brundtland changed one of the original premises of an organization designed as an intergovernmental agency. Although it was never officially stated, the members of the Executive Board and the traditional structure of assistant directors-general reflected a balance between the most powerful countries. Brundtland launched a vigorous in-house reform, starting with a cabinet system with executive directors selected because of their technical competence rather than their political connections. She met with her cabinet once a week. These directors were in charge of nine "clusters" that replaced the traditional technical programs (most of them responsible for disease control). Creation of clusters involved the reduction, merging, and transformation of 50 programs into 36 departments. Dozens of top officers were rotated to new assignments. In a dramatic change for the WHO, five of the new executive directors were women and three were from developing countries; Africans were appointed to high positions in the agency. It set as goals finding more qualified women from under-represented countries to appoint in directive positions at the WHO and to reach and surpass the UN target of 34 percent of women in professional and higher categories (in December of 2002 the agency had 33 percent of women in these categories, an improvement from the 22 percent of 1992). "Equitable geographical representation" in the recruitment of staff in headquarters, meaning more experts from developing areas of the world, was also eagerly pursued. To combat corruption, Brundtland implemented a code of conduct whereby high-level WHO officials, and their spouses and dependent children, disclosed financial interests in the private sector, including any possible conflicts of interest, ties with tobacco companies, patents, or participation in company directorships.

Most of Brundtland's high-level appointments – like herself – had little professional history within the WHO. She selected outsiders for leadership positions rather than choosing from within the ranks of the agency, allowing more latitude in making radical reforms. Among them was the Mexican public health scholar, Julio Frenk, in charge of the new cluster on "Evidence and Information for Policy." David Heymann, one of the few high-ranking officers who had worked under Nakajima, oversaw "Communicable Diseases." One of his tasks was to more fully integrate the semi-autonomous Special Program in Research and Training in Tropical Diseases, TDR, into the WHO and thus incorporate active research on therapies for the neglected diseases suffered by the world's poor. The Tunisian Souad Lyagoubi-Ouachi was named as the new head of "External Affairs and Governing Bodies," with responsibilities for managing the WHO's relationships with external partners. The environmentally oriented health scholar and administrator Poonam Khetrapal Singh, from India, was director for "Sustainable Development and Healthy Environments."

Singh had previously been an officer in the World Bank's Population, Health, and Nutrition program, and it was to be part of her new job to mainstream health into poverty reduction programs. Michael Scholtz, a German administrator from the private sector who had been at the pharmaceutical firm Smith-Kline Beecham, was to manage "Health Technology and Pharmaceuticals" and was instructed to work collaboratively with governments, consumers, and pharmaceuticals to provide access to high quality and affordable drugs for developing countries. The decision to work with pharmaceutical companies was contrary to the WHO's usual practice. Years of rancorous exchanges with brief moments of collaboration between officers and representatives of the pharmaceutical industry over the WHO's Action Programme on Essential Drugs and the list of drugs published in 1977 had by the mid-1990s ended all friendly communication, and many officers considered the pharmaceutical industry an enemy bound to sabotage the WHO's attempts to implement rational drug policies. Under Brundtland, however, the new leaders of the WHO believed it was possible to harness private pharmaceutical companies for the common good, convincing them to invest more in research and development for new drugs and vaccines for developing countries; maintain the independence of the agency; fulfill its normative and standard-setting functions; and work productively with the private sector.

Brundtland also shook up the structure of the agency by reducing administrative expenses by 15 percent, requiring program funds to be used in the field rather than in Geneva, and expecting regional offices to work closely with headquarters to produce – for the first time – a unified budget. She rotated the functions of 750 employees at headquarters. In addition, she tried to address one of the most controversial problems in the architecture of the agency: the relative autonomy of the regional offices. In several speeches, she referred to "WHO as One," meaning that it was not seven organizations (headquarters and the six regional offices) but a single, "harmonized" integrated unit. One of the agency's problems was that the Regional Offices did their own planning and decided on how to spend most of their resources independently from headquarters. Since 2002, Brundtland presented budgets for the whole agency in an effort to coordinate spending at both headquarters and regions. She frowned on the administrative, financial, and political autonomy of regional directors, whose allegiances were to the ministers of health who had elected them rather than to WHO headquarters. All these changes created disruption and distress. An American journal editor who visited Geneva after Brundtland's appointment reported that "speculation and debate about internal changes dominated conversation around the offices and in the WHO staff cafeteria."[5] Other

---

[5] Anthony Robbins, "Brundtland's World Health, a Test Case for United Nations Reform," *Public Health Reports* 114 (1999), 36.

observers supported these changes. An editorial in *Science* – cosigned by the economist Jeffrey Sachs and Barry R. Bloom, dean of the Harvard School of Public Health, among others – stated approvingly that Brundtland was "reinventing" the WHO, and called on the US government to pay its USD 35 million pending contribution to the agency as an investment in health.[6] The US and European governments and donors backed Brundtland's ambitious management reform and her plans to change the external policies and programs of the WHO. They hoped that the WHO's reorganization would set an example for other UN agencies and create a more constructive and business-friendly multilateral health agency. The Norwegian government awarded the WHO USD 7.5 million and the Rockefeller Foundation gave USD 2.5 million to a Global Health Leadership fund, to be used for internal changes and to recruit expert personnel from outside the WHO.[7]

Brundtland's reforms were linked to her goal of enhancing the WHO's global reach. In October 1998, she traveled to France to hold discussions with President Jacques Chirac and his prime minister, Lionel Jospin, and to Washington, DC, to meet with First Lady Hillary R. Clinton and James Wolfensohn, the president of the World Bank, to talk about the new structure and goals of the agency, especially in relation to TB and malaria.[8] In the United States, she also met with the CEO of Coca Cola in an effort to strengthen ties between the private sector and global health. As Mr. Douglas Ivester, an advisor to USAID who supported the director-general, put it: "In the good old days of WHO – by which I mean the 60s – WHO was the only actor on the world stage in terms of world health," but the agency had to reckon with the fact that "today, there are bilateral donors, multilateral donors, financial institutions like the World Bank, 'mega-foundations' such as the Bill and Melinda Gates Foundation, and non-governmental organizations."[9]

Brundtland went beyond the ministers of health – the usual heads of the country delegations to the world health assemblies who frequently had little power in their governments and were therefore often considered ineffective – and engaged in dialogues with presidents, prime ministers, and ministers of finance, all of whom outranked ministers of health and could directly fund health interventions. She also tried to reconceptualize global health as a tool for fighting poverty and a global responsibility of different actors because

---

[6] Barry R. Bloom, David E. Bloom, Joel E. Cohen, & Jeffrey D. Sachs, "Investing in the World Health Organization," *Science* 284:5416 (May 7, 1999), 911.

[7] Barbara Crossette, "New Leader of WHO Gets Big Grant to Hire Experts," *The New York Times*, July 21, 1998, A19.

[8] "Director-General: Five-Day Visit to France and the United States," October 27, 1998, Press Release WHO/70, Press Releases 1988.

[9] Nils Daulaire is cited in "What's Going on at the World Health Organization?" *The Lancet* 360:9340 (October 12, 2002), 118–120, p. 120.

globalization blurred the traditional responsibilities between government, the private sector, the international organizations, and civil society, urging them all to work together.

A decisive step in improving the WHO's international profile was enhancing the agency's capacity to respond rapidly and effectively to new epidemiological landscapes. The response envisioned by Brundtland was an echo of the health reforms promoted by the World Bank during the second half of the 1980s. Under these reforms, ministries of health would not spend their time and resources operating programs but would set standards, provide technical guidance, and where necessary, create alliances with the private sector. Under Brundtland, these alliances were better known as public-private partnerships, PPPs (the organizing principle of previous WHO programs such as TDR, the OCP, and UNAIDS). They brought together bilateral agencies, foundations, pharmaceutical companies, and the different administrative levels of the WHO, e.g., headquarters, regional offices, and country offices, to find the most effective way to address a particular health problem. Usually, PPPs had a board on which all stakeholders were represented and had the same power in terms of votes (contrary to the world health assemblies, dominated by ministers of health). The failure of national health systems to obtain new financial resources to control certain diseases or to have clear deadlines was stressed, to justify the PPPs. These partnerships appealed to private donors and private corporations because within them they enjoyed considerable influence, could oversee the progress of activities, and could direct their investments toward very specific goals. For example, the Global Alliance for Vaccines and Immunization, GAVI, created in 1999, had a board of 15 members, of whom two were permanent (the WHO and the Gates Foundation); the other memberships rotated among representatives of UNICEF, the World Bank, the Rockefeller Foundation, vaccine manufacturers, medical research institutes, and the governments of industrialized and developing countries. The mission of GAVI was the promotion of new, largely unused vaccines that were either too expensive or not a priority for developing countries struggling to enhance child development. One of its main challenges was to overcome the problems encountered by the Children Vaccine Initiative (CVI), created in the early 1990s but trapped for years in rivalries between UNICEF and the WHO.[10] The PPPs used a system of rewards based on performance to encourage superior results, resembling the bonuses paid in the private sector to productive employees.

---

[10] William Alan Muraskin, *The Politics of International Health: The Children's Vaccine Initiative and the Struggle to Develop Vaccines for the Third World* (Albany: State University of New York Press, 1998).

An important PPP was established shortly before Brundtland's election and received staunch support from the new director-general: the Roll Back Malaria (RBM) partnership. This was a global partnership between the WHO, the World Bank, UNICEF, the United Nations Development Program, USAID, and the British bilateral agency, DFID. The British provided the initial drive, much of the funding, and an engaging leader, David Nabarro, who was the former head of the health unit at DFID. The UK supported the WHO initiative shortly before it was announced in Geneva and included a line in the Birmingham G8 summit communique in 1998. The UK bilateral assistance agency provided USD 19 million in the first year, a significant amount for a global health program, and Nabarro helped shape a new philosophy for antimalaria work. This would not be an eradication campaign, nor a short-term effort; the goal was to cut malaria-associated mortality by half by 2010. The partnership set out to collaborate with research-based pharmaceutical companies to develop new drugs and improve control activities across health systems and to rely on civil society organizations as well as national health services, using a series of methods for prevention and control, and emphasizing that rural poverty was the real cause of the disease. In typical Brundtland style, her support to the program included a meeting in October of 1998 in the White House with Hillary Clinton, the director of USAID, the president of the World Bank, and the philanthropist George Soros to discuss increased funding for RBM and other health interventions (Soros was especially interested in the rising infection rates of TB in Eastern Europe and the countries of the former Soviet Union).[11]

RBM built upon efforts to reverse the trend among health systems to concede the fight against malaria after the failure of earlier malaria eradication programs initiated in the mid-1950's. Malaria had once again come to cause tragedy. By the early 1990s, the disease had resurfaced in almost all the regions where it had previously been controlled, and almost half of the world's population was living in malaria-risk areas. By 1993, of the estimated 300 million clinical cases worldwide, 80 percent were believed to occur in Africa and epidemic outbreaks were reported everywhere.[12] In 1996, AFRO launched a control program on malaria, and a year later, African medical scientists organized a meeting in Dakar that led to the Multilateral Initiative on Malaria, MIM, to increase research on the disease. The African scientists developed new control methods and, in partnership with researchers from the US National Institute of Allergy and Infectious Diseases, worked on a malaria vaccine,

---

[11] "Top-Level Meeting at White House on Tuberculosis," October 28, 1998, Press Release, WHO/79, Press Releases 1998.

[12] World Health Organization, *A Global Strategy for Malaria Control* (Geneva: World Health Organization, 1993), 19.

believing that this could soon be developed. Another significant program was the Medicines for Malaria Venture (MMV), launched in 1999 as a nonprofit foundation devoted to discovering and delivering new and affordable antimalarial drugs. Its members included the Rockefeller Foundation, the Wellcome Trust, and several pharmaceutical companies. This effort was motivated by the fact that chloroquine, the traditional drug of choice, had become largely ineffective in many parts of the world. Artemisinin, a Chinese plant extract long used in herbal medicine, came to be the core ingredient in a series of drugs that replaced chloroquine. It had the inconvenience of being expensive.

In 2000, RBM received further support in Africa. A meeting in Abuja, Nigeria, attended by 52 African heads of State, endorsed RBM, categorized malaria as a disease of poverty, and set interim targets for Africa. Following the Abuja meeting, April 25 was declared "Africa Malaria Day," and a UN resolution declared the period from 2001 to 2010 to be "the decade to Roll Back Malaria." Other meetings established RBM in the international agenda and contributed to a significant increase in international funding for malaria work (donations almost doubled in the first five years of RBM, from 67 million in 1997 to 130 million in 2002). This reversed the trend whereby medical scientists and pharmaceutical companies gave scant attention to the disease: between 1975 and 1999, only 4 of the approximately 1,400 new drugs launched worldwide were for treating malaria. However, around the turn of the twenty-first century, RBM moved away from its initially broad programs. Since then, it has focused more narrowly on the safe use of DDT as a means of prevention and on the distribution of bed nets impregnated with pyrethroids. Despite the Persistent Organic Pollutants Treaty, which aimed to phase out the use of insecticides because of their toxicity, the RBM partnership and the WHO began to promote DDT in 2006.[13] The RBM partnership came under criticism not only for putting too much emphasis on insecticide-impregnated bed nets, but also for its weak monitoring and evaluation systems and for paying too little attention to other components of a good program, such as microscopy services, reliable drug supplies, and community participation. A 2004 article critical of Roll Back Malaria asserted grimly that "the annual number of deaths worldwide from malaria is higher now than in 1998."[14]

After such criticism, RBM underwent a drastic restructuring and managed to retain the support of most of its partners. RBM created an independent governance board, increased its membership to about 90 multilaterals, bilaterals, NGOs, and other donors, and concentrated its work on prevention – redefining

[13] Christiane Rehwagen, "WHO Recommends DDT to Control Malaria," *British Medical Journal* 333:756 (2006), 622.
[14] "Editorial: Roll Back Malaria: A Failing Global Health Campaign," *British Medical Journal* 328 (2004), 1086–1087.

its goal as a reduction in malaria cases by 2015. There was still an emphasis on DDT, mainly through the distribution of insecticide-impregnated bed nets. Drug efficacy was a major problem. Unfortunately, the use of single-dose artemisinin, the new drug of choice, proved ineffective and contributed to parasite resistance. In 2006, the WHO announced that after considerable effort, it had convinced 13 pharmaceutical companies to phase out therapies based on a single drug, artemisinin, because of malaria-resistant parasites and to focus malaria-related marketing efforts primarily on artemisinin combination therapies (ACT), which were effective for uncomplicated cases of the disease. With these new drugs, malaria workers followed the example set for addressing tuberculosis, HIV, and leprosy, in which the combination of two drugs proved effective in preventing the evolution of resistant strains.

The response to malaria continued in the early twenty-first century with a new powerful bilateral. In 2005, the Bush administration launched the President's Malaria Initiative (PMI), providing about USD 1.2 billion to be spent in 15 high-burden countries in sub-Saharan Africa. The following year Rear Admiral Tim Ziemer was appointed as the US global malaria coordinator and would become head of the Initiative. In 2011, the WHO hailed as an important achievement a 26 percent decrease in malaria mortality since 2000, yet this achievement fell short of the 50 percent target set at the beginning of the century. A concern was the growing resistance of the mosquitoes to pyrethroids, the insecticide class used in insecticide-treated mosquito nets, ITNs (the new term for bed nets). In 2015, there were an estimated 446,000 deaths from malaria globally, of which about 90 percent occurred in Africa, and it was clear that critical political and social issues and anomalous climate patterns prevented the control of the disease.

At a time when tuberculosis was the largest and deadliest infection in the world, another public-private partnership was Stop TB. This was organized in 1998, a few years after the WHO had declared the disease a global health emergency, with an initial budget of more than USD 120 million, and involved more than 120 groups, including George Soros' Open Society Institute (a new global health philanthropy), the World Bank, USAID, and the Canadian International Development Agency. A Stop TB Secretariat was located at the Communicable Disease Cluster at the WHO, its head for the first years was the Japanese physician Arata Kochi, and the PPP was closer to the WHO than most other partnerships promoted by Brundtland. An important event that would occur later, in March 2000, was a ministerial TB conference in Amsterdam that called for the establishment of a TB Drug Purchasing Facility to be housed and administered by the WHO.

In the late 1990s, TB affected about a third of the world's population and killed more than 2 million of its victims every year. Poverty and uncontrolled urbanization intensified TB in developing countries. The disease was also prominent because it attacked vulnerable people living with HIV/AIDS. The situation was particularly acute among people from sub-Saharan Africa, Asia, and the Russian Federation, who were faced with misery, malnutrition, and a lack of proper shelter, social factors that were all contributing factors to the disease. In addition, Russia's health budgets were slashed and the supply of drugs was, at best, erratic. To make matters worse, it is likely that an additional 20 percent of Russian cases went undetected due to under-registration. Previous WHO achievements were not sufficient to stop the reemergence of the disease (the agency's Expert Committee on Tuberculosis in 1974 discouraged both traditional radiographic screening as well as isolation of patients in sanatoria).

In the United States, fears about TB outbreaks were intertwined with fears about immigration. In the late 1990s, about a quarter of the tuberculosis cases reported in the United States were in foreign-born individuals, many of them immigrants from developing countries. In affluent Japan, the disease also touched the lives of noblemen when an elderly attendant in the Imperial house of Prince Naruhito came down with tuberculosis. The number of new Japanese cases increased dramatically in 1999 and Japan's per capita infection rate was then the highest among industrial countries.[15] Other developed nations feared that the disease, which had been kept under control in the past, would reappear in their countries – as a result of a number of factors including immigrants, vulnerable communities of destitute people living in urban shelters, vulnerable aging populations, and widespread ignorance among health workers, who knew little about a disease uncommon in hospitals. Since the 1980s, most industrialized countries had given scant attention to tuberculosis under the false belief that TB was under control and would soon vanish. Instead, the growing menace of multidrug-resistant tuberculosis or MDR-TB, a form of the disease resistant to first line drugs (such as isoniazid and rifampin), was found in approximately 10 percent of TB cases across the globe. MDR-TB was ubiquitous and the result of poor, discontinued, and inappropriate treatment as well as difficulties in access to drugs.

Directly Observed Therapy, or DOTS, is a technique designed to monitor tuberculosis patients and thus ensure that they receive a full course of treatment. It was designed in the mid-1990s and became DOTS-Plus around 2000. DOTS-Plus consisted of careful supervision of tuberculosis patients and a greater consideration of other concomitant infections, which required a second line of powerful drugs taken daily in the presence of a health worker for a period of six to eight months. It also involved the use of second-line anti-TB drugs and a negotiation with pharmaceutical companies for reduced prices for

[15] "Tuberculosis on Rise in Japan for 3rd Year," *The New York Times*, November 29, 2000, p. 9.

drugs. DOTS-Plus was further supported by Stop TB, which emphasized prevention and logistical issues, early case detection, an adequate drug supply, and good reporting systems. The full implementation of DOT-Plus required firm commitments from governments. Health systems and local workers, supported by the PPP, were responsible for monitoring treatment and recovery, promoting adherence to treatment by patients, their families, and communities, and establishing an efficient case-detection system for microscopic examination of sputum. A problem for DOTs Plus programs was the need to obtain more expensive drugs and to sustain quality-controls. After 2006, the WHO redefined its work on tuberculosis to pay more attention to adequate health services and diagnosis, treatment and care for all patients including patients with drug resistant TB, and treatment for patients co-infected with HIV. This meant the increased interaction of DOTS Plus programs with other health programs. These goals were difficult to achieve because by 2004 the disease had reached monumental proportions such that about 9 to 10 million people developed active TB every year, about 80 percent of whom lived in Southeast Asia and sub-Saharan Africa. Reports of a deadlier version of the disease, Extensively Drug-Resistant TB (XDRTB), resistant to the second line of anti-TB drugs fluoroquinolones and parenteral agents, appeared around the world beginning in 2006. Criticism of the WHO's work on tuberculosis over the past few years also appeared. Between the early 1990s and 2002 the WHO, citing cost considerations, recommended unsound treatment for MDR-TB patients in poor countries, instead of the standard, more expensive treatment successfully used in rich countries.[16]

Another area where Brundtland enhanced the political meaning of public health was in the relationship between health and economics. In 2000, she recruited the American economist Jeffrey Sachs, a professor at Harvard University, to chair a WHO Commission on Macroeconomics and Health, which received support from the British, Norwegian, and Swedish bilateral agencies and the Rockefeller Foundation. Sachs had been advisor to economic "stabilization" programs in Bolivia, Peru, Russia, Poland, Slovenia, and Estonia but would later become a critic of the World Bank's orthodox stabilization plans. However, when Sachs collaborated with the WHO he had distanced himself from the neoliberal structural adjustment policies promoted by the World Bank. Sachs' Commission was composed of 18 heads of state and ministers of finance, foreign affairs, and planning, as well as well-known academics, economists, and health experts from around the world (absent among the commissioners were representatives of nongovernmental organizations that

---

[16] Thomas Nicholson, Catherine Admay, Aaron Shakow, & Salmaan Keshavjee, "Double Standards in Global Health: Medicine, Human Rights Law and Multidrug-Resistant TB Treatment Policy," *Health and Human Rights Journal* 18:1 (2016), 85–102.

criticized economic globalization). The goals of the Commission were to study the impact of ill health on economic development and to find evidence of ways in which sound economic investments in health could reduce poverty, especially in poor countries. After two years of work, the Commission's report, and the publicity campaign that followed, played a key role in placing health at the forefront of the development agenda.[17] Its rationale was much like that of the World Bank report, *Investing in Health*: Increased economic investment was a powerful driver of economic growth, and investing heavily in health was a sure ticket for an enormous payoff. It made a compelling case for specific health interventions against fatal diseases. These interventions should have well-targeted goals, clear measures, specific time-frames, and use the latest technology. The Commission also made a call to donors and governments from industrialized countries to increase their assistance for health to USD 27 billion by 2007 and asserted that the return on this investment would be more than USD 360 billion by 2015. The Commission on Macroeconomics and Health, which was later criticized for framing health solely as an economic input to productivity, advocated for a limited health package and copayment for additional health services, encouraged charity from the rich, and emphasized technical solutions.[18] It was a clear example of the second technocratic perspective that existed at the WHO.

Perhaps Brundtland's most important contribution was in the field of tobacco control: the creation and implementation of the Tobacco Free Initiative and the Framework Convention on Tobacco Control (FCTC) adopted by the 56th World Health Assembly held in 2003, discussed in the previous chapter. Brundtland said that tobacco was a "communicated disease" – communicated by the advertising and promotion strategies of the multinational tobacco companies.[19] The FCTC was unlike any other disease-control program and cast a very wide net; it was to address almost every aspect of tobacco and cigarettes: price and taxation, smuggling, duty-free sales, advertising and sponsorship, internet trade, package design and labeling, tobacco agriculture, and information sharing. No doubt because of Brundtland's experience with environmental control, the approach of the FCTC was modeled on the international treaties and conventions such as the United Nations Framework

---

[17] Jeffrey D. Sachs (ed.), *Macroeconomics and Health: Investing in Health for Economic Development: Report of the Commission on Macroeconomics and Health* (Geneva: World Health Organization, 2001).

[18] Howard Waitzkin, "Report of the WHO Commission on Macroeconomics and Health: A Summary and Critique," *The Lancet* 361:9356 (February 8, 2003), 523–526.

[19] World Health Organization, Tobacco Free Initiative, Framework Convention on Tobacco Control: *Report of the WHO Meeting of Public Health Experts, December 2–4, 1998* (Geneva: World Health Organization, 1998), p. 9, www.who.int/tobacco/media/en/vancouver.pdf, last accessed 21 October, 2017.

Convention on Climate Change, negotiated under her leadership at the Earth Summit in Rio de Janeiro in June 1992. Brundtland also made WHO one of the first major employers to make quitting smoking a condition of employment.

New Actors and Perspectives in Global Health

The symbolism of the turn of the millennium prompted international agencies to launch several important health and developmental initiatives. The most prominent was the Millennium Development Goals (MDGs), which were established at a meeting of heads of state and government and high-ranking officials at the UN Millennium Summit that took place in New York in September of 2000. Kofi Annan, the charismatic United Nations secretary-general during the years 1997 to 2006, who was carving out an independent space for his agency to launch ambitious proposals, authored a report entitled "We the people: The Role of the United Nations in the Twenty-First Century," that was the basis for these MDG. These consisted of eight goals, each with clear targets and measurable indicators of progress, which aimed to combine idealism and realistic precision in order to lift 1 billion people out of misery by 2015.[20] Among the goals were the eradication of extreme poverty and hunger, the achievement of universal primary schooling, the promotion of gender equality and women's empowerment, and the creation of partnerships for development. Specifically, targeted health goals were the reduction of under-five child-infant mortality by two-thirds, the reduction of the maternal mortality rate by three-quarters, and campaigns against HIV/AIDS, malaria, and other diseases which aimed to halve the number of cases by 2015. The tools in achieving the health goals included an increase in immunization, training of skilled child health workers, DOTS Plus and the provision of maternal care, insecticide-treated bed nets, condoms, and drugs such as ARVs. In 2002, the United Nations secretary-general created a commission headed by Sachs, then a professor at Columbia University, to recommend an action plan to implement the Millennium Development Goals. In the following years, all agencies recognized the legitimacy of the MDGs and contributed to their achievement. The WHO supported the MDGs and was considered a leader in the health field.

The Bill and Melinda Gates Foundation enthusiastically supported the MDGs in general, and especially focused their attention on reducing infant mortality. Shortly after its creation in 2000, the foundation joined the WHO's campaigns against TB and AIDS and vaccine-development studies and programs. Within

---

[20] See United Nations Development Group, *Indicators for Monitoring the Millennium Development Goals: Definitions, Rationale, Concepts and Sources* (New York: United Nations, 2003).

three years, the Foundation had committed more than USD 1.7 billion to health projects.[21] In 2005, in recognition of its Foundation that was key in setting global health priorities and awarding money, Bill Gates was a guest speaker at the World Health Assembly in Geneva, where he stated that thanks to new science, child mortality was declining significantly, and that within 10 years, everyone would recognize that the death of a child in the developing world was as tragic as the death of a child in an industrialized nation. The Gates Foundation brought huge sums of money into international health work against childhood diseases and transformed international health. Critics of the Foundation argued that it was driven by the promotion of science and technological breakthroughs, downplayed the importance of poverty and malnutrition as a cause of infant deaths, and dismissed the idea that money should be spent on more socially oriented campaigns.[22]

A new and powerful PPP, the Global Fund to Fight AIDS, Tuberculosis, and Malaria, established itself as the tool to achieve the MDGs in these disease-control campaigns. The Fund was designed in 2000 by the leading industrialized countries and worked on the assumption that existing bilateral and multilateral agencies would not by themselves eradicate the world's three most important diseases (initially, the participation of the United States was not too active because of the presidential election of 2000). The governments of these countries had a strong interest in living up to expectations, allaying anxieties caused by some critics of globalization, and minimizing the image of heartless rich countries using discourses on globalization as a smokescreen for continued hegemony. The final communiqué of the G8 meeting in Okinawa, Japan, announced: a "widespread agreement on what the priority diseases are and basic technologies to tackle . . . in place."[23] The subsequent G8 meeting in Genoa, Italy, in 2001 announced the Fund as a "public-private partnership marked by its "light governance with a strong focus on outcomes" and with participation of governments, donors, the pharmaceutical industry, foundations, and academic institutions.[24] Thus, the new Fund and major donations in global health directed to technological interventions became the "human face" of economic globalization. These governments believed, contrary to the

---

[21] Gordon Perkin & William Foege, "A Conversation with the Leaders of the Gates Foundation's Global Health Program: Gordon Perkin and William Foege," *The Lancet* 356:9224 (July 8, 2000), 356.

[22] See A. E. Birn, "Gates's Grandest Challenge: Transcending Technology as Public Health Ideology," *The Lancet* 366:9484 (August 6, 2005), 514–519.

[23] G8 Communiqué Okinawa, Japan, July 23, 2000, www.g8.utoronto.ca/summit/2000okinawa/finalcom.htm, last accessed February 18, 2018.

[24] Communiqué, Genova, Italy, July 22, 2001, www.g8.utoronto.ca/summit/2001genoa/finalcommunique.html, last accessed February 19, 2018.

first neoliberal governments, that markets most likely fail in providing health services and alleviating poverty, and that it was their responsibility to seek investments in health and other social programs. The Abuja African Summit of 2001 where Secretary-General Kofi Annan called for a mobilization to fight HIV/AIDS was also important for the validation of the Fund. Initially, a board, with two seats each for the private sector and civil society, and with the WHO and UNAIDS sidelined with just two nonvoting seats, was the main decision body of the Fund. The Global Fund was designed as a funding agency that did not involve itself in program operations. Its mission was to attract additional funding, to distribute grants in an open, transparent and accountable manner, and to create or support existing public-private partnerships (such as UNAIDS, Roll Back Malaria, and Stop TB). The Fund imitated GAVI in requesting applications to be reviewed by a panel that would make recommendations to the Fund's board. In 2001, commitments to the Global Fund had reached the figure of more than USD 1.5 billion. However, it was difficult to maintain support for the Fund because after September 11, 2001, and the US invasion of Afghanistan in October of the same year, the demands of military expenditures became a priority for industrialized countries.

In any case, with support from these donations, the Fund established its headquarters in Geneva with a board made up of members from multilaterals, private corporations, donors, and NGOs and legally had the status of a private foundation. The Swiss government granted it privileges like those it gave to foundations and multilateral agencies. In 2002, Richard Feachem, a former officer of the World Bank, was appointed as the first executive director of the Fund (a position he would hold until 2007, when he was replaced by French AIDS expert Michel Kazatchkine). Early in 2003, the US Secretary of Health and Human Services Tommy G. Thompson was elected chair of the Board of the Global Fund. Later that year, the US Congress approved significant sums to support the Fund, amounting to almost half of all the money to be disbursed by the organization. A congressional representative from California supported the Fund, using terms traditionally employed to validate international health: "Disease knows no borders ... and tuberculosis is arriving in America. Most of the cases in America ... are foreign-born people. So, if we want to eradicate tuberculosis in the United States, it must be an international effort."[25] In 2004, the Gates Foundation announced a gift of USD 50 million to the Global Fund, with most of the money going toward vaccine development. Altogether, about

---

[25] "Intervention of Lois Capps from California," in United States, Congress, HIV/AIDS, TB and Malaria: Combating a Global Pandemic, Hearing before the Subcommittee on Energy and Commerce, House of Representatives, One Hundred and Eight Congress, March 20, 2003 (Washington, DC: US Government Printing Office, 2003), 6.

USD 5 billion was committed to the Fund with 40 percent coming from the United States and the United Kingdom.[26]

The Fund had a novel approach to financing. Independent review processes were established to evaluate proposals and assess a country's ability to assume ownership of the project after funding had ended. The Global Fund aimed to strengthen local capacity, complement available resources, integrate prevention and treatment, promote the transparent use of financial resources, and encourage poor countries to buy inexpensive but good quality generic medicines instead of expensive brand-name ones. Global Fund grants were closely evaluated for good management practices and tangible outcomes, and the renewal of funding was based on the achievement of noteworthy results. The Fund hired independent accounting firms to oversee its distributions. One of the requirements of a Global Fund application was that the proposal made by a multi-sector Country Coordinating Mechanism (CCM), representing both the public and private sectors; it had to include nongovernmental organizations (NGOs) and groups of individuals affected by the disease. This gathering of diverse stakeholders was intended to improve coordination, avoid duplication of work, and develop a consensus on the country's programs. It was also an effort to establish the public-private partnerships model at the local level.

Between 2001 and 2007, the Fund attracted assets of USD 4.7 billion, to be spent through 2008. In its first two rounds of proposal evaluations, it committed USD 1.5 billion to support 154 programs in 93 countries. In these rounds of funding, 61 percent of the money awarded was directed to sub-Saharan Africa, where many of the world's poorest struggled to survive. Nearly two-thirds of this funding went to AIDS programs, with 17 percent to malaria and 14 percent to tuberculosis. The methods to control these diseases were those established previously by other PPPs: UNAIDS, Roll Back Malaria, and Stop TB. Most of the countries awarded HIV/AIDS funds intended to use a significant portion of their grants to provide antiretroviral treatment. Grants for malaria control both expanded the distribution of insecticide-treated bed nets and provided treatment for the sick. DOTS Plus was promoted in tuberculosis treatment programs.

After a few years of operations, the Fund faced a few challenges. The coordination with other UN agencies, such as the WHO, was considered insufficient, and frequently multilateral agencies perceived the Fund as a competition. Also, the amount of money used was high but still considered insufficient for the health needs of people in the world. In some nations, recipients were found to have misused financial resources, and their grants were suspended. The two acute cases were the Ukraine and Uganda. In

---

[26] Institute of Medicine, *President's Emergency Plan for AIDS Relief, PEPFAR Implementation: Progress and Promise* (Washington, DC: National Academies Press, 2007).

January 2004, the Fund decided to temporarily withdraw support to the Ukraine health program due to mismanagement and murky accounting practices. In Uganda more than USD 360 million awarded by the Global Fund was suspended, which affected the country's credibility, particularly in the fight against AIDS. The Fund asked the Ugandan Ministry of Finance to create a completely new structure to ensure the effective and transparent management of funds. Questions were also raised about the decision-making process at the Global Fund. In 2005, the US Government Accountability Office submitted a report to Congress arguing that the Global Fund, although doing a fine job, ought to have a better system for gathering information from recipient nations in order to make sound financial decisions.[27] The following year, the US Congress required that USD 20 percent of US contributions to the Fund be withheld until the secretary of state certified that the Fund had strengthened its oversight and spending practices.

At the same time, criticism of the techniques and methodologies used by the Fund emerged. For some critics, support to previous PPPs had several negative consequences, including: prioritizing those infectious diseases that were more popular in the media; sustaining "vertical" disease-specific control programs; seeking short-term results, while dismissing broader "horizontal" approaches and drawing away resources from public health systems; and paying little attention to Neglected Tropical Diseases (NTD). This line of thinking suggested that the Fund was adding to the problems of duplication and overlapping of the several PPPs, with little coordination or distribution of responsibilities between them, and that the Fund had also tense relations with UN agencies such as the WHO and UNAIDS. Another criticism was that the Fund gave too much attention to stand-alone interventions to control certain diseases, further drawing attention away from NTDs, and paying insufficient attention to improving the working conditions of health personnel or to building essential health infrastructure, water sanitation, and good housing and nutrition. The latter criticism asserted that local public-private partnerships were often formed too quickly, merely for the sake of submitting grant proposals to the Global Fund. Another question that was never fully answered was what would happen after the funding provided by the Fund came to an end (initially it was hoped that developing countries would take full financial responsibility for the programs after a few years, which was unlikely to happen).

These criticisms and questions came from a global network of scholars and health activists who were highly critical of the influence of neoliberalism on

---

[27] United States Government Accountability Office, *Global Health: The Global Fund to Fight AIDS, TB and Malaria Is Responding to Challenges but Needs Better Information and Documentation for Performance-Based Funding, Report to Congressional Committees* (Washington, DC: US Government Printing Office, 2005).

global health organizations. Many of them came together around the grassroots NGO the People's Health Movement, which was created in December 2000 in Bangladesh and began to issue critical commentaries on items coming before the World Health Assemblies and on decisions made by the Global Fund. Its organizing principle was that the holistic version of Primary Health Care should be the goal of health organizations. The Movement condemned neo-liberal economic policies promoted by the World Bank, the International Monetary Fund, and the World Trade Organization (WTO) and questioned a "naïve" assumption behind the MDGs, the Global Fund, and donors, namely that solving disease problems was just a matter of applying proper technology and convincing the rich to increase their donations to very poor nations. On the contrary, they argued that political and social exploitation were the main barriers to implementing long-term solutions and defended health as a human right for all people.

Criticisms made by the People's Health Movement were part of a broader critique of PPPs and their decisions. The points raised by such critics included: Rather than developing balanced health systems, public-private programs skewed national priorities to accommodate the agendas of international organizations; their performance was not always better than traditional public health services; and recipients had little participation in the design of programs. To some organizations, PPPs were wrong in principle. For the French-based NGO Doctors Without Borders (one of the NGOs working along with others such as Oxfam), since companies were drug suppliers "it did not make sense" that they were at the table with other decision-makers and created a conflict of interest.[28] This criticism was aimed directly at certain PPPs and the Macroeconomics Commission. Although Roll Back Malaria initially recognized some of the cultural dimensions of the disease, such as the need to dialogue with rural ethnic groups, it became in fact a vertical intervention, overemphasizing in many places bed nets and making them "magic bullets" against the disease. In the case of the DOTS technique used against tuberculosis, critics signaled that in shantytowns and rural areas it was very difficult to ensure good drugs, supervise treatment, and maintain a quality system of TB sputum microscopy to evaluate the advances of the program. (Figure 10.2 illustrates a treatment given at a Peruvian health center in the early twentieth century.) Poverty made it difficult for some patients to keep to the daily discipline of the program. Paraphrasing the title of an article, it said "The program was good but the disease was better." The meaning of this phrase was that although drugs were effective in individual cases, medicines and health workers could do little against the poor nutrition, bad housing, and precarious living conditions that

---

[28] Elizabeth Olson, "Changing of Guard at WHO," *The New York Times*, January 28, 2003, p. 11.

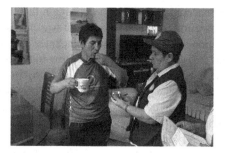

Figure 10.2 A lay health worker supervises the use of tuberculosis medication in a shantytown of Lima, Peru, one of the cities most affected by the disease. The activity was part of the campaign conducted in 2010 by the Pan American Health Organization, USAID, and the Peruvian Ministry of Health. Courtesy: World Health Organization Photo Library.

sustained TB. Poor compliance or insufficient surveillance were not the main drivers of tuberculosis.[29]

The most controversial decision taken by Brundtland was the 2000 WHO report entitled *Health Systems: Improving Performance* that ranked 191 countries on a "comparable" set of standards. It was done under the assumption that policy makers only pay attention to scorecards and the WHO should produce one similar to those in existence (such as UN Development Programme's Human Development Index developed in the 1990s and embraced by prestigious economists such as Amartya Sen, who had received the Nobel Prize in 1998). The report prompted debates in medical and health circles and attracted much media attention.[30] The standards used in the report included the overall level of population health, health inequalities, system responsiveness, and the distribution of the health system's financial burden among the population (i.e., who paid the costs) to establish a ranking. The report was the first of its kind. Some European nations such as France and Italy appeared at the top of the ranking, but the health systems of others, such as Sweden and Denmark (considered stellar models) ranked lower. The United States appeared in 37th place, below Greece and Portugal (the latter on spending less of their national resources on public health). Despite having excellent health indicators, Cuba and Brazil, which were thought to have the best health systems in Latin America,

[29] Sandy Smith-Nonini, "When the Program is Good but the Disease is Better: Lessons from Peru on Drug-Resistant Tuberculosis," *Medical Anthropology* 24 (2005), 265–296.

[30] World Health Organization, Evidence and Information for Policy, *Health Systems: Improving Performance* (Geneva: World Health Organization, 2000). A critical approach appears in Vicente Navarro, "The New Conventional Wisdom: An Evaluation of the WHO Report: Health Systems, Improving Performance," *International Journal of Health Services* 31:1 (2001), 23–33.

had a low ranking. The report encountered so much opposition that the WHO never tried another such ranking effort. About a year after it was published, the Pan American Health Organization held a meeting which included speakers that criticized the methodology and "absurd" ranking results. Brundtland conceded that it was necessary to revise notions and measures. The controversy would linger for years, with critiques and rebuttals. In 2010, a former economist of the WHO criticized the report for relying on estimates and noncompatible data and for ignoring all cultural, geographic, and historical factors.[31]

Brundtland was director-general only for one term. Late in 2002 she announced, to the surprise of many, that she would not run for reelection. Although it is not clear why she made the decision, it is possible that she sought another position in the UN system or was frustrated by her unsuccessful attempts to centralize the agency and restrict the powers of the WHO regional directors. It also appears that she was beginning to be isolated from her Geneva staff, who had initially been enthusiastic about her decisions on transparency at the agency and her prominent role as a world leader. Toward the end of her term she had little contact with the staff. Her organizational changes meant an effort to make the WHO a sort of business-efficient organization, which pleased donors and industrialized countries but was hard on staff. Her critics also accused her of having an authoritarian business-management style, seeking a collaboration with the private sector such as private pharmaceutical companies, or for saying too little about the impact of neoliberal economic policies on the deterioration of health. Anyway, in the competition for the position of director-general that would replace Brundtland, all contenders recognized that she had succeeded in shaking up the WHO's traditional structures and played a crucial role in making the WHO a player in international affairs.

In her final year as director-general, Brundtland faced an alarming and unexpected challenge: the outbreak of severe acute respiratory syndrome (SARS) in South-East Asia, which was initially identified as an atypical pneumonia in a province of China in late 2002 but was not reported to the WHO until early 2003. As it spread rapidly, there was clearly potential for a global pandemic. Brundtland and David Heymann, chief of the infectious disease section, instantly sounded the alarm to media and health authorities around the world. This was the first health emergency in which the WHO was to take full advantage of the internet. Virus experts communicated continually and constantly to share information and report progress. Within a month, they had identified the virus responsible for SARS, and within eight months, they had broken the chains of transmission and contained the disease, marking another success for the WHO.

---

[31] Philip Musgrove, "Letter to the Editor, Health Care System Rankings," *New England Journal of Medicine* 362 (2010), 1546–1547.

The WHO under Lee

The election process that followed the tenure of Brundtland was hotly disputed. Candidates included one of Brundtland's former associates, Julio Frenk, who was the WHO's executive director in charge of Evidence and Information for Policy; a UN officer she knew well, Peter Piot, who was the prestigious head of UNAIDS; Pascoal Mocumbi from Mozambique; Ismail Sallam from Egypt; and the soft-spoken Korean Jong-wook Lee – considered a dark horse in the race. In January 2003, Lee was nominated by the Executive Board for the post of director-general. During the campaign, Frenk was generally perceived as Brundtland's successor and his failure to win the election was interpreted by some as a criticism of Brundtland's policies, such as the "cluster" organizational system that was disbanded shortly after she left the WHO. Also against him was the fact that many saw Frenk as the force behind the controversial country-ranking of the 2000 report *Health Systems: Improving Performance.*

In May 2003, Lee, director of the WHO's Global Programme on Vaccines, who had never been a government official, was elected by the WHO Assembly to a five-year term as director-general. He was the first Korean national to head an international organization. Defending his candidacy, he argued in the Executive Board election:

I grew up in what was then an extremely poor country. The Republic of Korea today has become an industrial and economic power house, but during my early life, Korea faced the problems of a developing country. I have not forgotten that experience.[32]

Several anecdotes suggest he had a humble and compelling personality that attracted respect. One of the most colorful anecdotes was that in his official visits as director-general he received many gifts but never kept any. When a gift was received he would immediately have his staff store it without even unwrapping it. The exception was if the gift was food. Then it would be opened and shared with his staff. Unopened gifts, such as an expensive one given by the King of Spain, accumulated for a year and then sold at a year-end bazaar to raise funds for an orphanage in St. Petersburg, Russia, that cared for children whose parents had died of AIDS. Lee joked: "People know that if they give me a gift, it always goes to a bazaar, so who is going to give me gifts anymore?"[33]

---

[32] *Korea Foundation for International Healthcare, 2006–2016* (Seoul: Korea Foundation for International Healthcare, 2016), p. 15.
[33] *Korea Foundation for International Healthcare, 2006–2016* (Seoul: Korea Foundation for International Healthcare, 2016), p. 19.

Unlike Brundtland, the Korean, who was then 50 years old, was little known outside the WHO bureaucracy, where he had worked for more than 19 years. He was a graduate from Seoul Medical School and held a master's degree from Hawaii's school of public health. After heading the WHO Global Program for Vaccines and Immunizations and serving as senior policy advisor to Brundtland, in 2000 Lee was promoted to director of the Stop TB Program (considered the least controversial PPP). He had a reputation for being an effective communicator, establishing good rapport with his staff, and having a productive dialogue with pharmaceutical companies. He signed an agreement between the WHO and Novartis for a five-year donation for a tuberculosis treatment that would benefit half a million people. Lee was a pragmatic consensus builder who rapidly became a global leader. When Lee was speaker at the G8 Summit in Saint Petersburg in July 2004, he called on world leaders to "act as a global community" to strengthen health systems and support the UN and the WHO in their global efforts to "control communicable diseases."[34] He countered the aggressive questioning of UN agencies carried out under Reagan's administration in the 1980s.

Lee reversed some of Brundtland's reforms, reintroducing the traditional structure of assistant director-generals and restoring the power of regional offices in response to their resentment of the intrusions by headquarters into their power and activities, although he did also recentralize some decision-making processes. He believed that public-private partnerships had become an end in themselves and wanted them to be limited and refocused. Nonetheless, he followed some of the practices of his predecessor such as bringing outsiders into leading positions in the agency and tried to reorganize public-private partnerships and link them with some common goals. He met with presidents Chirac from France, Hu Jintao from China, and George W. Bush, with whom he gave an informal joint press conference at the White House (see Figure 10.3). He promoted programs that had been supported by Brundtland, such as the fight against tobacco, and, like Brundtland, had few problems in establishing dialogue with pharmaceutical and other industries concerned with individual health. Some relationships, however, were not easy. Lee confronted the fast food industry about their contribution to obesity – a serious global risk factor for heart disease, diabetes, and some forms of cancer – and launched a global strategy on diet, physical activity, and health based on a joint WHO/FAO 2003 scientific report on nutrition which argued that free (that is, added) sugar should be no more than 10 percent of

---

[34] Jong-wook Lee, "Meeting of the G8 Health Ministers, Moscow, Russian Federation, 28 April 2006," www.who.int/dg/lee/speeches/2006/g8_health_ministers_meeting/en/index.html, last accessed October 21, 2017.

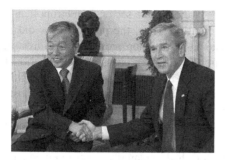

Figure 10.3 US President George W. Bush meets with World Health Organization Director-General Jong-wook Lee from Korea on December 6, 2005, at the Oval Office of the White House in Washington, DC. As director-general, Lee promoted three initiatives that would mark the agency in the twenty-first century: full access to antiretrovirals, the Commission on Social Determinants of Health, and Universal Health Coverage.
Credit AFP PHOTO/Mandel NGAN. Getty Images.

the calories in healthy daily food intake.[35] The American Sugar Association attacked the agency, asking US Health Secretary Tommy Thompson to use his influence to get the report withdrawn and demanding that the US Congress end its funding. The WHO held firm and opened a debate that continues to this day.

Another important goal for Lee was to improve the working conditions of health professionals in poor countries. This meant addressing the worldwide shortage of almost 4.3 million medical doctors, midwives, nurses, and lay health workers as well as the low salaries and insecurity of tenure of public health staff and the brain drain – all of which were acute problems in developing countries. It also meant to introduce some fairness and rationality to the unregulated medical job market where poor nations lost health professionals trained at home but attracted by offers in industrialized nations. Under his guidance, the WHO emphasized the quality and the appropriate distribution of health workers, whose numbers were associated with greater immunization coverage, better nutritional practices, promotion of primary care and infant survival, and positive outcomes in cardiovascular diseases. Even the WHO faced a critique of recruitment of professionals from developing countries thereby depleting staff from precarious health systems.

For Lee, one of the lessons from PPPs focused on control of specific diseases was that developing countries experienced an overall shortage of health personnel in public health systems and rural health because many

---

[35] Geoffrey Cannon, "Why the Bush Administration and the Global Sugar Industry Are Determined to Demolish the 2004 WHO Global Strategy on Diet, Physical Activity and Health," *Public Health Nutrition* 7:3 (2004), 369–380.

professionals preferred to work in the private sector, in metropolitan areas, or to migrate to industrialized countries. Thus, the public sector did not have enough trained health professionals to develop preventive and treatment programs. The WHO's annual report for 2006 emphasized that the critical factors for the success of health systems were not only scientific and technological breakthroughs, or well-designed disease-control programs, but most importantly, having a sufficient number of adequately trained medical personnel as well as active well-recognized teams of lay health workers and the political will to support them.[36]

As with other WHO leaders, Lee had to plan responses to emergencies. One of these was the 2004 tsunami in the Indian Ocean that devastated parts of Indonesia, Sri Lanka, India, and Thailand, affected many other countries, and led to hundreds of thousands of deaths and the homelessness of millions. The WHO rapidly set up a High-Level Task Force, with the close collaboration of the WHO South-East Asia Region, to deploy health experts and sanitation engineers and coordinate relief support. The focus was to be on preventing outbreaks of infectious water-borne diseases and providing safe water, surgical kits, oral rehydration salts, and medical supplies.

Lee made two lasting contributions that dominate the contemporary debate on global health: Universal Health Coverage and the Commission on Social Determinants of Health. Both proposals were the result of criticism of previous disease-control programs and growing skepticism that poor nations could reach the MDG targets by 2015. Some experts questioned the wisdom of simply pouring more money into developing countries with weak and inefficient public health systems and into public-private partnerships often characterized by fragmentation. Thus, after a wave of enthusiasm in embracing partnerships, health experts began to regard them with more caution. One learning experience was the 3 by 5 initiative (also promoted by Lee) that, not surprisingly, failed to reach 3 million people. Many countries found that as part of the neoliberal reforms of the 1980s and 1990s, poor patients had to pay user fees for drugs and other medical services. These copayments did not increase the budgets of public health systems and pushed aside poor people from medical services. In countries that had stopped using user fees, such as South Africa in the mid-1990s, outpatient attendance by public health services increased dramatically. The 3 by 5 initiative put a spotlight on the weaknesses of health systems in poor and middle-income countries: inadequate laboratory capacities, drug availability, protocols, and procurement; poorly balanced provision of services; and too few human resources devoted to health. It also demonstrated how difficult it was to sustain the global movement for universal access to ARVs.

[36] World Health Organization, *Working Together for Health: The World Health Report 2006* (Geneva: World Health Organization, 2006).

The two new proposals were also a consequence of political changes occurring outside the WHO. At the turn of the twenty-first century, anti-globalization movements blamed international corporations, bank conglomerates, the World Bank, bilateral agencies, and neoliberal governments for unemployment, environmental degradation, and failure to provide needed social programs for the middle classes and the poor. For the leaders of these movements, neoliberal reforms only made the rich richer, destroyed jobs, and promoted a privatization that did not improve public health services or people's health. The first major demonstration against globalization occurred in 1999. Angry massive street protests disrupted the meeting of the World Trade Organization in Seattle that overshadowed previous demonstrations against meetings of a "globalization" agency and masked the resentment of political leaders in developing countries that thought that economic globalization was widening the economic disparities between the north and south of the planet. Thereafter, riots occurred in many international meetings, including the G-8. The protest led the UN and other specialized agencies such as the WHO to rethink their mission. The criticism of globalization, embraced by some middle-income countries that challenged the power of governments of industrialized countries in the West, gave the WHO an opportunity and a necessity to promote comprehensive changes to health systems and address the complex relationships between health and society.

The Commission on Social Determinants of Health

The Commission on Social Determinants of Health was established in March 2005 as an independent unit within the WHO. Its goals were to gather evidence about the social determinants having an impact on health, to highlight inequalities within and between countries, and to identify ways of overcoming health inequities. Its chair was the renowned British epidemiologist, Sir Michael Marmot (Marmot received a knighthood in 2002, a rare distinction for a health researcher) and its 19 Commissioners were scientists from diverse disciplines, public health practitioners, and politicians who had little experience in working inside the WHO. Many of the Commissioners were known for their progressive and egalitarian ideas, such as Giovanni Berlinguer from Italy, Mocumbi from Mozambique, Ricardo Lagos from Chile, and Amartya Sen from India.

The appointment of the Commission was a response to criticism of the narrow health interventions promoted by disease-control PPPs. These interventions were said to place too much emphasis on technology, cost-effectiveness, and managerial capabilities and were said to have assumed that medical and health services were the primary determinants of the health of a population, contrary to the findings of previous work such as the Lalonde Report and the Declaration of Primary Health Care. A series of studies anticipated the theme of the Commission: health inequities. Among them was the UK report, *Inequalities in Health,* which was published in 1980 and known as the Black Report, (its main author was Scottish physician Douglas Black).[37] The British Department of Health and Social Security had commissioned the report in 1977 under the Labor government, based on the assumption that something was wrong with the National Health Service created in 1948. The report concluded that, although nothing was wrong with the NHS and, in fact, overall health had improved in England, there were discrepancies in the health of privileged and disadvantaged social groups. These gaps had to do with income, education, housing, diet, employment, and working conditions. The report recommended reforms in the provision of education, housing, and social welfare. Margaret Thatcher's conservative government dismissed the Black Report. Many British epidemiologists, including Marmot, continued to study the effects of, and to work against, the neoliberal reforms, while keeping a low profile (according to Marmot, they would let the evidence "speak for itself").

The Black Report had an impact on public health scholars and practitioners in Europe, Canada, the United States, the United Kingdom, and in developing countries. Marmot participated in a series of investigations, inspired by the report, that examined the relationship between chronic disease mortality and job hierarchy among British civil servants. These studies (known as the Whitehall studies) found that, as an individual's grade level within the hierarchy improved, so mortality declined. The published studies argued that the distribution of disease in the hierarchy, termed the "social gradient," was caused by acute inequities external to the health system and that these should be addressed by improving living conditions and reducing class inequality. The Whitehall Studies defined the distinction between health inequities and health inequalities. Health inequities were defined as differences in access to health services and differences in health outcomes that were socially produced, systemic, and unfair. Health inequalities indicated the diverse health status in society that were determined by biology or age (for example, on average, younger people fell sick less often than older people). Marmot hoped that governmental policies could reduce, if never eliminate, health inequities but could do little to change health inequalities. Marmot saw that there was a relationship between health inequities and the egalitarian ideas of the Indian economist, Amaryta Sen. According to Sen, freedom from want and poverty were essential for economic growth. Marmot knew Sen, and both were critical of Jeffrey Sachs's conception of health as merely an input to economic development. Based on Sen's ideas, Marmot argued that health was an

---

[37] Alastair Mcintosh Gray, "Inequalities in Health. The Black Report: A Summary and Comment," *International Journal of Health Services* 12:3 (1982), 349–380.

essential good that enabled individuals to function in society and that governments should ensure the access of all citizens to this good.

The Commission's work represented an effort to give new life to the holistic version of primary health care in the WHO and was a clear example of the socio-medical tradition that had existed in the agency. Except for the WHO Equity Initiative set up in 1995, the health agency did not work much on health inequity in the 1990s. Under Brundtland as director-general, a pragmatic approach predominated and social interventions were not a priority (an exception being the participation of Sen as a speaker in the World Health Assembly in 1999). Concern with health inequities revived under Lee. In 2004, he introduced the Commission to the World Health Assembly using language that recalled Mahler's vision of primary health care; Lee said that social determinants of health were part of a global effort to promote equity in a spirit of social justice.[38] He argued: "The Alma Ata goal of Health for All was right ... equitable access, community participation and intersectoral approaches to health improvement. These principles must be adapted to today's context."[39] Lee anticipated that by 2008 (the 38th anniversary of the Alma-Ata conference and the year of celebration of 60 years of the WHO Constitution), the Commission would publish its final report and indicate ways to translate its findings into policy.

The Commission had two secretariats: one in Geneva headed by the Chilean Jeanette Vega, who managed the meetings, especially with the UN agencies, and one in London where a team directed by Marmot concentrated on the scientific work. The dynamic was of debate, and if the rest of the commissioners proved Marmot wrong he was willing to change his mind (different from many health agencies where the director says something and other members just stamp it). Between 2005 and 2008, the Commission on Social Determinants of Health held consultations with representatives of civil society and NGOs, including the People's Health Movement. It also carried out a series of studies and established nine knowledge networks of researchers and advocates on child development, employment conditions, globalization, health systems, urban environments, methods, gender, social exclusion, and public health priorities), that enhanced the findings of previous work on social epidemiology, including the Black Report and the Whitehall Studies. The Commission adopted some terms from previous studies, such as the "social gradient," cited dramatic examples of global health inequities (such as the 43-year difference in life expectancy between Japanese and Sierra

[38] Jong-wook Lee, "Public Health Is a Social Issue," *The Lancet* 365 (March 19, 2005), 1005–1006.

[39] Jong-wook Lee, "Global Health Improvement and the WHO: Shaping the Future," *The Lancet* 362 (December 20, 2003), 2083–2088.

Leonean babies), and introduced a simple definition of social determinants: "the cause of causes." The definition conveyed the idea that poverty, stress, and discrimination – socioeconomic factors not targeted by health services – were the ultimate source of disease. These socioeconomic factors explained the main trends in morbidity and mortality.

The Commission's investigations can be summarized in three findings. First, while there have been improvements in health indicators and increases in life expectancy in most countries, there are considerable differences between people from different social classes, ethnic backgrounds, and genders. Second, discrimination against some of these groups has increased and inequalities heightened. Third, many of these disparities were related to social conditions that promoted health, chiefly: stress, early life, social exclusion, work, unemployment, social support, addiction, food, and transportation. Most of these differences were injustices. Overall, the Commission found that the benefits of economic globalization were good, but uneven, favoring the already rich and creating new social and health inequities. The policy implications of the work of the Commission were to improve the conditions in which people work and live, to diminish the discrimination of marginalized groups, and to promote equal opportunities and strong poverty reduction programs. In 2008, the final report of the Commission was issued, but its recommendations failed to become overriding priorities for the WHO.

Many medical doctors, perhaps not cognizant of nor interested in social epidemiology, believed that the issue of social and economic inequities determining individual health status was vague, and they considered Marmot's demands for healthy living and working conditions to be politically motivated and impossible to meet. At the same time, many conservative politicians considered Marmot's ideas for more egalitarian societies to be fanning the flames of anti-globalization movements. The final report of the Commission was criticized as "ideology with evidence" (a phrase that Marmot actually liked). *The Economist* published an article arguing that the report had some excellent ideas but was driven by a naïve egalitarian ideology of "quixotic determination" and that it was "baying at the moon when it attacks global imbalances in the distribution of power and money."[40] The statement was probably related to a sentence of the report that said implementing the Commission's recommendations would require "changes in the operation of the global economy."[41] The Commission's report achieved what few WHO

---

[40] "The Price of Being Well," *The Economist*, August 28, 2008, www.economist.com/node/12009974, last accessed October 21, 2017.

[41] *Closing the Gap in a Generation: Health Equity through Action on the Social Determinants of Health: Commission on Social Determinants of Health Final Report* (Geneva: World Health Organization, 2008), p. 54.

reports do – great visibility, influence outside Geneva, and in some places the facilitation of dialogue between scientists and policy makers. It also faced some criticism from left scholars and activists who argued that the report was "strong" in presenting evidence but "short" in its policy recommendations. According to this interpretation, the Report did not deal adequately with the greed of pharmaceutical companies and presented good ideals but did not explain how countries could mobilize political forces to correct the social determinants of ill health such as economic exploitation.[42]

The Commission's final report had a modest launch in August 2008 and did not garner sufficient support within the WHO to overcome the skepticism surrounding it. The agency was passing then through a period of considerable uncertainty. In May 2006, Lee had died unexpectedly; he had passed the midpoint of his term of office and many expected him to run for reelection as director-general in 2007. Shortly after Lee's death, the Swede Anders Nordström (see Figure 10.4), a physician from the Karolinska Institut and former interim executive director for the Global Fund to Fight AIDS, Tuberculosis, and Malaria as well as the WHO's assistant director-general for General Management, became Acting director-general. Nordström was very cautious about previous and future engagements of the agency and began the process of preparing for the election of a new director-general. In November 2006, the World Health Assembly approved the selection of the Executive Board: Margaret Chan from China. Jeanette Vega told Marmot that the future of the Commission was grim. Marmot did not have a "good meeting" with Chan, and she appeared uninterested in making the work of the Commission on the Social Determinants of Health a priority and did not fully grasp the dynamics of the Commission.[43] Chan allowed the work of the Commission on the Social Determinants of Health to continue but did not give it the prominence it had under Lee. Although Chan did little to enhance the Commission's role, some officers and country representatives worked hard to enhance its influence.

In the final report, Marmot introduced the idea of calling an international conference on social determinants with the help of northern European countries and Brazil – which had had a National Commission on Social Determinants on Health since 2006. Brazil provided 3 million dollars for a World Conference on Social Determinants of Health that took place in Rio de Janeiro in October 2011. Although there was some tension between WHO

---

[42] Carles Muntanera, Sanjeev Sridharana, Orielle Solarb, & Joan Benach, "Against Unjust Global Distribution of Power and Money: The Report of the WHO Commission on the Social Determinants of Health: Global Inequality and the Future of Public Health Policy," *Journal of Public Health Policy* 30:2 (2009), 163–175.

[43] Michael Marmot, Interview with Marcos Cueto, London, January 18, 2017.

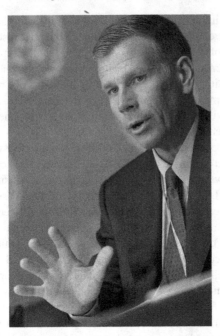

Figure 10.4 Anders Nordström of Sweden, interim executive director of the Global Fund to Fight AIDS, Tuberculosis and Malaria and WHO assistant director-general for General Management under Jong-wook Lee. Nordstrom became acting director-general in May 2006 following the sudden death of Lee. He served in this position until November 2006. AFP PHOTO FABRICE COFFRINI
Credit: FABRICE COFFRINI/AFP/Getty Images.

headquarters officers and the Brazilian organizers, the meeting approved a Rio de Janeiro Political Declaration on Social Determinants of Health; ultimately, however, the WHO headquarters lost interest in the work of the Commission. To further compound matters, in the following years the WHO documents coopted code words of the Commission's report but did not create mechanisms to address social and health inequities.

Margaret Chan and the WHO

Previously, for her election at the Board, Chan had close competition with other contenders, including Bernard Kouchner (the French founder of Méde-cins Sans Frontières); Kazem Behbehani, a senior WHO official from Kuwait; Elena Salgado, Spain's health minister; Shigeru Omi from Japan; and, once again, Julio Frenk, the Mexican health minister and former officer of the Gates

Foundation. Chan had trained at the Universities of Western Ontario and Singapore. In 1997, when Hong Kong was officially returned to China, she stayed on as director of Hong Kong's department of health, although many of her colleagues and relatives left. When she went to the WHO in 2005 as the agency's assistant director for communicable diseases, she had a reputation as a disciplined hard worker, a high-ranking officer who consulted science experts before making decisions, and a good administrator.

She was elected for reasons having little to do with the work on the social determinants of health. At a time when there was widespread fear of the potential for influenza to become a global pandemic, Chan had valuable experience in the control of Avian Influenza in 1997 and Severe Acute Respiratory Syndrome (SARS), which had come from mainland China in 2003. In fact, she was the only candidate who had been directly tested in these global health crises. Although there were no more cases after 2004, there was still a global concern over a possible SARS outbreak because it was thought that a new form of influenza could be the next pandemic. Many inside the WHO saw the response to SARS as a kind of dress rehearsal for the upcoming emergency. Thus, Chan was considered an expert in "pandemic preparedness" even though some thought she had made mistakes in handling the epidemic in China, such as not giving sufficient attention to the first outbreaks in mainland China. The People's Government of the People's Republic of China, which nominated and supported her, could point to a remarkable rate of economic growth and its efforts to compete for global leadership with the United States and Western Europe. It was also hoped that as director-general, Chan, considered a straight talker, could make China comply with the rules of global health; improve the sour relationship between China's government and the WHO, which could be traced to the SARS epidemic; and increase its contributions.

Under Chan, the WHO improved its finances as part of a general trend of more money for global health. (She appears in Figure 10.5 in her final General Assembly as director-general in 2017.) Previously, development assistance for global health had dramatically increased from USD 5.6 billion in 1990 to 21.8 billion in 2007.[44] The 2007 World Health Assembly approved a budget of USD 4.2 billion for the next biennium, the largest WHO budget ever adopted. The agency was still dependent on its extrabudgetary financial resources which comprised more than two-thirds of the total budget. These resources pay for specific, time-limited projects. Chan pursued several goals: promoting safer

---

[44] Nirmala Ravishankar, Paul Gubbins, Rebecca Cooley, Katherine Leach-Kemon, Catherine M. Michaud, Dean T. Jamison, & Christopher I. Murray, "Financing of Global Health: Tracking Development Assistance for Health from 1990 to 2007," *The Lancet* 373:9681 (June 20, 2009), 2113–2124.

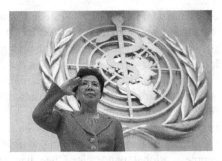

Figure 10.5 Margaret Chan from China was elected WHO director-general in 2006. She was appointed for a second five-year term in May 2012. Previously, she was director of health in Hong Kong and confronted the first human outbreak of H5N1 avian influenza in 1997. She joined the WHO in 2003 and in 2005 was appointed assistant director-general for Communicable Diseases.
Credit: FABRICE COFFRINI/AFP/Getty Images.

pregnancies, reducing the impact of childhood diseases, increasing immunization rates, and supporting the WHO reform process. Chan also played an important role in launching an Intensified Polio Eradication Effort that reinvigorated the Global Polio Eradication Initiative created in 1988 by a World Health Assembly. In 2009, she made an earnest effort at internal reform and modernization by fully supporting an independent evaluation prompted by the Executive Board's decision to create an Independent Expert Oversight. The mandate of this official body was to examine the financial statements and internal management systems of the agency. In 2011 she also presented a report to the 64th World Health Assembly on the future of the WHO's financing that identified two problems of the agency: it was overcommitted and overextended. She likewise promoted a much-needed meeting with representatives of NGOs in 2014 to discuss a draft document on how the WHO could engage with non-state actors.

Chan liked to describe herself as a "servant" of member states but there were doubts whether she would be able to streamline the complex structure of the WHO, establish a single budget, lead an internal, tough reform process, and become a visionary world leader. She showed little political astuteness when she visited and praised authoritarian regimes. She frequently visited China, meeting with top leaders including President Xi Jinping, congratulated the government for its health advances, and reiterated the agency's commitment to the One China policy, which does not recognize Taiwan as a sovereign country. Chan's other visits also generated controversy. Contrary to an Amnesty International report that denounced food shortages and poor medical care services in North Korea, she positively evaluated the medical care situation in North Korea and praised the authoritarian government for its tuberculosis program, its increase in the country's vaccination rate, and its decrease in the number of infections in hospitals. Chan likewise commended Russia's public health achievements without commenting on President Putin's disregard for human rights and asked if the country might be willing to produce an inexpensive vaccine to be used in developing countries. Chan also visited oil-rich Turkmenistan in Central Asia, a nation with a repressive human-rights record, and gave President Gurbanguly Berdymukhamedov, who rewrote the Constitution so he could rule for life, a special health award.[45]

Chan believed that it was possible to achieve the Millennium Development Goals by 2015 and launched a list of 24 "best buys" interventions (such as tobacco taxation, salt reduction in diets, and physical activity) to address Noncommunicable Diseases (NCDs), endorsed by the 2013 World Health Assembly, to control the growing rates of cardiovascular disease, diabetes, and cancer (It was estimated that more than 36 million people died annually as a result of NCDs). She invited Bill Gates to be speaker at the 2011 World Health Assembly (Gates had previously been a speaker at the Assembly in 2005, thanks to Lee. Melinda Gates, co-chair of the Bill and Melinda Gates Foundation, has also been an Assembly speaker) and subscribed to his call for a decade of vaccines and for the eradication of malaria – despite the reservations of some WHO officers who believed that the eradication goal was technologically impossible and that she failed to give the social determinants of disease proper attention.

Chan was not as committed to universal access to generic drugs as Lee. Representatives of developing countries were frustrated by the little progress made by an Intergovernmental Working Group on Innovation and Intellectual Property set up at the 2006 World Health Assembly. The Secretariat allocated meager resources to this group and did not appear very interested in doing more to assist developing countries to implement WTO's TRIPS "flexibilities" such as compulsory licensing to enable the supply of cheaper generic drugs. More criticism emerged when Chan visited Thailand in 2007 and criticized the Thai government for its compulsory licenses for three drugs (it was reported, however, that she apologized in a letter to the Thai health minister confirming that the licenses were a prerogative of Thai authorities).[46]

After a few years in office, Chan was able to obtain more control of the Geneva office and received recognition from other global institutions (in 2009

---

[45] Maria Cheng, "Outgoing WHO Head Practiced Art of Appeasement," May 23, 2017, www.apnews.com/590f2fa8ae9b423db7188b39f041f0de, last accessed March 1, 2018.

[46] "Countries Attending Global Fund Supporters Meeting 'Overlook Facts,' Only 'Inch Up' Their Contributions," *Kaiser Health News*, July 18, 2018, http://khn.org/morning-breakout/dr00018890/, last accessed April 20, 2018, & Bangkok Post February 2, 2007, "WHO Raps Compulsory Licensing Plan Govt Urged to Seek Talks with Drug Firms."

the WHO received, from Spain, the prestigious Prince of Asturias Award for International Cooperation) and emphasized one overarching objective as the organizing principle of the agency: Universal Health Coverage. (In 2012 she was reelected for a second five-year term with the stern support of China in an unchallenged election; no other candidate was proposed.)

Universal Health Coverage

WHO health economists had used the term "Universal Coverage" since mid-2003. Among them was Guy Carrin (1947–2011), a professor at the University of Antwerp who had published extensively on the economic and social aspects of social security. In 1990, he joined the WHO as senior health economist. Health economists were becoming more prominent, as many experts argued that bad management, unsound financial schemes, rapidly aging populations, and decreasing payroll contributions would soon make it impossible to afford traditional social security and national health systems. Health economists increased their status within the WHO with the creation of a Department of Health System Financing (HSF) in 2003. The Department was created by the merger of two preexisting units: one working on technical aspects of resource tracking, costing, and priority setting and the other on health-financing policy. Lee had supported the Department, in part because he was from South Korea, a country proud of its national health insurance, which required adequate financing and management. The Department was also strengthened by members of the WHO's Global Program on Evidence for Health Policy (GPE), including health economist David B. Evans. Two Rockefeller Foundation officials who had a keen interest in health equity added to the greater focus on health economics at the WHO: Ariel Pablos-Méndez, trained in medicine and public health, and Timothy Evans, trained in medicine and economics. In 2004, Pablos-Méndez led the Global Surveillance Project on Anti-Tuberculosis Drug Resistance and then became director of knowledge management. Tim Evans served as assistant director-general heading the Evidence, Information, Research, and Policy Clusters and overseeing the production of the annual World Health Report.

In 2003, the WHO Executive Board approved a document entitled "Social Health Insurance" that was seen as a means to reach universal health coverage. The term "Social Health Insurance" was on the agenda of the 2005 World Health Assembly and was expected to be approved as a resolution.[47] Most

---

[47] World Health Organization, "Social Health Insurance Document EB114/1," World Health Organization, Executive Board, 114th Session, May 26, 2004, apps.who.int/gb/archive/pdf_files/EB114/B114_PT2-en.pdf, last accessed October 21, 2017. World Health Organization, "Social Health Insurance, Report by the Secretariat," World Health Organization, Executive Board, 114th Session, May 26, 2004, apps.who.int/gb/archive/pdf files/EB114/B114_16-en.pdf, last accessed October 21, 2017.

members of the Assembly committee that discussed the document did not like its title and sought alternatives. These included "sustainable health financing," "universal coverage" and "sustainable health financing and universal insurance coverage."[48] US representatives preferred "universal insurance coverage," but this term was criticized by many European countries and by Brazil because it was perceived to mean the provision of medical services by a mix of private and public entities. They preferred a title that conveyed the idea of a public health system funded by the state that would include everyone, even those working in the informal sector. Finally, the 2005 Assembly approved Resolution WHA58.33 with a long title: "Sustainable Health Financing, Universal Coverage, and Social Health Insurance." The Resolution urged all member countries to establish prepayment financial contribution systems for health care and to plan the transition to universal coverage for their citizens to attain the MDGs and "Health for All." Also, in 2005, the WHO published the policy brief, *Achieving Universal Health Coverage: Developing the Health Financing System*, which argued in favor of reducing out-of-pocket payments and user fees that had been popular with the neoliberal health reformers of the 1980s.[49] After this publication, the term "universal health coverage" (UHC) became common, and "social health insurance" fell out of usage.

Before 2005, health economists used terms such as UHC to refer to an extension of private insurance and social security systems to the majority of people in developing countries who were uninsured and to the creation of a national health system in the only major industrial country that did not have one: the United States of America. After 2005, UHC conveyed three interconnected goals: first, coverage, or expanding high-quality health services; second, universality – providing access to these services to all; and third, making sure that accessing these services would not result in people falling into financial hardship or poverty. Initially, UHC supporters believed that a balance between these three goals was possible. Furthermore, some medical experts hoped that the "universality" goal of UHC could make it an entry point for the construction of integrated national health systems, where the state would play a prominent role. They believed that this could give everyone the same financial protection and access to the same range of high-quality services, regardless of employment status or ability to pay. It was an important distinction from the user-fees approach that was portrayed as a

---

[48] 58th World Health Assembly, May 16–25, 2005, Summary Records of Committees, Reports of Committees, WHA58/2005/REC/3 (Geneva: World Health Organization, 2005), apps.who.int/iris/handle/10665/20399, last accessed October 21, 2017.

[49] The 11-page document was intended for policy makers and was coauthored by Guy Carrin, Chris James, & David Evans, *Achieving Universal Health Coverage: Developing the Health Financing System* (Geneva: World Health Organization, 2005).

punishment of the poor.[50] Another important component was that good health services were no longer seen as a luxury in poor countries. Hopes were raised that the WHO would move beyond the disease-focused model and support interrelated prevention, treatment, and rehabilitation services. Some believed in a combination of UHC and the recommendations from the Commission on Social Determinants of Health, but it was not always clear how to combine UHC with anti-poverty programs. After 2008, the hopes for a holistic version of UHC began to wane.

The year 2008 was marked by the world economic crisis. It was the worst financial crisis since the Great Depression of the 1930s and a dramatic example of how unregulated markets can lead to stagnant economic growth, raise unemployment, produce misery, and cut government revenues and spending on public health. In the wake of the crisis, Chan expressed her profound disappointment with the business practices of globalization, which assumed that market forces were the perfect allocator of resources. Her words were strong and appeared dissonant to many of her earlier and more cautious statements:

Globalization was embraced as the rising tide that would lift all boats. This did not happen. Instead, wealth has come in waves that lift the big boats, but swamp or sink many smaller ones. Greater market efficiency, it was thought, would work to achieve greater equity in health. This did not happen ... I am not against free trade ... I am fully aware of the close links between greater economic prosperity, at household and national levels, and better health. But I do have to say this: the market does not solve social problems ... Globalization will not self-regulate in ways that favor fair distribution of benefits. Corporations will not automatically look after social concerns as well as profits.[51]

The governments of the United States and industrialized European nations chose to bail out banks despite protests from anti-globalization movements and resistance from much of their populations. This meant the loss of jobs and livelihoods and cutbacks in health spending and welfare programs that affected the poor. An article in *The Lancet* argued that the global financial crisis and subsequent austerity programs in high-income countries (the new code term for industrialized countries) resulted in a flatlining of development assistance for health (DAH) that had been growing consistently since the 1990s (with a dramatic surge since 2001). There was also a fear that this

---

[50] Robert Yates, "Universal Health Care and the Removal of User Fees," *The Lancet* 373:9680 (August 22, 2009), 2078–2081.

[51] Margaret Chan, "The Impact of Global Crises on Health: Money, Weather and Microbes, Address at the 23rd Forum on Global Issues," March 28, 2009, www.who.int/dg/speeches/2009/financial_crisis_20090318/en/, last accessed January 17, 2018.

assistance would decline.[52] More importantly, a global ideological shift to the right and a revival of conservatism occurred in many countries around the world, including low-income and middle-income countries (the new terms for developing nations). WHO officers feared that this shift would cause severe constraints on health spending and that any new plans for public health would have to be trimmed or shelved. In response to these concerns, the director-general convened a high-level consultation on the impact of the global financial and economic crisis. Ambitious proposals had to be postponed.[53]

The WHO tried to react to the crisis and beginning in 2009 appointed a panel of medical experts, academics, and health care officers. This panel asked industrialized countries to set aside fixed portions of their gross domestic product to finance global health, requested greater contributions from emerging industrial economies such as China and India, and entertained the idea of a global consumer tax on internet activity and financial transactions, such as paying bills online. (This was not the first time that global health tax ideas were discussed. UNITAID, which began in 2006 as an initiative of the governments of France, Brazil, Chile, Norway, and the UK to prevent, diagnose, and treat HIV/AIDS, tuberculosis, and malaria, was financed in part by a tax on airline tickets.) However, after being criticized by powerful financial institutions and governments, these ideas were dropped. According to the executive editor of *Fox News*, the real problem was tightwad middle-income economies, such as Brazil, Russia, India, China, and Saudi Arabia, that made small donations to the agency.[54]

In 2009, a landmark article, co-signed by Laurie Garrett, A. M. R. Chowdhury, and Ariel Pablos-Mendez, entitled "All for Universal Coverage," argued that UHC would help reduce poverty and promote human rights.[55] In the same year, the British prime minister, the director-general of the WHO, and the president of the World Bank met at the UN to support UHC and the commitment to free services at the point of delivery. In 2011, the 64th World Health Assembly approved another resolution (WHA64.9), entitled "Sustainable Health Financing Structures and Universal Coverage," part of a package of

[52] Dean Jamison, Lawrence H. Summers, George Alleyne et al., "Global Health 2035: A World Converging within a Generation," *The Lancet* 382:9908 (December 7, 2013), 1898–1955.
[53] Kammerle Schneider & Laurie Garrett, "The End of the Era of Generosity? Global Health amid Economic Crisis," *Philosophy, Ethics, and Humanities in Medicine* 4:1 (2009), 1–7.
[54] George Russell, "UN World Health Organization Faces Plague of Tightwads," *Fox News*, May 23, 2011, www.foxnews.com/world/2011/05/23/exclusive-world-health-organization-faces-plague-tightwads.html, last accessed May 1, 2018.
[55] Laurie Garrett, Mushtaque Chowdhury, & Ariel Pablos-Méndez, "All for Universal Health Coverage," *The Lancet* 374:9697 (October 10, 2009), 1294–1299.

five resolutions for strengthening health systems.[56] The WHO annual reports for 2010 and 2013 were devoted to UHC and entitled *Health Systems Financing: The Path to Universal Coverage* and *Research for Universal Health Coverage*.[57] The first report considered, as possible financial sources for UHC, new donations, a special levy on large profitable companies, a currency transaction levy, a financial transaction tax, and so-called sin taxes on alcohol and tobacco. A Conference on "Health Systems Financing - Key to Universal Coverage," convened by two German ministries on the occasion of the 2010 report, gathered almost thirty ministers of health from all over the world plus other government officials, politicians, and a few NGOs. The meeting promoted the idea of UHC not only as a package of limited medical services but of pooled funds. Chan insisted on getting rid of user fees and on the use of UHC for the strengthening of public health systems. Between the publication of these two reports, Margaret Chan made a decisive statement in 2012, shortly after she was elected for a second five-year term as head of the WHO: Universal health coverage was the most powerful concept that public health had to offer.[58] In 2013 at the 66th World Health Assembly, a passionate Jim Kim, the first non-economist to be president of the World Bank, supported UHC not only as a tool for better health services, but for inducing social change and the improvement of living conditions.

However, UHC has had its critics. Some argue that UHC wrongly overemphasizes health services and that after the economic crisis of 2008, UHC was reshaped as a "feasible" and decidedly cost-effective intervention. There was also an effort to pressure Michael Marmot to portray the social determinants of health as a subset of UHC, something he resisted. Marmot did not acquiesce and countered that full access to health services was good and necessary but by itself would not reduce health disparities.[59] Marmot also asked an essential question: How can an equality-inspired public good, such as UHC, flourish in societies where acute and unfair social inequalities are taken for granted? For one Indian researcher, Universal Health Coverage was a package that, instead of strengthening the full range of health services and emphasizing the change of living conditions where necessary, paid little

---

[56] Resolutions WHA64.6, WHA64.7, WHA64.8, WHA64.9, and WHA64.10, World Health Organization, *64th World Health Assembly, Geneva, 16–24 May 2011, Summary Records of Committees* (Geneva: World Health Assembly, 2011) [also available in WHA64/2011/REC/3], p. 338.

[57] World Health Organization, *World Health Report 2010: Health Systems Financing, Path to Universal Coverage* (Geneva: World Health Organization, 2010).

[58] Margaret Chan, "Universal Coverage Is the Ultimate Expression of Fairness, Acceptance Speech at the 65th World Health Assembly, Geneva, 23 May 2012," www.who.int/dg/speeches/2012/wha_20120523/en/index.html, last accessed October 21, 2017.

[59] Michael Marmot, "Universal Health Coverage and Social Determinants of Health," *The Lancet* 382:9900 (October 12, 2013), 1227.

attention to prevention and focused entirely on clinical care. In short, it was the "trojan horse" of blunt neoliberalism.[60] Of course, there were also critics on the right to whom UHC was a danger because it would mean more taxes, more governmental bureaucracy, and growing expenditures by governments. The issues surrounding UHC remain unresolved today.

---

[60] Imrana Qadeer, "Universal Health Care: The Trojan Horse of Neoliberal Policies," *Social Change* 43:2 (2013), 149–164.

11 The World Health Organization in the Second Decade of the Twenty-First Century

In the second decade of the twenty-first century, the World Health Organization was severely tested by an epidemic outbreak of Ebola in Africa. Not only was the WHO's ability to play a coordinating role in the global response to the epidemic widely questioned, but so was its very legitimacy as an international health agency. In the search for new approaches and institutional authority, the WHO appointed a new director-general from Africa and arrived at that outcome through a novel and transparent process that not only provided new leadership but attempted to address the current challenges of global health.

Ebola and the WHO's Controversial Response

In December 2013, a frightening hemorrhagic fever in West Central Africa attacked Guinea and some months later Liberia and Sierra Leone, eventually infecting more than 28,000 and killing more than 11,300. In March of 2014, it was scientifically confirmed that the hemorrhagic fever was Ebola, transmitted by the Zaire Ebolavirus. Scattered cases appeared in Mali, Nigeria, and Senegal and there was a danger that it could affect the rest of the world. Its swift and terrifying symptoms – internal and external bleeding and multiple organ failure – could kill in a few days. This outbreak would become the worst epidemic outbreak of Ebola virus ever known. The response was complicated from the outset because initially many suspected Lassa Fever, Yellow Fever, or some other disease since no previous major outbreak of Ebola had occurred in West Africa. Despite Ebola being known since 1976, existing medications were ineffective, and the disease was often misdiagnosed. There had been no investment in research to produce vaccines, specific antiviral drugs, or even point-of-care diagnostic tests. Little clinical training to treat the disease existed and the few previous studies by medical anthropologists detailing the risks involved in death burial practices (when the viral loads of the death were high) were not taken into account by health policy makers. Doctors could offer merely palliative care and were only certain of its mode of transmission: close contact with blood, secretions, or other body fluids of infected persons. Crucial aspects were left unexamined, such as characteristics of different Ebola virus species and the identification of an animal reservoir (African fruit bats were the most likely candidates).

To make matters worse, the affected African countries were all struggling economically and faced manpower shortages because they had endured harsh "structural adjustment" programs promoted by the World Bank that, among other things, eroded funding for public health. Other sociopolitical factors that explain the outbreak of the disease and the weak public health response were the protracted civil wars in Sierra Leone and Liberia, civil violence in Guinea, and massive migration from miserable rural areas to cities with little sanitation. In addition, a number of African-trained doctors had previously migrated to Europe and the United States to escape from low salaries and job insecurity. As a result, there was little health infrastructure and a severe shortage of health workers in the countries affected.

The first international responders were members of Doctors Without Borders, Oxfam, and other international NGOs, which mobilized both physicians and medical supplies such as face masks, boots, gloves, soap, and chlorine (used for disinfection). They also attended to water infrastructure, such as tanks and pipes. In June 2014, the head of Doctors Without Borders declared that the organization had reached its limits and was no longer able to send teams to new outbreak sites.[1] Developed countries were initially ambivalent about sending aid and then got caught up in the fear and anxiety that erupted when Ebola appeared among travelers. The first case of Ebola in the United States, the Liberian Thomas Eric Duncan, was identified in Dallas in late September and died in early October. In the weeks following Duncan's death, two health workers responsible for his care were both confirmed to be infected with Ebola.[2] Cases appeared in Spain, Italy, and the United Kingdom. Media around the world presented the dramatic cases of infected people and the equally dramatic medical paraphèrnalia of health workers protected from head-to-toe with goggles, aprons, taped closed gloves, and boots. Africans from south of the Sahara – it did not matter from what country – became targets of discrimination, as several airlines stopped flights to most of West Africa, disrupting business, trade, and tourism. (The camaraderie of health workers facing the ebola epidemic is suggested in Figure 11.1.)

It took until August 8, 2014, when the epidemic had already killed more than 1,000 people and was out of control in West Africa, for the WHO to declare Ebola a "Public Health Emergency of International Concern" (PHEIC), which meant that according to International Health Regulations it was a serious threat requiring a coordinated international response. The WHO sent

---

[1] "West Africa Ebola Epidemic Is 'out of control,'" *The Guardian*, June 23, 2014.
[2] Dorothy H. Crawford, *Ebola: Profile of a Killer Virus* (Oxford: Oxford University Press, 2016), p. 170.

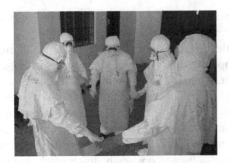

Figure 11.1 Health workers wearing protective equipment prepare to enter the Ebola treatment center at the Island Clinic in Liberia on September 30, 2014. They pray before starting their shift.
Credit WHO/Christopher Black. Courtesy: World Health Organization Photo Library.

experts, helped establish laboratories, supervised Ebola treatment centers, and tried its best at coordination. In August, and after some debate, the WHO also cautiously approved the use of experimental drugs to treat Ebola. The WHO's delay influenced other international organizations. Although before the WHO's intervention the World Bank made emergency funds available and USAID sent experts to West Africa, other donors did not appear until September and October when the situation was already critical. In mid-September 2014, when the death toll reached 3,091 of 6,574 suspected cases, Partners in Health provided medical assistance in Liberia and Sierra Leone and helped build rural health centers and train community health workers. Also in September, UNICEF mobilized an agency-wide response to Ebola, and the first-ever UN emergency mission, UN Mission for Ebola Emergency Response (UNMEER), was established. President Barack Obama sent US troops and health personnel to West Africa to build treatment centers and to supervise quarantines around these centers. The Americans joined health workers sent by the governments of Great Britain, Germany, China, France, Russia, Cuba, South Africa, Japan, and Germany. (An illustration of the work at the local level with the fatal victims of the disease is shown in Figure 11.2.)

In March 2015, Liberia was declared Ebola-free as part of a downward trend of the epidemic, which declined in Sierra Leone and Guinea as well. As the epidemic receded, the WHO came under heavy fire for not having reacted fast enough to the crisis when it had a better chance of controlling the outbreak. It was also criticized for failing to be a leader that avoided duplication of effort and for relying too heavily on International Health Regulations with no teeth. Many governments of industrialized and middle-income countries challenged the WHO's authority by imposing their own severe restrictions on travel and trade. For many, the agency and its Director-General

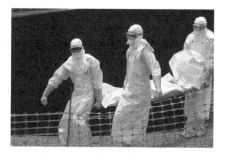

Figure 11.2 Staff of Doctors Without Borders carry the body of a person killed by Ebola in Guekedou, Guinea, on April 1, 2014.
Credit: SEYLLOU/AFP/Courtesy: Getty Images.

Margaret Chan in Geneva and the AFRO regional headquarters in Brazzaville proved inept and dysfunctional.

The relationship between Geneva and the WHO's African country offices, which were influenced by their national governments' fears of epidemic-related economic sanctions, was equivocal and sometimes confrontational. One African government, for example, decided to report only confirmed cases, not suspected and probable cases as formally required by the WHO. Yet the agency was portrayed as redundant because of the existence of other, better-funded global health organizations and at the same time was criticized for abandoning its responsibilities. For example, in September 2014, at the height of the epidemic, Chan downplayed the WHO's role in leading the fight against Ebola. In an interview with the *New York Times,* she declared that the WHO was not a "first responder" to epidemic outbreaks like Ebola because governments have "the first priority to take care of their people ... We are [also] not like international NGOs ... who are working on the ground." Although many believed that African countries were overwhelmed with chronic poverty and weak health systems, with hospitals often having no electricity and no isolation wards and generally ill-equipped to respond alone, Chan sometimes seemed to place the fault on Africa's "poor planning" in developing public health infra-structure and trained medical manpower.[3] Chan was portrayed in newspaper articles and academic reports as, at best, nothing more than a good "civil servant," not as a compelling world leader capable of inspiring or orchestrating other organizations in coordinated collective action.

Another explanation offered for the WHO's underestimation of the Ebola outbreak was that the agency was trying to avoid accusations of overreacting,

---

[3] Sheri Fink, "WHO Leader Describes the Agency's Ebola Operations," *The New York Times,* September 4, 2017.

as it was criticized for doing in 2009 when it too quickly designated the H1N1 flu pandemic a PHEIC. Furthermore, supporters of the WHO also argued that all global agencies underestimated the initial outbreak. In addition, they pointed out that the WHO was under-resourced because it had experienced severe cuts in its budget and staff; indeed, following the 2008 economic crisis it had reduced its staff by 20 percent, including a two-thirds cut to the emergency response staff.[4] According to Turshen and Gezmu, industrialized countries did not give the WHO the funds needed, instead favoring organizations that did not have long-term commitments to public health in the region. Moreover, they thought that the main problem of global epidemiological surveillance was the decline in financial resources received by the agency's regular budget since 1990. For example, the US government prioritized a bilateral response over a multilateral response and provided sizeable funds to NGOs. In August 2014, the WHO had requested USD 490 million from the international community to combat Ebola, but as of March 2015 the US government had only transferred a little more than USD 66 million to the health agency.[5] Thus, for some experts the main problem was the insufficient resources given to the WHO for surveillance. However, that was not the main conclusion of experts' panels that examined the response of the health agency during the epidemic.

At least four different major international panels came together to propose how the WHO should improve in response to the lessons of the Ebola epidemic. The first and least critical was established in 2015: the UN Panel on the Global Response to Health Crises. More critical was an independent commission on a "Global Health Risk Framework for the Future," created by the US National Academy of Medicine in 2015 with an international group of experts. Its members included Paul Farmer of Harvard's Medical School Department of Global Health and Social Medicine and cofounder of Partners in Health and Julio Frenk, then president of the University of Miami. As with other investigative commissions, one or more Africans were included. In this case it was Oyewale Tomori, president of the Nigerian Academy of Science. The National Academy's final report, "The Neglected Dimension of Global Security: A Framework to Counter Infectious Disease Crises," condemned the attitude for "waiting until the crisis hits" and criticized the WHO for doing little to help to solve the dramatic problem that less than a third of its members met the requirements of the 2005 International Health Regulations, and

---

[4] Kate Kelland, "The World Health Organization's Critical Challenge: Healing Itself," *Reuters*, February 8, 2016, www.reuters.com/investigates/special-report/health-who-future/, last accessed April 29, 2018.

[5] Meredeth Turshen & Tefera Gezmu, "The World Health Organization and the Ebola Epidemic," in Ibrahim Abdullah & Ismail Rashind (eds.), *Understanding West Africa's Ebola Epidemic; Towards a Political Economy* (London: Zed, 2017), p. 246.

because it did not have sound mechanisms to engage with non-state actors. The problem with the IHR requirements was that they were approved under the assumption that governments would develop robust national disease surveillance systems. However, there was no funding for this project and many developing countries simply could not afford the cost. The NAM report also identified the need to have clear criteria to specify what a Public Health Emergency of International Concern was. More importantly, it undermined the WHO's formal leadership in global heath by supporting the World Bank's proposal to create a new and independent Pandemic Emergency Financing Facility and recommended the creation of an autonomous Center for Health Emergency Preparedness and Response, overseen by a governing board possibly chaired by the WHO's DG but with members drawn from outside the WHO.[6]

A critical report also came from a third independent panel, this one convened by Harvard University and the London School of Hygiene and Tropical Medicine, in early 2015. It was chaired by Peter Piot who was then director of LSHTM and included Muhammad Pate, former Nigerian minister of state for health; Sophie Delaunay from Doctors Without Borders; Laurie Garrett, affiliated with the Council on Foreign Relations; and Lawrence O. Gostin of Georgetown University.[7] The panel issued a hard-hitting report in November of 2015, later published as an article in *The Lancet*. The report contained a proposal for a new WHO program on "Outbreaks and Emergencies," with a substantial budget and a unified workforce that would answer directly to the director-general. Toward the end of the article, criticism of Margaret Chan's non-assertive leadership style was included indirectly in comments about the forthcoming 2017 election of director-general: "Restoring credibility demands that WHO institutionalizes accountability mechanisms ... [M]ember states should insist on a dynamic leader ... with the character and capacity to challenge even the most powerful governments when necessary."[8]

Finally, the WHO itself set up an Independent Oversight and Advisory Committee in 2015 following a recommendation of a special session of the Executive Board. One of this committee's conclusions was that there were

---

[6] Commission on a Global Health Risk Framework, *The Neglected Dimension of Global Security: A Framework to Counter Infectious Disease Crises*, 2016, http://nam.edu/wp-content/uploads/2016/01/Neglected-Dimension-of-Global-Security.pdf, last accessed April 29, 2018.

[7] Lawrence O. Gostin was the author of influential studies on Ebola and the WHO, such as Gostin & Eric Friedman, "Ebola: A Crisis in Global Health Leadership," *The Lancet* 384 (October 8, 2014), 1323–1325, and Lawrence O. Gostin, "The Future of the World Health Organization: Lessons Learned from Ebola," *Milbank Quarterly* 93 (2015), 475–479.

[8] Suerie Moon, Devi Sridhar, Muhammad A. Pate et al., "Will Ebola Change the Game? Ten Essential Reforms before the Next Pandemic. The Report of the Harvard-LSHTM Independent Panel on the Global Response to Ebola," *The Lancet* 386 (November 22, 2015), 2204–2221, p. 2217.

unjustifiable delays in the WHO's declaration of a "Public Health Emergency of International Concern." The Committee called on wealthy states to provide funding to support the development of disease surveillance systems in poor countries and urged the WHO to create a "Multidisciplinary Global Health Emergency Workforce" and establish a "Contingency Fund for Emergencies" (CFE) as part of its process of internal reform. The other issue that was very much in mind in this report was how the WHO could dramatically improve its response to current epidemic outbreaks (In October of 2015, Brazil reported an epidemic of Zika, primarily transmitted by the bite of an infected mosquito *Aedes aegypti*, and an association between Zika virus infection and microcephaly.)

The Ebola outbreak exposed structural and financial weaknesses not only in the World Health Organization but in other global health organizations as well. For example, during the latter stages of the epidemic, US Democrats accused Republicans of having slashed the budget of the Centers for Disease Control and Prevention, thus preventing it from playing a greater role in the international response to the disease. But above all, the Ebola crisis exposed the result of years of first flatlining and then reducing resources for basic functions of the agency, namely global epidemiological surveillance, helping to improve and expand local laboratory capacities and establishing a staff ready for rapid response to outbreaks, and exposed the limits of the leadership style of the WHO director-general. Eventually, Margaret Chan took responsibility for the WHO's failures, in her last speech to the World Health Assembly in 2017: "WHO was too slow ... This happened on my watch, and I am personally accountable."[9]

The Budget and International Health Governance

The Ebola epidemic revealed the need to solve a series of the WHO's problems, notably how it finances its work and the limited control it has over how its money is spent. More than two-thirds of the money spent by the WHO in recent years came from earmarked voluntary "extrabudgetary" donations, which are very different from assessed contributions. The latter are dues determined by a country's wealth and population which the WHO can allocate as it sees fit. It is also important to note that 80 percent of WHO voluntary contributions come from just 20 sources and more than half of them are made by the governments of industrialized nations. The trend, transparency, pace, and size of these donations are generally unpredictable. Since 2012, the Bill and Melinda Gates Foundation has been the second largest contributor to the

---

[9] Margaret Chan, "Address to the Seventieth World Health Assembly," May 22, 2017, www.who.int/dg/speeches/2017/address-seventieth-assembly/en/, last accessed April 30, 2018.

WHO, after the United States government. Donations from powerful bilateral agencies and private foundations meant that important decisions about programs occur outside the realm of the World Health Assembly. The WHO has struggled unsuccessfully to increase assessed contributions and thus to have more autonomy in setting its own priorities.

Within the agency, extrabudgetary donations have created a competition among directors of WHO programs and between headquarters and the regional offices. Another effect has been that the agency is dominated by disease-control donations. In 2016, the WHO spent about USD 71 million on AIDS, USD 61 million on malaria, and USD 59 million on TB. Yet polio eradication was funded with more than USD 450 million, thanks to sizeable contributions from Gates, Rotary Clubs International, and other donors. Although the eradication of polio was a valuable effort, the disease only existed in a few countries, yet the polio funds were about a quarter of the WHO's overall budget. Even though the agency has been able to use some of these funds to cross-subsidize other activities – including using polio funds for 74 percent of all WHO salaried workers in Africa – and to use polio eradication infrastructure to stop outbreaks of yellow fever, cholera, and meningitis, it is possible that these funds will evaporate when the disease is eradicated with no other significant financial resources directly targeted to strengthen health systems.[10] Moreover, there was a general perception that the agency wasted its resources. According to newspaper accounts, the budget of the WHO was so carelessly administered that high officers of the WHO were allowed to spend far too much money on travel (USD 200 million in 2017). The WHO responded to criticism by saying that travel was an essential function of the agency and that in the future it was going to control the travel of its officers more strictly. The whole discussion had an aura of unfairness since the agency has a budget smaller than that of major hospitals in Western Europe or the United States.[11]

Funding problems were also related to the implementation of decisions. Before 1990, the World Health Assembly often approved resolutions with a rough estimate of the costs of implementation provided by the Secretariat, and there was confidence that funds would exist. However, in recent years it has not been clear if funds exist in the WHO's budget for resolutions that imply costs. As a result, there has been a frequent gap between expected deliverables and budget requirements, so that complementary funds need to

---

[10] Joshua Busby, Karen Grépin, & Jeremy Youde, "The World Health Organization Just Picked a New Leader. These are the Challenges He Faces," *The Washington Post,* June 15, 2017.

[11] "Report: Cash-Strapped UN Health Agency Spends about $200 million a Year on Travel," *CBS News,* May 21, 2017, www.cbsnews.com/news/world-health-organization-un-agency-spends-big-on-travel-report/, last accessed May 11, 2018.

be sought through donations – or certain resolutions just never come to fruition, whatever their political support.

The funding problem was also related to global health governance and leadership. The WHO's weak and unstable finances contributed to fragmented leadership in global health. Over the past few years, bilateral agencies such as USAID, private donors like the Gates Foundation, special multilaterals like UNAIDS and the World Bank, and public-private organizations like the Global Fund to Fight AIDS, Tuberculosis, and Malaria all outpaced the WHO in financial terms and challenged its traditional leadership role. Yet the decline of the WHO did not mean the emergence of a distinctive new leader or a new global health order. Paraphrasing Altman, the specific situation with the WHO and global health leadership is similar to what some critics denounce as a general consequence of economic globalization, namely the weakened power of national states and multilateral agencies without effective substitutes.[12]

Since 2007 a tentative solution to the problem of leadership in global health has been tried in the form of "H8," sometimes called "the Davos" of global health. It is an unofficial, non-voting, eight-member body made up of the heads of four UN agencies (the WHO, UNICEF, UNAIDS, and UNFPA), three health financing institutions (the World Bank, the Global Fund, and GAVI), and the Bill and Melinda Gates Foundation. H8 first tried to strengthen efforts to achieve the Millennium Development Goals (MDGs), but it has concentrated in the past few years on coordinating health initiatives and determining international priorities. However, there are questions about its transparency and fairness since the H8 holds meetings behind closed doors, does not keep a website, and the body is dominated by Americans (since only the WHO, UNAIDS, and UNFPA are not currently led by US nationals).

A New Director-General: Tedros from Ethiopia in Historical Context

In May of 2017, the WHO underwent an important change in the election of its eighth director-general. The election took place openly at the World Health Assembly, unlike previous elections in closed-door sessions of the Executive Board. The short list of candidates were: the British physician David Nabarro, Ethiopia's former minister of health Tedros Adhanom Ghebreyesus (who goes by "Tedros"), and the Pakistani physician Sania Nishtar. A veteran of the UN who recently had been UN secretary-general's special envoy on Ebola, Nabarro was supported by donor countries and Prime Minister Theresa May

---

[12] The idea is discussed in Dennis Altman, "Globalization, Political Economy and HIV/AIDS," *Theory and Society* 18:4 (1999), 559–584.

(however, a handicap for Nabarro was the 2016 vote of the UK electorate to leave the EU – known as the Brexit vote – which suggested that multilateralism was not going to be a value of the British government). Nominated candidates now made their electoral platforms available in a web forum and addressed the Health Assembly before the vote. The vote came out in favor of the 52-year-old Tedros, who became the first director-general from Africa.

The process and the outcome must be understood in historical context. Beginning in 1988, African candidates had attempted repeatedly to win the director-general position, but without success. One of the reasons was the dynamics of the non-transparent election process. The traditional procedure required member states to propose candidates between June and September of the year prior to the election. These candidates were then considered by the Executive Board, which in a private session that took place in January of the election year, nominated a single person by secret ballot. If necessary, voting by the EB continued in successive rounds – with fierce diplomatic intervention and negotiation at each step. The candidate with the fewest votes was eliminated at each stage until a winner emerged. Sometimes as many as five voting rounds were needed. The winner of the election was "recommended" to the World Health Assembly, which met in May and rubber-stamped the Board's choice. Although EB members were expected to vote as representatives of their governments, they had significant autonomy through the secret ballot system, and governments had little means of compelling their representatives to vote in accordance with official instructions. Ministries of foreign affairs tried to negotiate and would pledge to back another country's candidates for various UN positions in exchange for DG votes. The decisions also had an impact on other UN agencies (for example, the election of Candau as director-general ended the candidacy of another Brazilian, Paulo Carneiro, who was running to be head of UNESCO).[13] The candidates themselves relied on the financial resources and diplomatic connections of their governments to pay for country visits and aggressive lobbying campaigns in attempts to sway the EB vote. Behind-the-scenes political maneuvering for the DG post normally began up to two years in advance, even though the formal nomination period lasted only a few months.

Initially, African states had no influence as a separate group, but as decolonization proceeded in the 1950s and 1960s, newly independent African countries joined Asian and Latin American nations and gained influence. By the early twenty-first century, Africa with 40 member states had the largest number of members in the World Health Assembly. Affluent countries also promoted candidates or groomed other candidates if their first choice was

---

[13] "WHO Nomination," February 17, 1953, RFA, RG 2–1953, Series 100, Box 7, Folder 45, RAC.

defeated in the first round. A common trend in the EB elections was to oppose candidates who openly supported the "Health For All" Primary Health Care agenda, as many African candidates did before 2017.

In 1988, the Japanese Hiroshi Nakajima was elected in what *Le Monde* called the end of the Anglo-Saxon hegemony at the WHO. Nakajima's election took four rounds of voting in the Executive Board, and criticism of the DG election process was widespread afterwards.[14] Nakajima was regarded by many as a supporter of traditional biomedical interventions and an authoritarian manager. His competitors in 1988 were Carlyle Guerra de Macedo, a Brazilian physician heading the Pan American Health Organization and a champion of immunization programs; Gottlieb L. Monekosso of Cameroon, the regional director for Africa and a firm supporter of Primary Health Care; and Hussein A. Gezairy of Saudi Arabia, who promoted the modernization of medical education, and was the director of the WHO's Eastern Mediterranean Regional Office. Nakajima received 17 of the 31 votes cast by members of the EB who participated in the election.[15]

Nakajima's 1993 reelection campaign was dogged by his past missteps, especially the rude dismissal of the WHO's deputy director, Mohammed Abdelmoumene of Algeria, who had decided to run against him as a candidate, with the support of the United States, the European Community, and Canada. Also, there were accusations of generous contracts offered by the director-general to nationals of the countries represented on the Executive Board and promises of appointments in return for votes. An incident reported by Laurie Garrett suggests attempted bribery at WHO headquarters in Nakajima's reelection: A furious East African health minister flung a rug into a marbled hallway, shouting: "A rug? You think you can buy my vote with a rug?"[16] In May 1993, Nakajima was reelected for his second term as DG by a vote of 18 to 13. Rumors and accusations circulated within the agency, alleging under-the-table deals and Japanese promises of aid to developing countries. Nakajima's reelection was the only time that there was doubt that the EB vote would be ratified. The EB decision went to the General Assembly, where Nakajima won by a 93-to-58 margin.

Because of the controversy surrounding Nakajima's second-term election, changes were made in the bylaws. In 1996 it was decided to limit DGs to two terms and to establish a prior short list of eligible candidates. Even so, interviews and the vote itself still took place in private Executive Board

---

[14] Cited in "All the Change at WHO," *The Lancet* 331:8596 (May 28, 1988), 1201–1202.

[15] Ilona Kickbusch & Austin Liu, *Electing the WHO Director-General, Global Health Center Working Paper No 16* (Geneva: Graduate Institute of International and Development Studies, 2017), p. 24.

[16] Donald McNeill, "The Campaign to Lead the World Health Organization Global Health," *The New York Times*, April 3, 2017.

sessions. All DGs elected after Nakajima faced stiff challenges. Gro Harlem Brundtland of Norway was elected in 1998 with 18 votes of the 32 members of the Board in the fourth round, after a strong challenge from George Alleyne from Barbados, who was then director of the Pan American Health Organization. It is important to note that the Gambian candidate Ebrahim Samba, director of the WHO's prestigious Onchocerciasis Control Programme and regional director of AFRO from 1995 to 2005, was defeated in a previous round. In 2003 Jong-wook Lee became DG after beating the Belgian Peter Piot, head of UNAIDS, by one vote in the fifth round and outpacing Pascoal Mocumbi, the candidate from Mozambique who was a strong advocate of primary care and who had initially been the frontrunner.

By this time the election process had become increasingly controversial. One of the criticisms was that most candidates never published proposals for public scrutiny and there was no forum for debate. An editorial in *The Lancet* was eloquent: "This strangely closed process breeds ... intrigue."[17] In a 2002 radio conversation between David Nabarro, then a senior policy advisor at the WHO, and the editor-in-chief of *The Lancet*, Richard Horton, Horton described the DG election as:

a process typical of a totalitarian regime of 20 years ago. It's secret. It's non-transparent, it's non-accountable. There will be no formal debate associated with the election process. A group of men will meet in a room in January and cast a vote secretly. We have no idea what the criteria will be ... This is an antediluvian process.[18]

Nabarro, responded vaguely: "There are aspects of our organization in need of improvement."

The Lancet attempted to stimulate the transparency of the process by creating a section of the journal with articles about the different candidates that appeared before the decisive EB meeting in January 2003. Additionally, the WHO's World Health Channel organized a two-hour question and answer session with the candidates a few days prior to this meeting. This session was open to the public and the video was broadcast to sites in Brazil, Ethiopia, India, Japan, the United Kingdom, South Africa, and the United States. The WHO also changed some of its rules. The Executive Board drew up a short list. Of the initial eight candidates, those who failed to secure at least 10 percent of the Executive Board votes were excluded, resulting in a

---

[17] "The Future of the World Health Organization," *The Lancet* 360:9348, (December 7, 2002), 1798.

[18] "NewsHour BBC Guests David Nabarro and Richard Horton, editor-in-chief, *The Lancet*, moderator Owen Bennett-Jones" December 6, 2002 13.45 GB 0809 /4/2 2 of 2 2002–2003; Clare Kapp, "WHO's Executive Board Election Proceedings are Low-Key and Secretive," *The Lancet* 360:9347 (November 30, 2002), 1753.

short list of five candidates. Later, Board members interviewed the five candidates carefully and examined their platforms.

The three longest-lasting candidates in 2003 were Pascoal Mocumbi, Peter Piot, and Jong-wook Lee. The former prime minister of Mozambique, Mocumbi was opposed by the governments of some industrialized countries because he was a socialist. Lee had secured votes from Latin American countries, but he now also collected votes from African countries when Mocumbi fell in the fourth round. Victory went to the lesser-known South Korean candidate Lee, after a 16-to-16 tie with Piot was broken by the secret vote of one country (either the United States or the United Kingdom) that changed its vote from Piot to Lee.[19] The defeat of Mocumbi was viewed by African countries and several developing countries as a blow, and during Lee's term these nations tried to push for changes in how the DG would be chosen, including the possibility that geographical rotation should be a consideration in the next election. These efforts were cut short when Lee died suddenly.

After Lee's death in May 2006, the EB selected, by a majority vote, the Hong Kong–born physician Margaret Chan over four other candidates: Julio Frenk (who for *The Lancet* was "the objective frontrunner"), Shigeru Omi of Japan (the WHO's director for the Western Pacific), Bernard Kouchner (the French founder of Médecins Sans Frontières), and, again, Pascoal Mocumbi.[20] This final group had been short-listed from an original list of 13.[21] According to a critical article in *The British Medical Journal*: "In this contest, sadly, there seems to be no guarantee that the best person will necessarily win. Rather, it seems to be the most astute politician who will triumph ... [P]romises continue to be made and favors dangled by rich nations to their poorer fellow WHO members."[22]

Chan's candidacy was backed by significant Chinese promises to developing nations throughout the world, especially to African countries.[23] Chan was reelected for a second five-year term in 2012 in an unchallenged election (no other candidate was proposed). After Chan's reelection, new guidelines to

---

[19] Curtis F. J. Doebbler, "WHO's Reality Check: The Election of a New Director-General for the World Health Organization," INTLawyers, May 20, 2017, intlawyers.wordpress.com/2017/05/20/whos-reality-check-the-election-of-a-new-director-general-for-the-world-health-organization/, last accessed April 30, 2018.

[20] The reference to Frenk appears in David Brown, "Field of 11 Candidates Competes to Head WHO," *Washington Post,* November 5, 2006.

[21] David Brown, "Field of 11 Candidates Competes to Head WHO," *The Washington Post*, November 5, 2006.

[22] Anne Glusker, "Who Will Lead WHO?" *British Medical Journal* 333:7575 (November 4, 2006), 938.

[23] Laurie Garret, "Who's Going to Be the Next Leader of WHO?" *Foreign Policy,* May 22, 2017, policy.com/2017/05/22/whos-going-to-be-the-next-leader-of-who/, last accessed September 28, 2017.

promote "transparency and fairness" began to be introduced. The EB, which now had 34 members, would nominate three candidates in a secret ballot, and country representatives at the World Health Assembly would vote to choose the winner.[24] But there was now also a concern for the lack of transparency in the election of other officers at the WHO. Some regional offices had unlimited possibilities for reelection of their directors. An extreme example was Hussein A. Gezairy, who between 1982 and 2012 served for 30 years as regional director of the Eastern Mediterranean Office, and his predecessor, Abdul Hussein Taba from Iran, had served as regional director from 1957 to 1982. New codes of conduct for nomination of regional directors were now introduced. New rules standardized the submission of CVs and proposals, regulated the funding and conduct of candidates in electoral campaigns, and established disclosure of campaign activities like meetings, travel, and visits.[25]

In May 2017, the DG election took place at the 70th World Health Assembly following an unprecedented, one-country, one-vote, secret ballot procedure. For the first time, representatives from 194 countries elected a DG. The final three candidates, selected by the Executive Board from a longer list of six, were Nabarro, Tedros, and Nishtar, and each addressed the Health Assembly before the vote. According to a newspaper that sympathized with Tedros, it was time to break the "WHO's African leadership glass ceiling" and recognize that real progress could only be possible if "leaders of global institutions are from the communities most affected" by the problems those institutions try to address.[26] The final tally was 133 votes for Tedros (roughly two-thirds) versus 50 for Nabarro. Support from developing and middle-income countries was decisive in Tedros' victory. The selection of an African candidate from a poor developing country, the first DG from the Global South, was celebrated by cheerful African delegates with high-fives.

Tedros (see Figure 11.3) was the first health professional not trained as a physician to direct the WHO. He had a doctoral degree in community health from the University of Nottingham and a master of science in the immunology of infectious diseases from the University of London. He had political experience as a former health minister (2005–2012) and minister of foreign affairs

[24] Elizabeth Fee, "Whither WHO? Our Global Health Leadership," *American Journal of Public Health* 106:11 (2016), 1903–1904.

[25] "Annex 1: Code of Conduct for the Election of the Director General of the World Health Organization," in World Health Organization, Sixty-Sixth World Health Assembly, Resolutions and Decision, Geneva, May 20–27, 2013, WHA66/2013/REC/1, pp. 35–45, http://apps.who.int/gb/ebwha/pdf_files/WHA66-REC1/A66_REC1-en.pdf#page=57, last accessed March 10, 2018.

[26] Peter A. Singer & Jill W. Sheffield, "Breaking the WHO's Glass Ceiling," *Project Syndicate*, January 23, 2017, www.project-syndicate.org/commentary/who-director-general-ghebreyesus-africa-by-peter-a–singer-and-jill-w–sheffield-2017-01?barrier=accessreg, last accessed April 30, 2018.

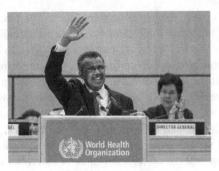

Figure 11.3 Tedros Adhanom Ghebreyesus of Ethiopia waves after his election as the WHO's director-general on May 23, 2017, in Geneva. Previously he served in the Government of Ethiopia as minister of health and minister of foreign affairs. He also had been board chair of The Global Fund to Fight AIDS, Tuberculosis and Malaria. He is the first African to head the World Health Organization.
Credit: FABRICE COFFRINI/AFP/Courtesy: Getty Images.

(2012–2016) in Ethiopia. He was also known among global health experts because in 2009 he was chairman of the board of the Global Fund to Fight AIDS, Tuberculosis, and Malaria and had previously served as chair of Roll Back Malaria. During his DG election campaign, Tedros said that he was a strong believer in Universal Health Coverage; rapid and focused response to health emergencies; women's, children's and adolescents' health; health impacts of climate and environmental change; and a reformed WHO. Tedros also embraced the agenda articulated in 2015 as the UN Sustainable Development Goals (SDGs) for 2030 which recognize the huge impact of noncommunicable diseases, climate change, and extreme poverty and supported Universal Health Coverage as one of the central health targets of the SDGs. Most experts celebrated Tedros' election as an opportunity for greater legitimacy and accountability for the WHO. However, he has had to face cuts in global health. In February 2018, the Trump administration released its proposed budget for Fiscal Year of 2019 with a 30 percent decrease in the foreign affairs activities, including programs managed by USAID and Department of State. At the same time, other industrialized countries have reduced or downgraded their development agencies, thus reducing funds for global health.

Tedros responded promptly to health emergencies, such as the 2017 cholera outbreak in Yemen and an epidemic of pneumonic plague in Madagascar, and was praised. In addition, under his command the WHO has promised to ensure timely and adequate responses to epidemic outbreaks and humanitarian emergencies by increasing the investment in the WHO Health Emergencies Program. But he has also been criticized for his decision to appoint 93-year-old

President Robert Mugabe, Zimbabwe's longtime dictator, as goodwill ambassador on non-communicable diseases for Africa (apparently in return for the African votes that made possible his election). After an outrage, Tedros changed his mind and rescinded the appointment. He has also been questioned on his appointment of a little-known Russian official to run the WHO's tuberculosis program one month after a meeting with President Vladimir Putin, using a fast-track process that circumvented the normal hiring process. His decision to appoint more women to the WHO's top management, including both of his deputy director-generals, has been greeted more favorably. Moreover, he has been criticized for his overemphasis on Universal Health Coverage instead of the support of universal and public health systems.

Tedros still has to do more work on contentious and disruptive institutional issues such as supporting a sustained process of internal reform, achieving better alignment between headquarters and regional offices, revising the functions of its more than 150 national offices, and enforcing enhanced performance mechanisms. Another critical issue is the composition of the WHO's professional staff, which is still dominated by physicians. In the view of some, the WHO has an insufficient number of social scientists and almost no health activists despite its recent adoption of the Framework for Engagement with Non-State Actors, which can bring to the WHO the concerns of marginalized people and health activists and hold governments accountable. On January 2018, the WHO's Executive Board approved a five-year work program containing three ambitious goals, the "Triple Billion" targets to be achieved by 2023: 1 billion more people with universal health coverage, 1 billion more people protected from health emergencies, and 1 billion more people enjoying better health. The WHO also organized in 2017 a major Global Conference on Primary Health Care, held at Astana, Kazakhstan, in Russia, to approve a Declaration where Universal Health Coverage appeared as the center of global and national health agendas.

Looking to the Past; Looking Ahead

The Executive Board's "Triple Billion" targets and Tedros' promise to revive Primary Health Care no doubt struck many in global health as the WHO's latest episode of starry-eyed idealism whose reappearance under Director-General Tedros casts a shadow over the future of the organization. But the organization now has 194 member states and a solid seventy-year history during which it has accomplished much. Despite its periods of challenge and crisis, the WHO has in fact played a decisive role in the substantial improvements in health indicators around the globe. The WHO has contributed to great advances in life expectancy, reductions in infant mortality, the eradication of smallpox, the spread of immunization, and the decline in the number of

Table I: *Election for Director-General of the World Health Organization, 1988–2017*

Year	Round	Winner	Closest competitor	Other candidates	Other
1988	4th	Hiroshi Nakajima (Japan)	Carlyle Guerra de Macedo (Brazil)	Gottlieb L. Monekosso (Cameroon) · Hussein A. Gezairy (Saudi Arabia)	
1993	?	Hiroshi Nakajima (Japan)	Mohammed Abdelmoumene (Algeria)		93/58 vote General Assembly
1998	4th	Gro Harlem Brundtland (Norway)	George Alleyne (Barbados)	Ebrahim Samba (The Gambia) · Uton Muchtar Rafei (Indonesia)	Nafis Sadik (Pakistan)
2003	5th	Jong-wook Lee (S. Korea)	Peter Piot (Belgium)	Awa Marie Coll-Seck (Senegal) · Pascoal Mocumbi (Mozambique)	Julio Frenk (Mexico)
2006		Anders Nordström (Sweden) Acting DG			
2007	4th	Margaret Chan	Julio Frenk (Mexico)	Kazem Behbehani (Kuwait) · Elena Salgado (Spain)	Shigeru Omi (Japan) · Pascoal Mocumbi
2012		Margaret Chan	Only one candidate proposed		
2017	General Assembly	Tedros Adhanom Ghebreyesus (Ethiopia)	David Nabarro (UK)	Sania Nishtar (Pakistan)	

Sources: "WHO Director-General – The Candidates," *BBC News*, Monday, January 26, 1998, last accessed September 10, 2017, http://news.bbc.co.uk/2/hi/special_report/1998/health/47205.stm, Donald McNeill and notes 579–592.

endemic communicable diseases. In addition, the WHO has helped to control neglected tropical diseases, drastically limited the consumption of tobacco, and helped to provide anti-AIDS drugs to millions of people living with HIV. The WHO has also been a clearinghouse for epidemiological information, provided emergency relief in crisis situations, launched ambitious disease-control programs, constructed a network of medical scientists and public health experts around the globe, supported the right to health of postcolonial nations, promoted links between human rights and health, championed medications as global public goods, and produced stirring proposals for social and health changes. In addition, although the WHO has worked mostly by consensus among governments, it has enjoyed considerable moral authority and many of its recommendations have been implemented in national legislation.

Some have written the history of the WHO quite differently and focus on a narrative of decline from an earlier "golden age" to its current much-diminished state. This declension narrative presumes that during its first decades through the 1970s, the WHO was the unquestioned leader of international health, yet it slipped seriously in authority and influence beginning in the 1980s.[27] But, in fact, an unchallenged WHO that singlehandedly set the agenda for international health never existed. The agency was shaped from its early years by political entanglements and budgetary constraints that compromised its work and restricted its autonomy. Heavy-handed influence by the United States and European colonial powers was clear in the late 1940s and 1950s. In the first World Health Assembly of 1948, the US delegation set out strict boundaries to restrict the activities of the agency: "The WHO should concentrate its efforts on a limited number of major public health problems of international importance for which scientific knowledge and practical experience justify a hope of early positive results at a minimum cost of money and of personnel."[28] In 1949, a worried US surgeon general wrote to Martha Eliot, assistant director-general of the WHO from 1949 to 1951, complaining that the UN and the WHO were "featherbedding" their administrative structures and asserting that the United States should impose a ceiling on its contribution to the health agency and that it would be "folly" for the WHO to "embark on any program which attempts to cover every conceivable area of medicine and public health."[29]

---

[27] As argued in José Carlos Escudero, "What Is Said, What Is Silenced, What Is Obscured: The Report of the Commission on the Social Determinants of Health," *Social Medicine* 4:3 (2009), 183–185.

[28] "General Statement on Program of WHO by USA Delegation, First World Health Assembly," Folder 743, Box 55, Marta M. Eliot Papers [AESL].

[29] Leonard A. Scheele to Marta M. Eliot, August 29, 1949, Folder 753, Box 56, Martha M. Eliot Papers [AESL].

The US government had specific ideas about which programs the WHO should pursue. Malaria eradication was a major one, and in 1960 when the WHO's regular budget was USD 16,330,900, the largely US-funded and separately administered Malaria Eradication Special Account was budgeted for USD 18,197,726.[30] When the WHO disengaged from malaria eradication, the United States invested its considerable resources differently. In the late 1970s, USD 650 million of US donations to international health went to several organizations and hundreds of different programs, meaning that the pressure and influence of industrialized donor countries and especially the United States existed well before the supposed loss of WHO autonomy in the 1980s.[31]

The WHO's twists and turns were part of a set of internal gyrations along a path marked by the changing fortunes of two perspectives, neither of which achieved complete dominance inside or outside the agency. Their relative usefulness and comparative effectiveness have been matters of debate throughout the WHO's history. The first perspective presumes that changes in health require large social transformations and views health as an essential right of citizenship and one of the fundamental duties of nation states. The second perspective emphasizes technologically driven health interventions and programs organized around disease control and, in the rare case, eradication. In this perspective, public health is validated as a tool for economic productivity and national security, in contrast to the first perspective, which links public health to the goals of solidarity and equity. In the second perspective, patients and their families are primarily passive recipients of health programs, and their active participation is not necessarily required. A few WHO programs, such as smallpox eradication and the Global Program on AIDS, successfully blended these two perspectives, but the WHO's major programs have tended to reflect one agenda or the other.

The WHO was created in the 1940s when the influence of European social medicine, at its peak in the 1930s, was still strong. This broad vision was incorporated into the Preamble to the 1948 WHO Constitution but downplayed in the eradication initiatives of the 1950s and 1960s that reflected the rise to dominance of the biomedical view, which glorified technical interventions as the answer to all health problems. The social medicine perspective was strongly revived in 1978 with the Declaration of Alma-Ata and the launching of the Primary Health Care movement. In the 1980s the Global AIDS Program

[30] Lee, "WHO and the Developing World," pp. 24–45, p. 29.
[31] Peter Bourne, Memorandum for the President November 17, 1977, *Jimmy Carter Presidential Library, Collection: Office of Staff Secretary*; Series: Presidential Files; Folder: 11/18/77; Container 51, www.jimmycarterlibrary.gov/digital_library/sso/148878/51/SSO_148878_051_08.pdf, last accessed April 30, 2018.

asserted a close link between public health and human rights, and since then strong voices within the WHO have insisted that social reform and human rights be at the forefront of all global health initiatives. In the early twenty-first century, the Commission on Social Determinants of Health advocated interventions to end unjust social relations and political realities that lead to poor health and massive health disparities. The ideas and work of the Commission continue to influence public health professionals both inside and outside of the WHO, showing clearly the persisting influence of the social medicine perspective.

The technocratic perspective was hegemonic in the disease-control and eradication campaigns of the 1950s and 1960s, the population control and family-planning programs of the 1970s, and the Selective Primary Health Care interventions of the 1980s. Supporters of this perspective portray disease and extreme poverty as "natural" conditions that new technologies, good administration, charitable funding, and intelligently cost-effective programs can control. Advocates of this perspective criticize advocates of the first for being too idealistic and for asking public health workers to solve problems beyond their reach, such as poverty and seemingly unbridgeable gaps between poor and rich nations.

The WHO's ambivalent and shifting embrace of the social-medical and technocratic perspectives has shaped the organization internally but has also influenced its ability to deal with dramatically changing external realities. In the late twentieth century, the agency had difficulty adapting to the end of the Cold War. It simultaneously began to lose power and was trapped by the growing weight of bureaucratic procedures. It also had to contend with a new external reality of "economic globalization" with links to neoliberal politics. This new political-economic context was dramatically different from what prevailed during early years when it operated with nation states confident in UN agencies. Another important external change that came in the wake of the AIDS epidemic was a dramatic increase in health activism. As it was built to deal with governments, the WHO lacked the flexibility to deal with civil society organizations. Then with the turn of the twenty-first century, the proliferation of non-state actors, the relative disempowerment of nation states, and the growing hegemony of global caretaker organizations like the World Bank, the International Monetary Fund, the World Trade Organization, and new transnational philanthropies have compromised the UN system as a whole. To make matters more difficult, the emergence of authoritarian governmental and political reforms and neoliberalism are dangerously challenging multilateralism, democracy and global health governance. One result is that global economic and health policies are now frequently in conflict.

What should be the role of the WHO in the future? How can its leaders and staff advocate for democratic decisions as well as community participation in global health in the face of modern trends? How can the agency confront the recent losses of positive aspects of globalization such as the care of immigrants, transnational cooperation, and the availability of financial resources for health? How can it promote solidarity and collective action in an increasingly socially fractured and politically divided world? How can the WHO respond rapidly to epidemic outbreaks and at the same time sustain preventive efforts and robust institution-building processes? These are serious questions that must be addressed.

If this historical account can help in any way to answer these questions we would urge our readers to draw lessons from history. This means, in part, to recover the value and true meaning of health multilateralism that sustains the beliefs that any individual in the world has the right to physical and mental health and that free and open collective cooperation between nations is an imperative and that it is an obligation of all countries to make these health and social rights realities and promote health in the face of states unwilling to fulfill their obligations. We also urge readers to commit to the value of a holistic understanding of health, sometimes but not consistently championed by the WHO. In the past few decades, grassroots health activists have kept alive that holistic vision and we believe that their continuing commitment will also contribute to the reinvention of the WHO.

Bibliography

1 Primary Sources

1.1 Archives and Special Collections

Archives and Special Collections. Columbia University Health Sciences Libraries. New York.
    Frank A. Calderone Papers.
The Arthur and Elizabeth Schlesinger Library on the History of Women in America, Radcliffe Institute for Advanced Study at Harvard University, Cambridge, Massachusetts [AESL].
    Martha M. Eliot Papers, MC 229.
    Interview with Martha A. Eliot, November 1973–May 1974, Family Planning.
    Oral History Project, Cartoon 2, Schlesinger Library.
Center for the History of Medicine. Francis A. Countway Library of Medicine. Harvard University. Cambridge, Massachusetts.
    American Society of Tropical Medicine and Hygiene, Records. HMSc192.
Harry S. Truman Presidential Library and Museum. Independence, Missouri.
League of Nations Archives. United Nations Archives. Geneva [LNA-UNG].
    Series Health 8A. Years 1920–1942.
    Series Personnel S. Years 1919–1946.
National Archives and Records Administration. College Park, Maryland [NARA].

US Department of State records. Record Group 59. Years 1946–1962.

National Library of Medicine, History of Medicine Division, Archives and Modern Manuscripts. Bethesda, Maryland [NLM].

Eugene P. Campbell Papers. Years 1941–1986. MS C 467.

Howard B. Calderwood, World Health Organization Development Collection. Years 1945–1963. MS C 171.

Fred Lowe Soper Papers. Years 1919–1975. MS C 359.

Princeton University Library, Department of Rare Books and Special Collections. Princeton, New Jersey [PUL].

Collection Henry R. Labouisse Papers, MC199, Mudd Manuscript Library.

Rockefeller Archive Center. Sleepy Hollow, New York [RAC].

Rockefeller Foundation Archives. Record Group 1.1. Record Group 2, Record Group 6.1. Years 1922–1939.

Collection Population Council, Series Administration Files. Year 1968.

United Nations Archives. New York [UN-NY].

Series 0544. Year 1948.

Wellcome Library. Archives and Manuscripts. London [WLAM].

Melville Douglas Mackenzie papers.

Leonard J. Bruce-Chwatt papers.

Carl Wahren, Secretary-General, International Planned Parenthood. Federation papers. Years 1973–1984.

World Health Organization Archives. Geneva. [WHO]

Archives of the *Office International d'Hygiène Publique* (OIHP). Years 1907–1946.

Archives of the United Nations Relief and Rehabilitation Administration (UNRRA). Years 1943–1946.

Brock Chisholm papers. Years 1948–1953.

Halfdan Mahler papers. Years 1977–1988.

Hiroshi Nakajima papers. Years 1988–1998.

First Generation Files. Years 1945–1955.

Second Generation of Files. Years 1950–1955.

Third Generation of Files. Years 1955–1983.

Fourth Generation of Files. Years 1985–1996.

1.2 Official Journals and Periodical Publications

Bulletin of the World Health Organization. Years 1937–1946; 1847–1989.

Chronicle of the Health Organization. Years 1939–1981.

Department of State Bulletin. Years 1939–1989.

Monthly Letter. Division of Malaria Eradication. WHO. Years 1955–1955.

Official Records of the World Health Organization, 1946–1999.

Press Releases. World Health Organization. Years 1954–2002.

Public Health Reports. Years 1950–1995.

Quarterly Bulletin of the Health Organisation of the League of Nations. Years 1933–1937.

Sante du Monde. Years 1958–1959.
United Nations Bulletin. Years 1948–1954.
World Health. Years 1957–1998.
World Health Forum. Years 1980–1998.
World Health Organization Newsletter. Years 1947–1955.

1.3 Official Publications

Most of these publications can be found in the libraries of the World Health
  Organization (Geneva), the Wellcome Library (London), the National Library of
  Medicine (Bethesda), the Library of Congress (Washington, DC), and the Library
  of Columbia University (New York).
*A World Summit of Ministers of Health and Programmes for AIDS Prevention, London
  26–28, January 1988* (Geneva: Pergamon Press, 1988).
Akin, John S. *Financing Health Services in Developing Countries: An Agenda for
  Reform* (Washington, DC: World Bank, 1987).
Basu, R. N., Z. Jezek, & N. A. Ward. *The Eradication of Smallpox from India*
  (New Delhi: World Health Organization, South-East Asia Regional Office,
  1979).
Bruce-Chawtt, Leonard J. *Malaria at the Rio Congresses 1963: A Review of Papers on
  Malaria Presented at the Seventh International Congresses on Tropical Medicine
  and Malaria, Rio de Janeiro, September 1963* (Geneva: World Health
  Organization, 1963).
Canada. Department of National Health and Welfare. *A New Perspective on the
  Health of Canadians/Nouvelle Perspective de la Sante des Canadiens* (Ottawa:
  n.p., 1974).
Carrin, Guy, Chris James, & David Evans. *Achieving Universal Health Coverage:
  Developing the Health Financing System* (Geneva: World Health Organization,
  2005).
Djukanovic, Vojin & Edward P. Mach (eds.). *Alternative Approaches to Meeting Basic
  Health Needs of Populations in Developing Countries: A Joint UNICEF/WHO
  Study* (Geneva: World Health Organization, 1975).
Egypt. Ministry of Public Health. *Annual Report of the Department of Laboratories for
  the Year 1948* (Cairo: Government Printing Press, 1951).
Fenner, F., D. A. Henderson, I. Arita, Z. Jezek, & I. D. Ladnyi. *Smallpox and Its
  Eradication* (Geneva: World Health Organization, 1988).
Fleming, Alan F., Manuel Carballo, David W. FitzSimons, Michael R. Bailey, &
  Jonathan Mann (eds.). *The Global Impact of AIDS* (New York: Liss, 1988).
Francis, Rene. *Public Health in Egypt* (Cairo: n.p., 1951).
*Global Challenge of AIDS-Ten Years of HIV/AIDS Research, Proceedings of the Tenth
  International Conference on AIDS/International Conference on STD, Yokohama,
  August 7–12, 1994* (Tokyo: Karger, 1991).
Institute of Medicine. *America's Vital Interest in Global Health: Protecting Our
  People, Enhancing Our Economy, and Advancing Our International Interests*
  (Washington, DC: National Academy Press, 1997).
*President's Emergency Plan for AIDS Relief, PEPFAR Implementation: Progress
  and Promise* (Washington, DC: National Academies Press, 2007).

International Health Conference, New York, 19 June to 22 July 1946, Report of the United States Delegation, Including the final Acts and Related Documents (Washington, DC: US Government Printing Office, 1947).

Joarder, A. K., D. Tarantola, & J. Tulloch. *The Eradication of Smallpox from Bangladesh* (New Delhi: World Health Organization, South-East Asia Regional Office, 1980).

Joseph, S. C. *Bellagio, Conference to Protect the World's Children: Rapporteur's Summary* (New York: Rockefeller Foundation, 1984).

Kaprio, Leo. *Forty Years of WHO in Europe: The Development of a Common Health Policy* (Copenhagen: World Health Organization Regional Publications, 1991).

League of Nations. *Pan-African Health Conference (1935, Johannesburg)* (Geneva: League of Nations, 1936).

League of Nations Secretariat, Information Section. *The Health Organization of the League of Nations* (Geneva: n.p., 1923).

Staff List' of the Secretariat, Showing Nationalities and Salaries for 1932 (Geneva: League of Nations, 1932).

McDonald, Larry. "WHO Infant Formula Code," 2 August 1982. United States of America, Congressional Record, Proceedings and Debates of the 96th Congress, First Session, vol. 128, Part 14, 29 July to 5 August 1982 (Washington, DC: US Government Printing Office, 1982), p. 18928.

Memorandum Prepared in the Department of State for the White House, 29 May 1953. In William Z. Slany & Ralph R. Goodwin (eds.), *Foreign Relations of the United States, 1952–1954, vol. III United Nations Affairs* (Washington, DC: US Government Printing Office, 1979), pp. 70–73.

Ministry of Public Health. *Egypt Annual Report of the Department of Laboratories for the Year 1947* (Cairo: Government Press, 1950).

Office International d'Hygiène Publique. *Vingt-cinq ans d'activité de l'Office International d'Hygiène Publique, 1909–1933* (Paris: The Office, 1933).

Session Ordinaire du Comité Permanent (Paris: Office International d'Hygiene Publique, 1947).

Ottawa Charter for Health Promotion (Ottawa, Ontario: n.p., 1986).

Pampana, Emilio. *A Textbook of Malaria Eradication* (London: Oxford University Press, 1963).

Proceedings of the International Sanitary Conference, Fifth, Washington, DC, 1881 (Washington, DC: US Government Printing Office, 1881).

Proceedings of the Sixth International Congresses on Tropical Medicine and Malaria, Lisbon, September 5–13, 1958 (Lisbon: Instituto de Medicina Tropical, 1959).

Roemer, Ruth. *Legislative Action to Combat the World Tobacco Epidemic* (Geneva: World Health Organization, 1993).

Rubenson, Brigitta. "What the World Council of Churches is doing about AIDS," *Contact A bi-monthly publication of the Christian Medical Commission, World Council of Churches, Geneva 117* (December 1990).

Sachs, Jeffrey D. (ed.). *Macroeconomics and Health: Investing in Health for Economic Development: Report of the Commission on Macroeconomics and Health* (Geneva: World Health Organization, 2001).

Salas, Rafael M. *International Population Assistance: The First Decade: A Look at the Concepts and Policies which Have Guided the UNFPA in its First Ten Years* (New York: Pergamon Press, 1979).

Shell Oil Company. *Annual Report 1956* (New York: Shell Oil Company, 1956).

The Global Eradication of Smallpox: Final Report of the Global Commission for the Certification of Smallpox (Geneva: World Health Organization, 1980).

United Nations Development Group. *Indicators for Monitoring the Millennium Development Goals: Definitions, Rationale, Concepts and Sources* (New York: United Nations, 2003).

Population Program Assistance, United States Aid to Developing Countries (Washington, DC: US Government Printing Office, 1974).

United States. Agency for International Development. *Population Program Assistance, Annual Report 1975* (Washington, DC: USAID, 1976).

United States. Central Intelligence Agency. *Global Infectious Disease Threat and Its Implications for the United States* (Washington, DC: Central Intelligence Agency, 2000).

United States of America. Committee on Foreign Affairs House of Representatives. *Eightieth Congress, First Session, Hearings before Subcommittee No.5 – National and International Movements: A Joint Resolution Providing for Membership and Participation by The United States in the World Health Organization and Authorizing an Appropriation Therefore, 13, 17 June and 3 July 1947* (Washington, DC: US Government Printing Press, 1947).

United States. Congress. *Congressional Record, Proceedings and Debates of the 83rd Congress Second Session, Vol. 100—Part 5, 29 April 1954 to 25 May 1954* (Washington, DC: US Printing Gov. Office, 1954).

Congressional Record, Proceedings and Debates of the 83rd Congress, Second Session Volume 100-Part 4, April 1, 1954 to April 28, 1954 (Washington, DC: US Government Printing Office, 1954).

United States. Congress, Senate. *Committee on Labor and Human Resources. Subcommittee on Public Health and Safety. Global Health: U.S. Response to Infectious Diseases: Hearing Before the Subcommittee on Public Health and Safety of the Committee on Labor and Human Resources* (Washington, DC: US Government Printing Office, 1988).

Senate. *Committee on Government Operations. Subcommittee on Foreign Aid Expenditures. Population crisis: Hearings, Eighty-Ninth Congress, First Session 5 vols* (Washington, DC: US Government Printing Office, 1966).

HIV/AIDS, TB and Malaria: Combating a Global Pandemic, Hearing before the Subcommittee on Energy and Commerce, House of Representatives, One Hundred and Eight Congress, 20 March 2003. (Washington, DC: US Government Printing Office, 2003).

United States. Department of State. *American Foreign Policy, Current Document, 1956* (Washington, DC: US Government Printing Office, 1959).

The Foreign Assistance Program, Annual Report to the Congress, Fiscal Year 1968 (Washington, DC: US Government Printing Office, 1968).

World Health Organization (Washington, DC: Department of State, 1987).

United States Participation in the UN, Report by the President to the Congress for the year 1987 (Washington, DC: US Government Printing Office, 1988).

United States Participation in the UN, Report by the President to the Congress for the Year 1989 (Washington, DC: US Government Printing Office, 1990).

United States Participation in the UN, Report by the President to the Congress for the Year 1991 (Washington, DC: US Government Printing Office, 1992).

United States Participation in the UN, report by the President to the Congress for the year 1992 (Washington, DC: US Government Printing Office, 1993).

United States Participation in the United Nations, Report by the President to the Congress for the Year 1993 (Washington, DC: US Government Printing Office, 1994).

United States Participation in the United Nations, A Report to the President for the Year 1995 (Washington, DC: US Government Printing Office, 1995).

United States. Environmental Protection Agency. *DDT: a Review of Scientific andEconomic Aspects of the Decision to Ban Its Use as a Pesticide: Preparedfor Committee on Appropriations, U.S. House of Representatives* (Washington, DC: U.S. Environmental Protection Agency, 1975).

United States. General Accounting Office. *Report to Congressional Requesters, July 1998* "HIV/AIDS, USAID and UN Response to the Epidemic in the Developing World", GAO/NSIAD-98–202 (Washington, DC: The Office, 1998).

United States Government. Accountability Office. *Global Health: The Global Fund to Fight AIDS, TB and Malaria is responding to Challenges but needs Better Information and Documentation for Performance-based Funding, Report to Congressional Committees* (Washington, DC: US Government Printing Office, 2005).

United States. House of Representatives. *Hearings before the subcommittee on Africa of the Committee of Foreign Affairs, House of Representatives, One Hundred First Congress, First Session, June 14 and July 1989* (Washington, DC: US Government Printing Office, 1990).

United States, National Intelligence Council. *The Global Infectious Disease Threat and Its Implications for the United States, No. NIED 99–17D* (Washington, DC: National Intelligence Council, 2000).

Van Zile Hyde, Henry. *World Health Organization – Progress and Plans* (Washington, DC: US Government Printing Office, 1948).

Challenges and Opportunities in World Health: The First World Health Assembly (Washington, DC: US Government Printing Office, 1948).

World Bank. *World Development Report 1993. Investing in Health* (New York: Oxford University Press, 1993).

Confronting AIDS: Public Priorities in a Global Epidemic (New York: Oxford University Press, 1997).

Division of Public Information. WHO Special Features (Geneva: World Health Organization, 1953).

Expert Committee on Malaria. Malaria Terminology: Report of a Drafting Committee Appointed by WHO (Geneva: World Health Organization, 1953).

World Health Organization. *First International Symposium on Yaws Control* (Geneva: World Health Organization, 1953).

The First Ten Years of the World Health Organization (Geneva: World Health Organization, 1958).

The Second Ten Years of the World Health Organization, 1958–1967 (Geneva: World Health Organization, 1968).

People Report on Primary Health Care (1985), 6–9 (Geneva: World Health Organization, 1985).

From Alma-Ata to the Year 2000: Reflections at the Midpoint (Geneva: World Health Organization, 1988).

A Global Strategy for Malaria Control (Geneva: World Health Organization, 1993).

The World Health Report 1995 - Bridging the Gaps (Geneva: World Health Organization, 1995).

"Rapid Response to Emerging Disease," *World Health Forum* 17 (1996).

World Health Organization, *The World Health Report 1996 - Fighting Disease, Fostering Development* (Geneva: World Health Organization, 1996).

Division of Emerging and other Communicable Diseases Surveillance and Control, EMC. Annual Report 1997 (Geneva: World Health Organization, 1997).

Publishing for a Purpose: Fifty Years of Publishing by the World Health Organization (Geneva: World Health Organization, 1998).

Evidence and Information for Policy. Health Systems: Improving Performance (Geneva: World Health Organization, 2000).

The Onchocerciasis Control Programme, Success in Africa: The Onchocerciasis Control Programme in West Africa, 1974–2002 (Geneva: World Health Organization, 2002).

The World Health Report 2002 – Reducing Risks, Promoting Healthy Life (Geneva: World Health Organization, 2002).

Department of Reproductive Health and Research. *Reproductive Health Strategy, to Accelerate Progress towards the Attainment of International Development Goals and Targets* (Geneva: World Health Organization, 2004).

The World Health Report 2004 – Changing History (Geneva: The World Health Organization, 2004).

The World Health Report – 2005: Make Every Mother and Child Count (Geneva: The World Health Organization, 2005).

Working Together for Health: The World Health Report 2006 (Geneva: World Health Organization, 2006).

The Third Ten Years of the World Health Organization, 1968–1977 (Geneva: World Health Organization 2008).

World Health Report 2010 – Health Systems Financing, Path to Universal Coverage (Geneva: World Health Organization, 2010).

The Fourth Ten Years of the World Health Organization, 1978–1987 (Geneva: World Health Organization, 2011).

Resolutions WHA64.6, WHA64.7, WHA64.8, WHA64.9, and WHA64.10. World Health Organization, Sixty-Fourth World Health Assembly, Geneva, 16–24 May 2011, Summary Records of Committees (Geneva: World Health Organization, 2011).

Fifty-Eight World Health Assembly, 16–25 May 2005, Summary Records of Committees Reports of Committees, WHA58/2005/REC/3 (Geneva: World Health Organization, 2005) [apps.who.int/iris/handle/10665/20399 last accessed 7 September 2017].

Health for all in the 21st Century (Geneva: World Health Organization, 1998).

Department of Women's Health. Review of WHO's Work Related to the Implementation of the Program of Action of the International Conference on Population and Development (ICPD) (Geneva: World Health Organization, 1999).

World Health Organization, Regional Committee for Africa, Summary of Statement made by Brock Chisholm, 31 July 1952, p. 21, Second Session, Monrovia, Regional Committee & Report of the Regional Director 4 August 1952, Third Session, Kampala, Regional Committee, 13 August 1953.

World Health Organization. Regional Office for the Eastern Mediterranean. Summary minutes, 7 February 1949, Cairo, First Session, Regional Committee.

Regional Office for South-East Asia. "Conditions of Service of Public Health Personnel," August 4, 1949, New Delhi, Second Session, Regional Committee.

Regional Office for South-East Asia. Report of the Regional Director, 17 August 1950, New Delhi, Third Session, Regional Committee.

Regional Committee for Africa. Annual Report of the Regional Director, 13 August 1952. Third Session, Kampala, Regional Committee.

Regional Committee for Africa. Annual Report of the Regional Director, 1 July 1956–30 June 1957 15. Seventh Session, Brazzaville, Regional Committee.

Regional Office for South-East Asia. *Twenty Years in South-East Asia, 1948–1967* (New Delhi: World Health Organization, 1967).

Regional Office for South-East Asia. *A Decade of Health Development in South Asia 1968–1977* (New Delhi: World Health Organization, Regional Office for South-East Asia, 1980).

Regional Office for Europe. *Concepts and Principles of Health Promotion: Report on a WHO Meeting, Copenhagen, 9–13 July 1984* (Copenhagen: World Health Organization, 1984).

Regional Office for the Western Pacific Region. *Fifty Years of the World Health Organization in the Western Pacific Region* (Manila: WHO Regional Committee for the Western Pacific, 1988).

Regional Office for South-East Asia. *Health Care in South-East Asia* (New Delhi: World Health Organization Regional Publications South-East Asia Series No 14, 1989).

3 by 5 December 2003 through June 2004 Progress Report (Geneva: World Health Organization, 2004).

Western Pacific Region, SARS, How a Global Epidemic Was Stopped (Geneva: World Health Organization, 2006).

1.4 Internet

Bourne, Peter. Memorandum for the President November 17, 1977. *Jimmy Carter Presidential Library, Collection: Office of Staff Secretary*; Series: Presidential Files; Folder: 11/18/77; Container 51, www.jimmycarterlibrary.gov/digital_library/sso/148878/51/SSO_148878_051_08.pdf, last accessed April 30, 2018.

Chan, Margaret. "The Impact of Global Crises on Health: Money, Weather and Microbes, Address at the 23rd Forum on Global Issues, March 28, 2009," www.who.int/dg/speeches/2009/financial_crisis_20090318/en/, last accessed January 17, 2018.

"Universal Coverage is the Ultimate Expression of Fairness. Acceptance speech at the Sixty-fifth World Health Assembly Geneva, 23 May 2012," www.who.int/dg/speeches/2012/wha_20120523/en/index.html, last accessed February 3, 2017.

"Address to the Seventieth World Health Assembly," May 22, 2017, www.who.int/dg/speeches/2017/address-seventieth-assembly/en/, last accessed April 30, 2018.

A Conversation between Mahendra Dutta and Bill Foege, July 10, 2008, David J. Sencer CDC Museum at the Centers for Disease Control and Prevention and Emory University, www.globalhealthchronicles.org/items/show/3537, last accessed March 17, 2017.

Doebbler, Curtis F. J. "WHO's Reality Check: The Election of a New Director-General for the World Health Organization," INTLawyers, May 20, 2017, intlawyers.wordpress.com/2017/05/20/whos-reality-check-the-election-of-a-new-director-general-for-the-world-health-organization/, last accessed April 30, 2018.

Fink, Sheri. "WHO Leader Describes the Agency's Ebola Operations," *The New York Times*, September 4, 2017, www.nytimes.com/2014/09/04/world/africa/who-leader-describes-the-agencys-ebola-operations.html, last accessed April 22, 2018.

Garret, Laurie. "Who's Going to Be the Next Leader of WHO?" *Foreign Policy,* May 22, 2017, policy.com/2017/05/22/whos-going-to-be-the-next-leader-of-who/, last accessed September 28, 2017.

Interview with Dr. William Foege by Victoria Harden, July 13, 2006, David J. Sencer CDC Museum at the Centers for Disease Control and Prevention and Emory University, www.globalhealthchronicles.org/items/show/3516, last accessed March 1, 2017.

Interview with Zafar Husain, Smallpox Campaigner, India, *PBS* Series, www.pbs.org/wgbh/peoplescentury/episodes/livinglonger/husaintranscript.html, last accessed July 18, 2017.

Kelland, Kate. "The World Health Organization's Critical Challenge: Healing Itself," *Reuters*, February 8, 2016, www.reuters.com/investigates/special-report/health-who-future/, last accessed April 29, 2018.

Lee, Jong-wook. "Meeting of the G8 Health Ministers, Moscow, Russian Federation, 28 April 2006," www.who.int/dg/lee/speeches/2006/g8_health_ministers_meeting/en/index.html, last accessed October 21, 2017.

Lee, Jong-wook & Peter Piot. "3 by 5" Progress report, December 2004, www.who.int/3by5/progressreport05/en/, last accessed May 30, 2017.

Office International d'Hygiène Publique. *Vingt-Cinq Ans D'Activite de L'Office International d'Hygiene Publique, 1909–1933* (Paris: Office International d'Hygiene Publique, 1933), www.who.int/library/collections/publique_hygiene_1909_1933.pdf, last accessed April 25, 2017.

Oral History Interview with Henry Van Zile Hyde, July 14 and 16, 1975, www.trumanlibrary.org/oralhist/hydehvz.htm, last accessed December 3, 2016.

"Report: Cash-Strapped UN Health Agency Spends about $200 Million a Year on Travel," *CBS News*, May 21, 2017, www.cbsnews.com/news/world-health-organization-un-agency-spends-big-on-travel-report/, last accessed May 11, 2018.

Russel, George. "UN World Health Organization Faces Plague of Tightwads," *Fox News*, May 23, 2011, www.foxnews.com/world/2011/05/23/exclusive-world-health-organization-faces-plague-tightwads.html, last accessed May 1, 2018.

Transcript of an oral interview with Professor Milton P. Siegel by Mr Gino Levy with the participation of Norman Howard-Jones. Tape One, November 15, 1982, www.who.int/archives/fonds_collections/special/milton_siegel_tapes.pdf, last accessed September 19, 2017.

"The Price of Being Well," *The Economist,* August 28, 2008, www.economist.com/node/12009974, last accessed October 21, 2017.

The Vatican and World Population Policy: An Interview with Milton P. Siegel by Stephen D. Mumford, www.population-security.org/29-APP3.html, last accessed September 19, 2017.

World Health Organization. First World Assembly, Provisional Verbatim Records of the Eleventh Plenary Meeting, July 10, 1948, A/VR/11. Corr.1, apps.who.int/iris/bitstream/10665/98641/1/WHA1_VR-11_eng.pdf, last accessed November 25, 2017.

Regional Office for Europe. "The Charter against Tobacco, 1988," www.euro.who.int/__data/assets/pdf_file/0003/115338/E93946.pdf, last accessed February 3, 2017.

Tobacco Free Initiative, Framework Convention on Tobacco Control: Report of the WHO Meeting of Public Health Experts, December 2–4, 1998 (Geneva: World Health Organization, 1998), www.who.int/tobacco/media/en/vancouver.pdf, last accessed October 21, 2017.

Secretariat to the Fifty-Sixth World Health Assembly, March 31, 2003, Provisional agenda item 14.4, A56/12, apps.who.int/iris/bitstream/10665/78238/1/ea5612.pdf, last accessed August 20, 2017.

"Global Health-Sector Strategy for HIV/AIDS," Fifty-Sixth World Health Assembly, May 28, 2003. Agenda Item 14.4, WHA56.30, apps.who.int/iris/bitstream/10665/78339/1/ea56r30.pdf, last accessed August 20, 2017.

Social Health Insurance Document EB114/1. World Health Organization, Executive Board, 114th Session, May 26, 2004, apps.who.int/gb/archive/pdf_files/EB114/B114_PT2-en.pdf, last accessed October 21, 2017.

Social Health Insurance, Report by the Secretariat. World Health Organization, Executive Board, 114th Session, April 29, 2004, apps.who.int/gb/archive/pdf_files/EB114/B114_16-en.pdf, last accessed February 1, 2017.

Progress on Global Access to HIV Antiretroviral Therapy, an Update on "3 by 5" June 2005 (Geneva: The World Health Organization, 2005), www.who.int/3by5/publications/progressreport/en/, last accessed March 1, 2017.

Fifty-Ninth World Health Assembly. Resolution: Implementation by WHO of the Recommendations of the Global Task Team on Improving AIDS Coordination among Multilateral Institutions and International Donors. May 27, 2006. WHA59.12, apps.who.int/iris/bitstream/10665/21437/1/A59_R12-en.pdf, last accessed March 1, 2017.

Sixty-Sixth World Health Assembly, Resolutions and Decision, Geneva, May 20–27, 2013. WHA66/2013/REC/1, pp. 35–45, http://apps.who.int/gb/ebwha/pdf_files/WHA66-REC1/A66_REC1-en.pdf#page=57, last accessed March 10, 2018.

1.5 Newspapers

The Boston Globe, 1988–1990.
The Economist, 2008.
The Guardian, 2014.
The New York Times, 1946; 2017.
The Wall Street Journal, 1975–1979.
The Washington Post, 1977–1979; 2017.

1.6 Interviews

Marmot, Michael. Interview with Marcos Cueto, London, January 18, 2017.

2 Secondary Sources

2.1 Books and Articles

Abbassi, Kamran. "Education and Debate. The World Bank and World Health: Interview with Richard Feachem," *British Medical Journal* 318 (1999), 1206–1208.
Abel, Emily K., Elizabeth Fee, & Theodore M. Brown. "Milton I. Roemer: Advocate of Social Medicine, International Health, and National Health Insurance," *American Journal of Public Health* 98:9 (2008), 1596–1597.
Aguayo, Sergio. *Myths and [mis]Perceptions: Changing US Elite Visions of Mexico* (San Diego: Center for US-Mexican Studies at the University of California, 1998).
Ahluwalia, Sanjam & Daksha Parmar. "From Gandhi to Gandhi: Contraceptive Technologies and Sexual Politics in Post-Colonial India, 1947–1977," in Rickie Solinger & Mie Nakachi (eds.), *Reproductive States: Global Perspectives on the Invention and Implementation of Population Policy* (New York: Oxford University Press, 2016), pp. 124–155.
"All the change at WHO," *The Lancet* 331:8596 (28 May 28, 1988), 1201–1202.
Altman, Dennis. "Globalization, Political Economy and HIV/AIDS," *Theory and Society* 18:4 (1999), 559–584.
Amrith, Sunil S. *Decolonizing International Health, India and South Asia, 1930–1965* (Hapshire: Plagrave, 2006).
Anciaux, Alain. *Le Docteur Rene Sand ou la Culture des Valeurs Humaines* (Bruxelles: Universitaires de Bruxelles, 1988).
"Annexe II Au Procès-Verbal de la 10e Séance-Jeudi 31 Octobre 1946," in Office International d'Hygiene Publique, *Session Ordinaire du Comité Permanent* (Paris: Office International d'Hygiene Publique, 1947).
Arita, Isao, John Wickett, & Frank Fenner. "Impact of Population Density on Immunization Programs," *Journal of Hygiene* 96 (1986), 450–466.
Balińska, Marta A. *For the Good of Humanity: Ludwik Rajchman, Medical Statesman* (Budapest: Central European University Press, 1998).
Barona Vilar, Josep L. "International Organisations and the Development of a Physiology of Nutrition during the 1930s," *Food and History*, 6:1 (2008), 129–162.
Barros, James. *Betrayal From Within: Joseph Avenol, Secretary-General of the League of Nations, 1933–1940* (New Haven: Yale University Press, 1969), pp. 185–188.
Bashford, Alison (ed.). *Medicine at the Border: Disease, Globalization and Security, 1850 to the Present* (New York: Palgrave Macmillan, 2006).
Baxby, Derrick. "Should Smallpox Virus be Destroyed? The Relevance of the Origins of Vaccinia Virus," *Social History of Medicine* 9:1 (1996), 117–119.
Beigbeder, Yves. *The World Health Organization* (The Hague: M. Nijhoff, 1998).
Bellamy, Carol, Peter Adamson, Sheila B. Tacon et al. (eds.). *Jim Grant: UNICEF Visionary* (Florence, Italy: UNICEF, 2001).

Berkov, Robert. *The World Health Organization: A Study in Decentralized International Administration* (Geneva: Droz, 1957).

Le Berre, Ronan, J. Frank Walsh, Bernard Philippon et al. "The WHO Onchocerciasis Control Programme: Retrospect and Prospects," *Philosophical Transactions of the Royal Society of London. Series B, Biological Sciences*, 328:1251 (June 30, 1990), 721–727.

Berridge, Virginia. *AIDS in the UK: The Making of policy, 1981–1994* (New York: Oxford University Press, 1996).

Bhattacharya, Sanjoy (ed.). *Expunging Variola: The Control and Eradication of Smallpox in India, 1947–1977* (New Delhi: Orient Longman, 2006).

"The World Health Organization and Global Smallpox Eradication," *Journal of Epidemiological Community Health* 62:10 (2008), 909–912.

Bhattacharya, Sanjoy & Sharon Messenger (eds.). *The Global Eradication of Smallpox* (New Delhi: Orient BlackSwan, 2010).

Biraud, Yves & P. M. Kaul. "World Distribution and Prevalence of Cholera in Recent Years," *Epidemiological and Vital Statistics Report, Monthly Supplement to the Weekly Epidemiological Records* 1:7 (1947), 141–152.

Birn, Anne-Emanuelle. "Gates's Grandest Challenge: Transcending Technology as Public Health Ideology," *The Lancet* 366:9484 (March 11, 2005), 514–519.

"The Stages of International (Global) Health: Histories of Success or Successes of History?" *Global Public Health* 4:1 (2009), 50–68.

"Backstage: The Relationship between the Rockefeller Foundation and the World Health Organization, Part I: 1940s–1960s," *Public Health* 128:2 (2014), 129–140.

Black, Maggie. *Children First: The Story of UNICEF, Past and Present* (Oxford: Oxford University Press, 1996).

Borowy, Iris. *Coming to Terms with World Health: The League of Nations Health Organization, 1921–1946* (Frankfurt am Main: Peter Lang, 2009).

Uneasy Encounters: The Politics of Medicine and Health in China, 1900–1937 (Frankfurt am Main; Peter Lang, 2009).

Bloom, Barry B., David E. Bloom, Joel E. Cohen, & Jeffrey D. Sachs. "Investing in the World Health Organization," *Science* 284:5416 (May 7, 1999), 911.

Børdahl, Per E. "Tubal Sterilization. A Historical Review," *Journal of Reproductive Medicine* 30:1 (1985), 18–24.

Boudreau, Frank G. "International health," *American Journal of Public Health and the Nation's Health* 19:8 (1929), 863–878.

"Health Work of the League of Nations," *The Milbank Memorial Fund Quarterly* 13:1 (1935), 3–7.

Brand, Jeanne L. "The United States Public Health Service and International Health, 1945–1950," *The Bulletin of the History of Medicine* 63 (1989) 579–598.

Brandt, Allan M. *The Cigarette Century: The Rise, Fall and Deadly Persistence of the Product That Defined America* (New York: Basic Books, 2006).

Breman, Joel G. "A Miracle Happened There: The West and Central African Smallpox Eradication Programme and Its Impact," in Sanjoy Bhattacharya & Sharon Messenger (eds.), *The Global Eradication of Smallpox* (New Delhi: Orient BlackSwan, 2010) pp. 36–60.

Brown, Theodore M. & Marcos Cueto "The World Health Organization and the World of Global Health", in Richard Parker & Marni Sommer (eds.), *Routledge Handbook in Global Public Health* (London: Routledge, 2011) pp. 18–30.

Brown, Theodore M. & Elizabeth Fee. "The Bandoeng Conference of 1937: A Milestone in Health and Development," *American Journal of Public Health* 98:1 (2008), 42–43.

"Ludwig Teleky (1872–1957), A Leader in Social and Occupational Medicine", *American Journal of Public Health* 102 (2012), 1107–1107.

"Ludwik Rajchman (1881–1965), World Leader in Social Medicine and Director of the League of Nations Health Organization," *American Journal of Public Health* 104:9 (2014), 1638–1639.

"Cognitive Dissonance in the Early Thirties: The League of Nations Health Organization Confronts the Worldwide Economic Depression," *American Journal of Public Health* 105 (2015), 65–65.

Brown, Theodore M., Marcos Cueto, & Elizabeth Fee. "The World Health Organization and the Transition from "International" to "Global" Public Health," *American Journal of Public Health* 96:1 (2006), 62–72.

Brown, Theodore M, Elizabeth Fee, & Victoria Stepanova. "Halfdan Mahler: Architect and Defender of the World Health Organization 'Health for All by 2000' Declaration of 1978," *American Journal of Public Health* 196 (2016), 38–39.

Malaria at the Rio Congresses 1963: A Review of Papers on Malaria Presented at the Seventh International Congresses on Tropical Medicine and Malaria, Rio de Janeiro, September 1963 (Geneva: World Health Organization, 1963).

Bruce-Chwatt, Leonard J. "Malaria Eradication at the Crossroads," *Bulletin of the New York Academy of Medicine* 45:10 (1969), 999–1012.

Brundtland, Gro Harlem. *Madam Prime Minister: A Life in Power and Politics* (New York: Farrar, Straus and Giroux, 2002).

Bryant, John H. *Health and the Developing World* (Ithaca: Cornell University Press, 1969).

Burci, Gian Luca & Claude-Henri Vignes. *World Health Organization* (The Hague: Kluwer Law International, 2004).

Bynum, William F. "Policing Hearts of Darkness: Aspects of the International Sanitary Conferences," *History and Philosophy of the Life Sciences*, 15 (1993), 421–434.

Calderwood, Howard B. "The World Health Organization and Its Regional Organizations," *Temple Law Quarterly* 37:1 (1963), 15–27.

Callahan, Michael D. *A Sacred Trust, the League of Nations and Africa, 1929–1946* (Brighton Portland: Academic Press, 2004).

Cannon, Geoffrey. "Why the Bush Administration and the Global Sugar Industry Are Determined to Demolish the 2004 WHO Global Strategy on Diet, Physical Activity and Health," *Public Health Nutrition* 7:3 (2004), 369–380.

Cambournac, Francisco. J. "Health in Africa," *American Journal of Public Health and The Nation's Health*, 50:5 (1960), 13–19.

Campbell, Eugene P. "The Role of the International Cooperation Administration in International Health," *Archives of Environmental Health* 1:6 (1960), 502–511.

Campos, Cristina. *São Paulo pela lente da Higiene: as Propostas de Geraldo Horácio de Paula Souza para a Cidade (1925–1945)* (São Paulo: Rima, 2000).

Chadarevian, Soraya de. "Human Population Studies and the World Health Organization," *Dynamis* 35 (2015), 359–388.

Challenor, Bernard D. "Cultural Resistance to Smallpox Vaccination in West Africa," *Journal of Tropical Medicine and Hygiene* 73:3 (1971), 57–59.

Chin, James & Jonathan Mann. "Global Surveillance and Forecasting of AIDS," *Bulletin of the World Health Organization* 67:1 (1989), 1–7.

Chisholm, Brock. "The World Health Organization," *International Conciliation* 437 (1947), 111–116.

"Social Medicine," *Scientific American* 180:4 (1949), 11–14.

"Cholera and Hysteria," *The Lancet* 250:5483 (November 29, 1947), 797–798.

"Cholera in Egypt," *The Lancet* 250:6479 (November 1, 1947), 657–658.

Claeson, Marian, Joy de Beyer, Prabhat Jha, & Richard G. Feachem. "The World Bank's Perspective on Global Health," *Current Issues in Public Health* 2:5–6 (1996), 264–269.

Chorev, Nitsan. *The World Health Organization between North and South* (Ithaca: Cornell University Press, 2012).

Cohen, J. "Editorial: WHO: Power and Inglory," *The Lancet*, 341:8840 (January 30, 1993), 277–278.

Cook, Rebecca J. & Mahmoud F. Fathalla. "Advancing Reproductive Rights beyond Cairo and Beijing," *International Family Planning Perspectives* 22:3 (1996), 115–121.

Cooper, Frederick. *Decolonization and African Society: The Labor Question in French and British Africa* (New York: Cambridge University Press, 1996).

Crane, B. & J. Dusenberry. "Power and Politics in International Funding for Reproductive Health: The US Global Gag Rule," *Reproductive Health Matters* 12:24 (2004), 128–137.

Crawford, Dorothy H. *Ebola: Profile of a Killer Virus* (Oxford: Oxford University Press, 2016).

Cueto, Marcos. "The Origins of Primary Health Care and Selective Primary Health Care," *American Journal of Public Health* 94:11 (2004), 1864–1874.

Cold War and Deadly Fevers: Malaria Eradication in Mexico, 1955–1970 (Baltimore: Johns Hopkins University Press, 2007).

The Value of Health: A History of the Pan American Health Organization. (Rochester: Rochester University Press, 2007).

Dobson, Mary, Maureen Malowany, & Robert W. Snow. "Malaria Control in East Africa: The Kampala Conference and the Pare-Taveta Scheme: A Meeting of Common and High Ground," *Parassitologia* 42:1/2 (2000), 149–166.

Donnelly, John. "The President's Emergency Plan for AIDS Relief: How George W. Bush and Aides Came to 'Think Big' on Battling HIV," *Health Affairs* 31:7 (2012), 1389–1396.

Drew, Barbara. "World AIDS Day, Essay Contest," *Canadian Medical Association Journal* 139 (1988), 1031.

Dubin, Martin D. "The League of Nations Health Organization," in Paul Weindling (ed.), *International Health Organizations and Movements, 1918–1939* (Cambridge: Cambridge University Press, 1995), pp. 56–80.

Dubos, Rene. "Human Ecology," *The Chronicle of the World Health Organization* 23:11 (1969), 499–504.

Echenberg, Myron. *Plague Ports: The Global Urban Impact of Bubonic Plague, 1894–1901* (New York: New York University Press, 2007).

"Editorial, Maintaining Anti-AIDS Commitment post "3 by 5," *The Lancet* 366:9500 (November 26, 2005), 1828.

"Editorial: Roll Back Malaria: A failing Global Health Campaign," *British Medical Journal* 328 (2004), 1086–1087.

Elrich, Paul E. *The Population Bomb* (New York, Ballantine Books, 1968).

"Emerging Infectious Diseases: Memorandum from a WHO meeting," *Bulletin of the World Health Organization* 72:8 (1994), 845–850.

Engel, Jonathan. *The Epidemic: A Global History of AIDS* (New York: Harper and Collins, 2006).

"Editorial, Epitaph for Global Malaria Eradication?" *The Lancet* 306:7923 (July 5, 1975), 15–16.

Ersoy, Nermin, Yuksel Gungor, & Aslihan Akpinar. "International Sanitary Conferences from the Ottoman Perspective (1851–1938)," *Hygiea Internationalis* 10:1 (2011), 53–79.

Escudero, José Carlos. "What Is Said, What Is Silenced, What Is Obscured: The Report of the Commission on the Social Determinants of Health," *Social Medicine* 4:3 (2009), 183–185.

Espinosa, Mariola. *Epidemic Invasions: Yellow Fever and the Limits of Cuban Independence, 1878–1930* (Chicago: University of Chicago Press, 2009).

Etheridge, Elizabeth. *Sentinel for Health: A History of the Centers for Disease Control* (Berkeley: University of California Press, 1992).

Evans, Hughes. "European Malaria Policy in the 1920s and 1930s: The Epidemiology of Minutiae," *Isis* 80 (1989) 45–49.

Evans, Richard J. "Epidemics and Revolutions: Cholera in Nineteenth Century Europe," *Past and Present* 120 (1988), 123–146.

Farley, John. *To Cast Out Disease: A History of the International Health Division of the Rockefeller Foundation, 1913–1951* (New York: Oxford University Press, 2004).

   Brock Chisholm, the World Health Organization and the Cold War (Vancouver: UBC Press, 2008).

Farmer, Paul. "Social Inequalities and Emerging Infectious Diseases," *Emerging Infectious Diseases* 2:4 (1996), 259–269.

Fee, Elizabeth. "Whither WHO? Our Global Health Leadership," *American Journal of Public Health* 106:11 (2016), 1903–1904.

Fee, Elizabeth & Daniel M. Fox (eds.). *AIDS: The Burdens of History* (Berkeley: University of California Press, 1988).

Foege, William Herbert. *House on Fire: The Fight to Eradicate Smallpox* (Berkeley: University of California Press, 2011).

Foege, William Herbert, John Donald Millar, & Donald Ainslie Henderson. "Smallpox Eradication in West and Central Africa," *Bulletin of the World Health Organization* 52 (1972), 209–222

Fox, Annette Baker. "The United Nations and Colonial Development," *International Organization* 4:2 (1950), 199–218.

Gallagher, Maureen. "The World Health Organization: Promotion of US and Soviet Foreign Policy Goals," *Journal of the American Medical Association* 186:1 (1963), 29–34.

Garrett, Laurie. *The Coming Plague: Newly Emerging Diseases in a World out of Balance* (New York: Farrar, Straus and Giroux, 1994).

Betrayal of Trust: The Collapse of Global Public Health (New York: Hyperion, 2000).

Garrett, Laurie, Mushtaque Chowdhury, & Ariel Pablos-Méndez. "All for Universal Health Coverage," *The Lancet* 374:9697 (August 20, 2009), 1294–1299.

Garthoff, Raymond L. *The Great Transition: American Russian Relations and the End of the Cold War* (Washington, DC: Brookings Institution, 1994).

Détente and Confrontation: American-Soviet Relations from Nixon to Reagan (Washington, DC: The Brookings Institution, 1994).

Gear, Harry S. "Ten Years of Growth of the World Health Organization," *The Lancet* 272:7037 (July 12, 1958), 85–88.

Giles-Vernick, Tamara, & James L. A. Webb, Jr. (eds.). *Global Health in Africa: Historical Perspectives on Disease Control* (Athens, Ohio: Ohio University Press, 2013).

Glusker, Anne. "Who Will Lead WHO?" *British Medical Journal* 333:7575 (November 4, 2006), 938.

Godlee, Fiona. "WHO's Election Throws Agency into Bitter Turmoil," *British Medical Journal* 306 (1992), 161.

"WHO at the Crossroads," *British Medical Journal* 306 (1993), 1143–1144.

"The World Health Organization in Africa," *British Medical Journal* 309 (1994), 553–554.

"WHO in Crisis," *British Medical Journal* 309 (1994), 1424–1428.

"WHO in Retreat; Is it Losing its Influence?" *British Medical Journal* 309 (1994), 1491–1495.

"The Regions – Too Much Power, Too Little Effect," *British Medical Journal* 309 (1994), 1566–1570.

"The World Health Organization: Interview with the Director General," *British Medical Journal* 310 (1995), 583–588.

Goodman, Neville M. *International Health Organizations and Their Work* (London: Churchill Livingstone, 1952).

Gostin, Lawrence O. "International Infectious Disease Law: Revision of the World Health Organization's International Health Regulations," *Journal of the American Medical Association* 291:21 (2004), 2623–2627.

"The Future of the World Health Organization: Lessons Learned from Ebola," *Milbank Quarterly* 93 (2015), 475–479.

Gostin, Lawrence O. & Eric Friedman. "Ebola: A Crisis in Global Health Leadership," *The Lancet* 384 (October 8, 2014), 1323–1325.

Gray, Alastair Mcintosh. "Inequalities in Health. The Black Report: A Summary and Comment," *International Journal of Health Services* 12:3 (1982), 349–380.

Green, Marshall. "The Evolution of US International Population Policy, 1965–92: A Chronological Account," *Population and Development Review* 19:2 (1993), 303–321.

Greenhalgh, Susan. "The Social Construction of Population Science: An Intellectual, Institutional, and Political History of Twentieth-Century Demography," *Comparative Studies in Society and History* 38:1 (1996), 26–66.

Greenough, Paul. "Intimidation, Coercion, and Resistance in the Final Stages of the South Asian Smallpox Eradication Campaign, 1973–1975," *Social Science and Medicine*, 41:5 (1995), 633–645.

"'A Wild and Wondrous Ride': CDC Field Epidemiologists in the East Pakistan Smallpox and Cholera Epidemics of 1958," *Ciência & Saúde Coletiva*, 16:2 (2011), 491–500.

Hankins, R. "The World Health Organization and Immunology Research and Training, 1961–1974," *Medical History* 45 (2001), 243–266.

Harrison, Mark. *Contagion: How Commerce Has Spread Disease* (New Haven: Yale University Press, 2012).

Harkavy, Oscar, Lyle Saunders, & Anna L. Southam. "An Overview of the Ford Foundation's Strategy for Population Work," *Demography*, 5:2 (1968), 541–552.

Hayland, William G. *Clinton's World: Remaking American Foreign Policy* (Westport, CT: Praeger, 1999).

"Health and Social Conditions in China," in Mirko Drazen Grmek (ed.), *Serving the Cause of Public Health: Selected Papers of Andrija Stampar* (Zagreb: University of Zagreb, 1966), pp. 123–151.

"Health Work of the League." *The British Medical Journal* 2: 2826 (1934), 72.

Heiser, Victor G. "The Health Work of the League of Nations," *Proceedings of the American Philosophical Society*, 65:5, Supplement (1926), 1–9.

Henderson, Donald A. *Smallpox: The Death of a Disease – The Inside Story of Eradicating a Worldwide Killer* (Amherst, MA: Prometheus Books, 2009).

Heymann, David L., Mary Kay Kindhauser, & Guénaël Rodier. "Coordinating the Global Reponse," in World Health Organization, Western Pacific Region, *SARS, How a Global Epidemic Was Stopped* (Geneva: World Health Organization, 2006), pp. 49–55.

"Les Six Conférences Sanitaires internationales de 1851 a 1885 Prémices de l'organisation Mondiale de la Santé (OMS)," *Histoire des Sciences Médicales* 47 (2013), 37–44.

Hillemand, Bernard & Alain Ségal. "Les Six Conférences Sanitaires Internationales de 1851 a 1885 Prémices de l'Organisation Mondiale de la Santé (OMS)," *Histoire des Sciences Médicales* 48 (2014), 131–138.

"History at Geneva," *The Lancet* 252:6514 (July 3, 1948), 17–18.

Hochman, Gilberto. "Priority, Invisibility and Eradication: The History of Smallpox and the Brazilian Public Health Agenda," *Medical History* 53 (2009), 229–252.

Hoen, Ellen 't, Jonathan Berger, Alexandra Calmy, & Suerie Moon. "Driving a Decade of Change: HIV/AIDS, Patents and Access to Medicines for all," *Journal of the International AIDS Association* 14:15 (2011), 1–12.

Holland, Walter W. "Karel Raška – The Development of Modern Epidemiology, the Role of the International Epidemiology Association," *Central European Journal of Public Health* 18:1 (2010), 57–60, [www.szu.cz/svi/cejph/archiv/2010-1-11-full.pdf, last accessed 10 August 10, 2017].

Hoopes, Townsend & Douglas Brinkley, *FDR and the Creation of the U.N.* (New Haven: Yale University Press, 1997).

"Hopes and Fears of International Health." *The Lancet* 250:6474 (September 27, 1947), 474–475.

Hopkins, Donald R. *Princes and Peasants: Smallpox in History* (Chicago: University of Chicago Press, 1983).

Howard-Jones, Norman. *International Public Health between the Two World Wars: The Organizational Problems* (Geneva: World Health Organization, 1978).
    "The World Health Organization in historical perspective," *Perspectives in Biology and Medicine*, 24:3 (1981), 467–82.

Humphreys, Margaret. *Malaria: Poverty, Race, and Public Health in the United States* (Baltimore: Johns Hopkins University Press, 2001).

Hutchinson, John F. *Champions of Charity: War and the Rise of the Red Cross* (Boulder, CO: Westview Press, 1996).

Illich, Ivan. *Medical Nemesis: The Expropriation of Health* (New York: Pantheon Books, 1976).

Immerman, Richard H. (ed.) *John Foster Dulles and the Diplomacy of the Cold War* (Princeton: Princeton University Press, 1990).

"In memoriam, Jonathan Mann 1947–1998," *Health and Human Rights, an International Journal* 3:2 (1998), 1–2.

Iriye, Akira. *Global Community: The Role of International Organizations in the Making of the Contemporary World* (Berkeley: University of California Press, 2002).

Jamison, Dean T., Lawrence H. Summers, George Alleyne et al. "Global health 2035: A World Converging within a Generation," *The Lancet* 382 (December 7, 2013), 1898–1955.

Johnson, Donald & Roy Fritz. "Status Report on Malaria Eradication," *Mosquito News* 22:2 (1962), 80–81.

Johnson, Stanley P. *World Population and the United Nations: Challenge and Response* (Cambridge: Cambridge University Press, 1987).

Jones, Joseph M. *Does Overpopulation Mean Poverty? The Facts about Population Growth and Economic Development* (Washington, DC: Center for International Economic Growth, 1962).

Kark, Sidney & Emily Kark. *Promoting Community Health: From Pholela to Jerusalem* (Johannesburg: Witwatersrand University Press, 2001).

Kaul, Inge & Michael Faust. "Global Public Goods and Health: Taking the Agenda Forward," *Bulletin of the World Health Organization* 79:9 (2001), 869–874.

Keating, Conrad. "Ken Warren and the Rockefeller Foundation's Great Neglected Diseases Network, 1978–1988: The Transformation of Tropical and Global Medicine," *Molecular Medicine* 20 (2014), S24–S30.

Kent, John. *The Internationalization of Colonialism: Britain, France and Black Africa, 1939–1956* (Oxford: Clarendon Press, 1992).

Kessler, Alexander. "Family Planning and the Role of WHO," *World Health Organization* 47:3 (1994), pp. 4–6.

Kessler, Alexander, Gordon W. Perkin, & Constance C. Standley. "The WHO Expanded Research Programme in Human Reproduction," *Contraception* 5:5 (1972), 423–428.

Kraut, Alan M. *Silent Travelers: Germs, Genes, and the "Immigrant Menace"* (Baltimore: Johns Hopkins University Press, 1995).

Kickbusch, Ilona. "Issues in Health Promotion," *Health Promotion* 1:4 (1987), 437–442.

Kickbusch, Ilona & Austin Liu. *Electing the WHO Director-General, Global Health Center Working Paper No 16* (Geneva: Graduate Institute of International and Development Studies, 2017).

Koivusalo, Meri & Eeva Ollila. *Making a Healthy World: Agencies, Actors and Policies in International Health* (London: Zed Books, 1997).

Korea Foundation for International Healthcare, 2006–2016 (Seoul: Korea Foundation for International Healthcare, 2016).

Laurell, Asa Cristina & Oliva López Arellano. "Market Commodities and Poor Relief: The World Bank Proposal for Health," *International Journal of Health Services* 26:1 (1996), 1–18.

Lebeuf, Jean Paul. "Sociology as the Basis of Health Education," *Health Education Journal* 13 (1955), 232–238.

Lederberg, Joshua, Robert E. Shope, & Stanley C. Oaks, Jr. (eds.). *Emerging Infections: Microbial Threats to Health in the United States* (Washington, DC: National Academy Press, 1992).

Lee, Jong-wook. "Global Health Improvement and the WHO: Shaping the Future," *The Lancet* 362 (December 20, 2003), 2083–2088.

    "Public Health is a Social Issue," *The Lancet* 365: 9464 (March 19, 2005), 1005–1006.

Lee, Kelley. *Historical Dictionary of the World Health Organization* (London: The Scarecrow Press, Inc., 1998).

    The World Health Organization (WHO) (New York: Routledge, 2009).

Lee, Sung. "WHO and the Developing World: The Contest for Ideology," in Andrew Cunningham & Bridie Andrews (eds.), *Western Medicine as Contested Knowledge* (Manchester: Manchester University Press), 24–45.

Lidén, Jon. "The World Health Organization and Global Health Governance: Post-1990," *Public Health* 128 (2014), 141–147.

Litsios, Socrates. "The Christian Medical Commission and the Development of the World Health Organization's Primary Health Care Approach," *American Journal of Public Health* 94 (2004), 1884–1893.

    "The Health, Poverty and Development Merry-Go-Round, the Tribulations of WHO," in S. William A. Gunn (ed.), *Understanding the Global Dimensions of Health* (New York: Springer, 2005), pp. 15–34.

    "Selskar Gunn and China: The Rockefeller Foundation's "Other" Approach to Public Health," *Bulletin for the History of Medicine* 79:2 (2005), 295–318.

    "Revisiting Bandoeng," *Social Medicine* 8:3 (2014), 113–128.

Lucas, Adetokunbo O. *It Was the Best of Times, from Local to Global Health: The Autobiography of Adetokunbo Olumide Lucas* (Ibadan: Bookbuilders, Editions Africa, 2010).

Mackay, Judith. "The Making of a Convention on Tobacco Control," *Bulletin of the World Health Organization* 81:8 (2003), 551–551.

Mahler, Hafdan. "Health – A Demystification of Medical Technology," *The Lancet* 306:7940 (November 1, 1975), 829–833.

"A Social Revolution in Public Health," *Chronicle of the World Health Organization* 30:12 (1976), 475–480.

Manderson, Lenore. "Wireless Wars in the Eastern Area: Epidemiological Surveillance, Disease Prevention and the Work of the Eastern Bureau of the League of Nations Health Organization, 1925–1942," in Paul Weindling (ed.), *International Health Organizations and Movements, 1918–1939* (Cambridge: Cambridge University Press, 1995), pp. 109–133.

Manela, Erez. "A Pox on Your Narrative: Writing Disease Control into Cold War History," *Diplomatic History* 34: 2 (2010), 299–323.

Mann, Jonathan. "Global AIDS: Critical Issues for Prevention in the 1990s," *International Journal of Health Services* 21:3 (1991), 553–539.

Marks, Harry M. "Epidemiologists Explain Pellagra: Gender, Race, and Political Economy in the Work of Edgar Sydenstricker," *Journal of the History of Medicine*, 58 (2003), 34–55.

Marmot, Michael. "Universal Health Coverage and Social Determinants of Health," *The Lancet* 382:9900 (October 12, 2013), 1227.

The Health Gap, the Challenge of an Unequal World (London: Bloomsbury Publishing, 2015).

Mass, Bonnie. "A Historical Sketch in the American Population Control Movement," *International Journal of Health Services* 4:4 (1974), 651–676.

Mateos Jiménez, Juan B. "Actas de las Conferencias Sanitarias Internacionales (1851–1938)," *Revista Española de Salud Pública* 79:3 (2005), 339–349.

McDougall, J. B. "Editorial: The World Health Organization and Tuberculosis, Aims, Objects and Accomplishments," *The American Review of Tuberculosis* 64:2 (1951), 218–222.

McKeown, Thomas. *The Modern Rise of Population* (New York: Academic Press, 1976).

Merson, Michael. "Global Status on HIV/AIDS," in *Global Challenge of AIDS: Ten Years of HIV/AIDS Research, Proceedings of the Tenth International Conference on AIDS/International Conference on STD, Yokohama, August 7–12, 1994* (Tokyo: Karger, 1991), pp. 3–11.

Merson, Michael and Stephen Inring. *The AIDS Pandemic, Searching for a Global Response.* (Cham, Switzerland: Springer, 2018).

Misra, Babagrahi. "Sitala: The Smallpox Goddess of India," *Asian Folklore Studies* 28:2 (1969), 133–142.

Moon, Suerie, Devi Sridhar, Muhammad A. Pate et al. "Will Ebola Change the Game? Ten Essential Reforms before the Next Pandemic. The Report of the Harvard-LSHTM Independent Panel on the Global Response to Ebola," *The Lancet* 386 (November 22, 2015), 2204–21.

Morel, Carlos M. "Reaching Maturity: 25 Years of TDR," *Parasitology Today* 16:12 (2000), 2–8.

Murard, Lion. "Health Policy between the International and the Local: Jacques Parisot in Nancy and Geneva," in Iris Borowy & Wolf Gruner (eds.), *Facing Illness in Troubled Times, 1918–1939* (Frankfurt am Main: Peter Lang, 2005), pp. 207–245.

"Social Medicine in the Interwar Years. The Case of Jacques Parisot (1882–1967)," *Medicina nei Secoli 20*:3 (2008), 871–890.

Muraskin, William. *The Politics of International Health: The Children's Vaccine Initiative and the Struggle to Develop Vaccines for the Third World*. (New York: State University of New York Press, 1998).

Murray, Christopher J. L. & Alan D. Lopez (eds.). *The Global Burden of Disease: A Comprehensive Assessment of Mortality and Disability from Diseases, Injuries, and Risk Factors in 1990 and Projected to 2020* (Cambridge.: Harvard University Press, 1996).

Mutundwa, Andrew. "International Partnerships in the Fight against AIDS," *AIDS Analysis Africa* 10:3 (1999), 15–16.

Navarro, Vicente. "The New Conventional Wisdom: An Evaluation of the WHO Report: Health Systems, Improving Performance," *International Journal of Health Services* 31:1 (2001), 23–33.

Neelakantan, Vivek. "Eradicating Smallpox in Indonesia: The archipelagic challenge," *Health & History* 212: 1 (2010), 61–87.

"New Director-General for the World Health Organization," *The Lancet* 331:8579 (February 6, 1988), 291.

Newell, Kenneth (ed.). *Health by the People* (Geneva: World Health Organization, 1975).

"Selective Primary Health Care: The Counter Revolution," *Social Science and Medicine* 26:9 (1988), 903–906.

Nicholas, Ralph W. "The Goddess Sitala and Epidemic Smallpox in Bengal," *Journal of Asian Studies* 41:1 (1981), 21–45.

Noah, Norman D. "Key Figure in World Smallpox Eradication Receives Jenner Medal," *Journal of the Royal Society of Medicine* 78:4 (1985), 344–345.

Nunn, Amy. *The Politics and History of AIDS Treatment in Brazil* (New York: Springer, 2009).

"Obituary Raymond Gautier, MD," *British Medical Journal*, 1:5027 (1957), 1127.

Oestrich, Joel E. *Power and Principle: Human Rights Programming in International Organizations* (Georgetown University Press, 2007).

Ogden, Horace G. *CDC and the Smallpox Crusade* (Washington, DC: US Department of Health and Human Services, 1987).

Packard, Randall M. "'No Other Logical Choice': Global Malaria Eradication and the Politics of International Health in the Post-War Era," *Parassitologia* 40:1–2 (1998), 217–229.

The Making of a Tropical Disease: A Short History of Malaria (Baltimore: Oxford University Press, 2007).

A History of Global Health: Interventions into the Lives of other Peoples (Baltimore: Johns Hopkins University Press, 2016)

Paillette, Céline. "Épidémies, Santé et Ordre Mondial. Le Rôle des Organisations Sanitaires Internationales, 1903–1923," *Monde(s): Histoire, Espaces, Relations* 2:2 (2012), 235–256.

Pankhurst, Richard. "The History and Traditional Treatment of Smallpox in Ethiopia," *Medical History* 9:4 (1965), 343–55.

Patel, Maurice. "An Economic Evaluation of Health for All," *Health and Policy and Planning* 1 (1986), 37–47.

Paterson, Gillian. "The CMC Story, 1968–1998," *Contact* 161–162 (1998), 3–18.

Pendergrast, Mark. *Inside the Outbreaks: The Elite Medical Detectives of the Epidemic Intelligence Service* (Boston: Houghton Mifflin Harcourt, 2010).

Perkin, Gordon & William Foege. "A Conversation with the Leaders of the Gates Foundation's Global Health Program: Gordon Perkin and William Foege," *The Lancet* 356:9224 (July 8, 2000), 153–155.

Piot, Peter. *No Time to Lose: A Life in Pursuit of Deadly Viruses* (New York: W.W. Norton and Company, 2012).

AIDS, between Science and Politics (New York: Columbia University Press, 2015).

Pisani, Elizabeth. *The Wisdom of Whores, Bureaucrats, Brothels and the Business of Aids* (New York: W. W. Norton & Company, 2008).

Pollitzer, Robert. *Cholera* (Geneva: World Health Organization, 1959).

Qadeer, Imrana. "Universal Health Care: The Trojan Horse of Neoliberal Policies," *Social Change* 43: 2 (2013), 149–164.

Quinn, Thomas C. "AIDS in Africa: A Retrospective," *Bulletin of the World Health Organization* 79:12 (2001), 1156–1158.

Rajchman, Ludwig. "United Nations Health Organization," *The Lancet* 247:6399 (April 20, 1946), 584–585.

Ravishankar, Nirmala, Paul Gubbins, Rebecca J. Cooley, Katherine Leach-Kemon, Catherine M. Michaud, Dean T. Jamison, & Christopher Murray. "Financing of Global Health: Tracking Development Assistance for Health from 1990 to 2007," *The Lancet*, 373:9681 (June 20, 2009), 2113–2124.

Rehwagen, Christiane. "WHO Recommends DDT to Control Malaria," *British Medical Journal* 333:756 (2006), 622.

Reinhardt, Bob H. *The End of a Global Pox: America and the Eradication of Smallpox in the Cold War Era* (Chapel Hill: University of North Carolina Press, 2015).

Reinisch, Jessica. "Internationalism in Relief: The Birth (and Death) of UNRRA," in Mark Mazower, Jessica Reinisch, & David Feldman (eds.), *Past and Present Supplements, Supplement Post-War Reconstruction in Europe: International Perspectives, 1945–1949* 6 (2011), 258–289.

Reynolds, Lois A. & Elisabeth M. Tansey (eds.). *WHO Framework Convention On Tobacco Control: The Transcript of a Witness Seminar Organized by the Wellcome Trust Centre for the History of Medicine at UCL, in Collaboration with the Department of Knowledge Management and Sharing, WHO, held in Geneva, on 26 February 2010* (London: The Wellcome Trust, 2012).

Ringen, Knut. "Karl Evang: A Giant in Public Health," *Journal of Public Health Policy* 11:3 (1990), 360–367.

Robbins, Anthony. "Brundtland's World Health, a Test Case for United Nations Reform," *Public Health Reports* 114 (1999), 30–39.

"Roche gives in to Brazil over AIDS drug," *The Lancet Infectious Diseases* 1:3 (October 2001), 138.

Rodman, Peter W. *More Precious than Peace, the Cold War and the Struggle for the Third World* (New York: Charles Scribner's Son, 1994).

Ruger, Jennifer P. "The Changing Role of the World Bank in Global Health," *American Journal of Public Health* 95:1 (2005), 60–70.

Ruger, Jennifer P. & Derek Yach. "The Global Role of the World Health Organization," *Global Health Governance* 1:2 (2009), 1–11.

Ruxin, Joshua. "Magical Bullet: The History of Oral Rehydratation Therapy," *Medical History* 38 (1991), 363–397.

Samamé, Guillermo E. "Treponematosis Eradication, with Special Reference to Yaws Eradication in Haiti," *Bulletin of the World Health Organization* 15:6 (1956), 897–910.

Satcher, David. "Global Health at the Crossroads Surgeon General's Report on the 50th World Health Assembly," *Journal of the American Medical Association* 281 (1999), 942–943.

Schwartländer, Bernhard, John Stover, Neff Walker, L. Bollinger, Juan-Pablo Gutierrez, William McGreevey, Marjorie Opuni, Steve Forsythe, Lilani Kumaranayake, Charlotte Watts, & Stefano Bertozzi. "Resource Needs for HIV/AIDS," *Science* 292:3326 (June 29, 2001), 2434–2436.

Sealey, Anne. "Globalizing the 1926 International Sanitary Convention," *Journal of Global History* 6:3 (2011), 431–455.

Seytre, Bernard & Mary Shaffer. *The Death of a Disease: A History of the Eradication of Poliomyelitis* (New Brunswick: Rutgers University Press, 2005).

Shack, Reneé, Alan P. Kendal, Lars R. Haaheiim, & John Wood. "The Next Influenza Pandemic: Lessons from Hong Kong, 1997," *Emerging Infectious Diseases* 5:2 (1999), 195–203.

Sharma, Vinod Prakash. "Re-Emergence of Malaria in India," *Indian Journal of Medical Research*, 103 (1996), 26–45.

Schneider, Kammerle & Laurie Garrett. "The End of the Era of Generosity? Global Health Amid Economic Crisis," *Philosophy, Ethics, and Humanities in Medicine*, 4:1 (2009), 1–7.

Shubber, Sami. *The International Code of Marketing of Breast-Milk Substitutes: An International Measure to Protect and Promote Breastfeeding* (The Hague: Kluger Law International, 1983).

Siddiqi, Javed. *World Health and World Politics: The World Health Organization and the UN System* (Columbia: University of South Carolina Press, 1995).

Simon, Julian L. *The Ultimate Resource* (Princeton: Princeton University Press, 1981).

Smith-Nonini, Sandy. "When the Program is Good but the Disease is Better: Lessons from Peru on Drug-Resistant Tuberculosis," *Medical Anthropology* 24 (2005), 265–296.

Soetopo, Mas & Raden Wasito. "Experience with Yaws Control in Indonesia; Preliminary Results with a Simplified Approach," *Bulletin of the World Health Organization* 8:1–3 (1953), 273–295.

Staples, Amy L. S. *The Birth of Development: How the World Bank, Food and Agriculture Organization and World Health Organization, Changed the World, 1945–1965* (Kent, Ohio: The Kent State University Press, 2006).

"The Future of the World Health Organization," *The Lancet* 360:9348 (December 7, 2002), 1798.

"The International Office of Public Health," *The British Medical Journal*, 2:2548 (October 30, 1909), 1297–1298.

"The World's Health," *The Lancet* 255:6611 (May 13, 1950), 920.

Taylor, Carl E. (ed.). *Doctors for the Villages: Study of Rural Internships in Seven Indian Medical Colleges* (New York: Asia Publishing House, 1976).

Tenover, Fred C. & James M. Hughes. "WHO Scientific Working Group on Monitoring and Management of Bacterial Resistance to Antimicrobial Agents," *Emerging Infectious Diseases* 1:1 (1995), 37.

Tipps, Dean C. "Modernization Theory and the Comparative Study of Societies: A Critical Perspective," *Comparative Studies in Society and History* 15:2 (1973), 199–226.

Towers, Bridget. "Red Cross Organizational Politics, 1918–1922: Relations of Dominance and the Influence of the United States," in Paul Weindling (ed.), *International Health Organizations and Movements, 1918–1939* (Cambridge: Cambridge University Press, 1995), pp. 36–55.

Turshen, Meredeth & Tefera Gezmu. "The World Health Organization and the Ebola Epidemic," in Ibrahim Abdullah & Ismail Rashind (eds.), *Understanding West Africa's Ebola Epidemic; Towards a Political Economy* (London: Zed, 2017).

Vaughan, J. Patrick, Sigrun Møgedal, Gill Walt, Stein-Erik Kruse, Kelley Lee, & Koen de Wilde. "WHO and the Effects of Extrabudgetary Funds: Is the Organization Donor Driven?" *Health Policy and Planning* 11:3 (1996), 253–264.

Waitzkin, Howard. "Report of the WHO Commission on Macroeconomics and Health: A Summary and Critique," *The Lancet* 361:9356 (February 8, 2003), 523–526.

Wallace S. Jones. "Italy, International Sanitary Conference," *Public Health Reports* 12:19 (1897), 452–459.

Walsh, Julia A. & Kenneth S. Warren. "Selective Primary Health Care, an Interim Strategy for Disease Control in Developing Countries," *New England Journal of Medicine* 301 (1979), 967–974.

Walt, Gill. "WHO under Stress: Implications for Health Policy," *Health Policy* 24 (1993), 125–144.

Walters, Francis Paul. *A History of the League of Nations* (London: Oxford University Press, 1952).

Warren, Kenneth S. "The Evolution of Selective Primary Health Care," *Social Science and Medicine* 26 (1988), 891–898.

"What's Going on at the World Health Organization?" *The Lancet* 360:9340 (October 12, 2002), 118–120.

Webb Jr., James L. A. "The First Large-Scale Use of Synthetic Insecticide for Malaria Control in Tropical Africa, Lessons from Liberia," in Tamara Giles-Vernick & James L. A. Webb Jr. (eds.), *Global Health in Africa, Historical Perspectives on Disease Control* (Athens, Ohio University Press, 2013), pp. 42–69.

Weindling, Paul. "From Infectious to Chronic Diseases: Changing Patterns of Sickness in the Nineteenth and Twentieth Centuries," in Andrew Wear (ed.), *Medicine in Society* (Cambridge: Cambridge University Press, 1992), pp. 303–316.

"Social Medicine at the League of Nations Health Organization and the International Labour Office Compared," Paul Weindling (ed.), *International Health Organizations and Movements, 1918–1939* (Cambridge: Cambridge University Press, 1995), pp. 134–153.

Epidemics and Genocide in Eastern Europe, 1890–1945 (London: Oxford University Press, 2000).

Weir, David & Mark Schapiro. *Circle of Poison, Pesticides in a Hungry World* (San Francisco: Institute for Food and Development Policy, 1981).

Werner, David & David Sanders. *Questioning the Solution: The Politics of Primary Health Care and Child Survival, with an In-Depth Critique of Oral Rehydration Therapy* (Palo Alto: Health Rights, 1997).

White, Tyrene. *China's Longest Campaign: Birth Planning in the People's Republic, 1949–2005* (Ithaca: Cornell University Press, 2006).

"WHO's African Regional Office Must Evolve or Die," *The Lancet* 364:9433 (August 7, 2004), 475–476.

"WHO's Executive Board Election Proceedings are Low-Key and Secretive," *The Lancet* 360:9347 (November 30, 2002), 1753.

"WHO Regional Director Dismisses 'Bleak Picture' of his Work in Africa," *Bulletin of the World Health Organization* 82:9 (2004), 717–718.

Widdus, R. "Public-Private Partnerships for Health Require Thoughtful Evaluation," *Bulletin of the World Health Organization* 81:4 (2003), 235.

Wilcox, Francis O. "International Organizations: Aid to World Trade and Prosperity," *The Department of State Bulletin* 37 (1957), 749–754.

Wildschut, Hajo I. J. & Wilma Monincx. "Vasectomy and the Risk of Prostate Cancer," *The Bulletin of the World Health Organization* 72:5 (1994), 777–778.

Winslow, Charles-Edward Amory. "International Health," *American Journal of Public Health* 41:12 (1951), 1455–1482.

Wisner, Ben. "GOBI versus PHC? Some Dangers of Selective Primary Health Care," *Social Science and Medicine* 26:9 (1988), 963–969.

Woodbridge, George. *UNRRA: The History of the United Nations Relief and Rehabilitation Administration Vol 1* (New York: Columbia University Press, 1950).

Worboys, Michael. "The Emergence of Tropical Medicine: A Study in the Establishment of a Scientific Speciality," in Gerard Lemaine, Roy MacLeod, Michael Mulkay & Peter Weingart (eds.), *Perspectives on the Emergence of Scientific Disciplines* (The Hague: Mouton and Co., 1976), pp. 75–98.

Wu, Harry Yi-Jui. "World Citizenship and the Emergence of the Social Psychiatry Project of the World Health Organization, 1948-c.1965," *History of Psychiatry* 26 (2015), 166–181.

Yates, Robert. "Universal Health Care and the Removal of User Fees," *The Lancet* 373:9680 (August 22, 2009), 2078–2081.

Zinder, Lynne Page. "New York, the Nation, the World, The Career of Surgeon General Thomas J. Parran Jr. MD (1892–1968)," *Public Health Reports* 110 (1995), 630–632.

Zse, Simon. *The Origins of the World Health Organization: A Personal Memoir 1945–1948* (Boca Raton: L.I.S.Z. Publications, 1982).

Zelizer, Julian E. (ed.). *The Presidency of George W. Bush: A First Historical Assessment* (Princeton: Princeton University Press, 2010).

Zubok, Vladislav & Constantine Pleshavok. *Inside the Kremlin's Cold War, From Stalin to Khrushev* (Cambridge: Harvard University Press, 1996).

Zylberman, Patrick. "Fewer Parallels than Antitheses: René Sand and Andrija Stampar on Social Medicine, 1919–1955," *Social History of Medicine* 17:1 (2005), 77–92.
  "Civilizing the State: Borders, Weak States and International Health in Modern Europe," in Alison Bashford (ed.), *Disease, Globalization and Security, 1850 to the Present* (New York: Palgrave Macmillan, 2006), 21–40.

2.2 Unpublished Theses and Dissertations

Kyzr-Sheeley, Gary R. "The Evolution of Population Policies in the World Health Organization, the World Bank and the United Nations Fund for Population Activities," unpublished PhD dissertation, Indiana University (1980).
Macfayden, David. "The Genealogy of WHO and UNICEF and the Intersecting Careers of Melville Mackenzie (1889–1972) and Ludwik Rajchman (1881–1965)," unpublished PhD dissertation, University of Glasgow (2014).
Rana, Zeeshan A. "The Evolution of the World Health Organization's Policy Response to the HIV/AIDS Crisis," unpublished master of science thesis, University of Toronto (2006).
Reinhardt, Robert H. "Remaking Bodily Environments: The Global Eradication of Smallpox," unpublished PhD dissertation, University of California, Davis (2012).
Scales, David A. "The World Health Organization and the Dynamics of International Disease Control: Exit, Voice, and Trojan Loyalty," unpublished PhD dissertation, Yale University (2009).

Index